PEDIATRIC HOSPITAL MEDICINE BOARD REVIEW

EDITED BY

Deepa Kulkarni, MD

PEDIATRIC HOSPITAL MEDICINE FELLOWSHIP PROGRAM
DIRECTOR, ASSISTANT CLINICAL PROFESSOR OF
PEDIATRICS, DAVID GEFFEN SCHOOL OF MEDICINE,
UNIVERSITY OF CALIFORNIA, LOS ANGELES (UCLA),
LOS ANGELES, CA, USA

Audrey Kamzan, MD

PEDIATRIC HOSPITAL MEDICINE DIVISION CHIEF,
ASSISTANT CLINICAL PROFESSOR OF PEDIATRICS,
DAVID GEFFEN SCHOOL OF MEDICINE, UNIVERSITY OF
CALIFORNIA, LOS ANGELES (UCLA), LOS ANGELES, CA, USA

Charles A. Newcomer, MD

UCLA MATTEL CHILDREN'S HOSPITAL ASSOCIATE
MEDICAL DIRECTOR, ASSISTANT CLINICAL PROFESSOR
OF PEDIATRICS, DAVID GEFFEN SCHOOL OF MEDICINE,
UNIVERSITY OF CALIFORNIA, LOS ANGELES (UCLA),
LOS ANGELES, CA, USA

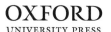

OXFORD
UNIVERSITY PRESS

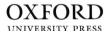

OXFORD
UNIVERSITY PRESS

Oxford University Press is a department of the University of Oxford. It furthers
the University's objective of excellence in research, scholarship, and education
by publishing worldwide. Oxford is a registered trade mark of Oxford University
Press in the UK and certain other countries.

Published in the United States of America by Oxford University Press
198 Madison Avenue, New York, NY 10016, United States of America.

Library of Congress Cataloging-in-Publication Data
Names: Kulkarni, Deepa, author. | Kamzan, Audrey, author. |
Newcomer, Charles A., author.
Title: Pediatric hospital medicine board review / Deepa Kulkarni,
Audrey Kamzan, and Charles A. Newcomer.
Other titles: Medical specialty board review.
Description: New York, NY : Oxford University Press, [2022] |
Series: Medical specialty board review series |
Includes bibliographical references and index.
Identifiers: LCCN 2021056054 (print) | LCCN 2021056055 (ebook) |
ISBN 9780197580196 (paperback) | ISBN 9780197580219 (epub) |
ISBN 9780197580226 (online)
Subjects: MESH: Pediatrics | Inpatients | Diagnosis, Differential |
Examination Questions
Classification: LCC RJ102 (print) | LCC RJ102 (ebook) | NLM WS 18.2 |
DDC 362.1989200076—dc23/eng/20220119
LC record available at https://lccn.loc.gov/2021056054
LC ebook record available at https://lccn.loc.gov/2021056055

DOI: 10.1093/med/9780197580196.001.0001

3 5 7 9 8 6 4 2

Printed by Marquis, Canada

CONTENTS

CONTRIBUTORS

Namrata Ahuja, MD
Assistant Professor of Clinical Pediatrics, Associate Fellowship
    Program Director
Division of Hospital Medicine, Department of Pediatrics
Children's Hospital Los Angeles, University of Southern
    California
Los Angeles, CA, USA

Gal Barak, MD, MEd
Assistant Professor
Department of Pediatrics
Baylor College of Medicine, Texas Children's Hospital
Houston, TX, USA

Daxa Clarke, MD
Chief Medical Information Officer and Pediatric Hospitalist
Information Technology and Hospital Medicine
Phoenix Children's Hospital
Phoenix, AZ, USA

Michelle Essig, MD
Clinical Assistant Professor of Pediatrics
Division of Hospital Medicine
Children's Hospital Los Angeles; USC Keck School of
    Medicine
Los Angeles, CA, USA

Anand Gourishankar, MBBS, MRCP, MAS
Associate Professor of Pediatrics
Pediatrics/Division of Hospital Medicine
Children's National Hospital
Washington, DC, USA

Elisa Hampton, MD
Assistant Professor
Department of Pediatrics
University of Virginia
Charlottesville, VA, USA

Dan Herchline, MD, MSEd
Assistant Professor
Department of Pediatrics
Cincinnati Children's Hospital
Cincinnati, OH, USA

Esther Jun-Ihn, MD
Clinical Instructor
Department of Pediatrics
University of California, Los Angeles
Los Angeles, CA, USA

Jennifer Kaczmarek, MD, MSc
Pediatric Hospital Medicine Fellow
Cleveland Clinic Children's
Cleveland, OH, USA

Audrey Kamzan, MD
Assistant Clinical Professor
Department of Pediatrics
University of California, Los Angeles
Los Angeles, CA, USA

Mikelle Key-Solle, MD
Assistant Professor
Department of Pediatrics
Duke Children's Hospital
Durham, NC, USA

Anjali Kirpalani, MD
Pediatric Hospitalist, PHM Fellowship Program Director
Department of Pediatrics
Emory, Children's Healthcare of Atlanta
Atlanta, GA, USA

Sangeeta Krishna, MD
Associate Professor, Fellowship Director
Pediatric Hospital Medicine
Cleveland Clinic
Cleveland, OH, USA

John Kulesa, MD
Department of Hospital Medicine
Children's National Hospital
Washington, DC, USA

Deepa Kulkarni, MD
Assistant Clinical Professor
Department of Pediatrics
University of California Los Angeles
Los Angeles, CA, USA

Nancy Liao, MD
Assistant Professor
Department of Pediatrics
Nationwide Children's Hospital
Columbus, OH, USA

Jamie Librizzi, MD, MSHS
Assistant Clinical Professor
Pediatric Hospital Medicine
Phoenix Children's Hospital
Phoenix, AZ, USA

James Lin, MD
Assistant Clinical Professor and Medical Director
Department of Pediatrics
University of California, Los Angeles
Los Angeles, CA, USA

Jasen Liu, MD
Assistant Clinical Professor
Department of Pediatrics
University of California Los Angeles
Los Angeles, CA, USA

Jessica Lloyd, MD
Associate Clinical Professor
Department of Pediatrics
University of California, Los Angeles
Los Angeles, CA, USA

Michelle Lopez, MD, MPH
Associate Professor
Department of Pediatrics and Center for Medical Ethics and
    Health Policy
Baylor College Medicine
Houston, TX, USA

Patrick McCarthy, MD, MME
Assistant Professor; Program Director, Pediatric Hospital
    Medicine Fellowship
Section of Hospital Medicine, Department of
    Pediatrics
Medical College of Wisconsin
Milwaukee, WI, USA

Elisha McCoy, MD
Associate Professor and Division Chief of Pediatric Academic
    Hospital Medicine
Department of Pediatrics
University of Tennessee Health Science Center, Le Bonheur
    Children's Hospital
Memphis, TN, USA

Kira Molas-Torreblanca, DO
Clinical Associate Professor of Pediatrics
Department of Pediatrics
University of Southern California/Children's Hospital Los Angeles
Los Angeles, CA, USA

Kristina Nazareth-Pidgeon, MD
Pediatric Hospitalist
Department of Pediatrics
Duke University
Durham, NC, USA

Adin Nelson, MD, MHPE, FAAP
Assistant Professor
Department of Pediatrics
Weill Cornell Medicine
New York, NY, USA

Charles A. Newcomer, MD
Assistant Clinical Professor
Department of Pediatrics
University of California, Los Angeles
Los Angeles, CA, USA

Elayna Ng, MD
Clinical Instructor
Department of Pediatrics
University of California, Los Angeles
Los Angeles, CA, USA

Maren Olson, MD, MPH, MEd
Assistant Professor
Department of Pediatrics
University of Minnesota
Minneapolis, MN, USA

Sonya Patel-Nguyen, MD
Medical Instructor
Department of Medicine and Department of Pediatrics
Duke University
Durham, NC, USA

Michael F. Perry, MD
Assistant Professor
Department of Pediatrics
Nationwide Children's Hospital
Columbus, OH, USA

Michael B. Pitt, MD
Associate Professor
Department of Pediatrics
University of Minnesota
Minneapolis, MN, USA

Michael Platt, MD
Pediatric Hospitalist
Division of Hospital Medicine
Children's Mercy Kansas City
Kansas City, MO, USA

Kyle Pronko, MD
Assistant Professor
Department of Pediatrics
Medical College of Wisconsin
Milwaukee, WI, USA

Hanna Siddiqui, MD, MPH
Assistant Clinical Professor
Department of Pediatrics
University of California, Los Angeles
Los Angeles, CA, USA

Ankit Singla, MD
Pediatric Hospital Medicine Fellow
Department of Pediatrics
University of California, Los Angeles
Los Angeles, CA, USA

Brooke Spector, MD
Assistant Professor
Department of Pediatrics
New York Presbyterian Hospital–Weill Cornell
New York, NY, USA

Rebecca Tenney-Soeiro, MD, MSEd
Associate Professor of Pediatrics
Department of Pediatrics
Children's Hospital of Philadelphia
Philadelphia, PA, USA

Nehal Thakkar, MD, MBA
Pediatric Hospitalist, Associate Program Director Pediatric
    Hospital Medicine Fellowship
Department of Pediatric Hospital Medicine
Phoenix Children's Hospital
Phoenix, AZ, USA

Margaret Trost, MD, MS
Clinical Associate Professor of Pediatrics
Pediatric Hospital Medicine
University of Southern California Keck School of Medicine;
    Children's Hospital Los Angeles
Los Angeles, CA, USA

Sarah Varghese, MD
Assistant Professor
Department of Pediatrics
Emory University School of Medicine
Atlanta, GA, USA

Jacqueline Walker, MD, MHPE
Pediatric Hospital Medicine Fellowship Director, Associate
    Professor of Pediatrics, Associate Dean for Clinical
    Medical Education
Department of Pediatrics
Children's Mercy Hospital, University of Missouri–Kansas
    City School of Medicine
Kansas City, MO, USA

Evan Wiley, MD
Pediatric Hospital Medicine Fellow
Department of Pediatrics
University of California Los Angeles
Los Angeles, CA, USA

Jeffrey C. Winer, MD, MA, MSHS, FAAP
Associate Professor
Department of Pediatrics
University of Tennessee Health Science Center, Le Bonheur
    Children's Hospital
Memphis, TN, USA

Sarah Yale, MD
Assistant Professor
Department of Pediatrics
Medical College of Wisconsin
Milwaukee, WI, USA

1.

COMMON CLINICAL DIAGNOSES AND CONDITIONS

QUESTIONS

1. A 15-year-old male presents to the emergency department with 2 weeks of bloody mucoid diarrhea and lower abdominal pain. He reports an unintentional 5-kilogram weight loss over the last 3 months. Which test is most likely to confirm the diagnosis in this patient?

    A. Stool culture
    B. Abdominal ultrasound
    C. Stool guaiac
    D. Upper gastrointestinal (GI) series with small bowel follow-through
    E. Endoscopy/colonoscopy

2. A 9-month-old boy with a history of eczema, recurrent otitis media, and three hospitalizations for pneumonia is admitted to the hospital for abnormalities on a routine blood test. On examination, he has numerous petechiae scattered across his chest, abdomen, and back. The results of his laboratory testing are as follows:

White blood cells: 6820/μL
Hemoglobin: 11.3 g/dL
Hematocrit: 34.1
Platelets: 12 × 103/μL
Peripheral blood smear: small, rare platelets
Blood type: A+
Direct antiglobulin test: negative

Which of the following treatments is most likely to be curative for this patient?

    A. Anti-D immune globulin
    B. Methylprednisolone
    C. Intravenous immune globulin (IVIG)
    D. Hematopoietic stem cell transplant
    E. Clarithromycin, omeprazole, and metronidazole

3. A 13-year-old obese male presents following an episode of chest pain after a 3-mile run that resolved after rest. He reports a similar episode 1 month ago while playing soccer. His family history includes an uncle who died suddenly of unknown causes during college.

The patient's physical examination is normal other than a systolic ejection murmur over the left sternal border that is louder with the Valsalva maneuver. An electrocardiogram (ECG) at admission shows increased voltages in the precordial leads, left-axis deviation, and deep Q waves in the inferior and lateral leads. Which of the following would be the next best step?

    A. Serial troponins
    B. Initiation of β-blockers
    C. Placement of an automatic implantable cardioverter defibrillator (AICD)
    D. Initiation of amlodipine
    E. Reassurance

4. A 15-year-old boy is brought to the emergency department immediately after a suicide attempt. He reportedly ingested a bottle of acetaminophen but regrets his actions and is no longer suicidal. His initial hepatic function panel and acetaminophen level are normal, and he is currently asymptomatic. You are contacted for possible admission. Which of the following do you recommend?

    A. Admit and initiate treatment based on the current acetaminophen level
    B. Obtain new laboratory tests 4 hours after ingestion to determine disposition
    C. Discharge the patient home with psychiatric follow-up
    D. Admit the patient for observation and obtain new laboratory tests based on clinical symptoms
    E. Medically clear the patient for admission to psychiatry

5. A 7-year-old developmentally delayed female presents to the emergency department (ED) with new onset wheezing. Her parents reports that she was playing with her sister when she suddenly started to wheeze. The patient has no prior history of wheezing or asthma. In the ED, the patient is given three albuterol nebulizer treatments and corticosteroids without any improvement. The ED physician consults the pediatric hospitalist to help with further management for this patient.

The hospitalist recommends obtaining a chest radiograph. Which of the following findings would most likely be seen on imaging?

    A. Posterior rib fractures of the eighth and ninth ribs
    B. Asymmetric air trapping
    C. Bilateral symmetrical peribronchial thickening and cuffing
    D. Right middle lobar consolidation
    E. Enlarged cardiac silhouette

6. A 13-year-old previously healthy female presents with acute onset facial weakness involving the entire right side of the face, fatigue, and myalgia. Her neurologic examination is otherwise normal with intact reflexes, normal strength and sensation, normal gait, and no cerebellar dysfunction. Her vital signs are within normal limits. Which of the following is the most likely diagnosis?

    A. Cerebrovascular accident
    B. Lyme disease
    C. Bell's palsy
    D. Ramsay Hunt syndrome
    E. Guillain-Barré syndrome

7. A 7-year-old male presents to the emergency department with concern for fevers, decreased oral intake, and unilateral testicular swelling. The parents report that his symptoms started about 1 week prior to presentation and have been associated with myalgia, malaise, and headaches. His parents brought him in today for concern that his symptoms were getting worse. They note that he is incompletely vaccinated. Which of the following is the most common presenting feature of this condition?

    A. Parotitis
    B. Periorbital swelling
    C. Pedal edema
    D. Truncal rash
    E. Conjunctivitis

8. A 45-day-old, full-term male presents to the emergency department after an episode of unresponsiveness. Parents report that 25 minutes following a feed they noted his face turned red, and he appeared to stop breathing and seemed "out of it." The episode lasted approximately 30 seconds, and then he cried and return to his baseline. On examination, the infant appears vigorous with a normal examination and vital signs for age. Based on the current guidelines for a brief resolved unexplained event (BRUE), this patient would be classified as "higher risk" due to

    A. Color change noted during the event
    B. The duration of the event lasting greater than 20 seconds

    C. The patient's age being less than 60 days
    D. A change in breathing pattern during the event
    E. A change in level of consciousness during the event

9. While rounding in the newborn nursery, you note a term male baby with a large tongue. The baby weighs 4.5 kg. The nurses note that he has been having difficulty maintaining blood glucose levels. Which of the following tumors is this baby at increased risk for?

    A. Thyroid cancer
    B. Insulinoma
    C. Retinoblastoma
    D. Wilms tumor
    E. Brain tumor

10. A 12-year-old female with a history of constipation and encopresis is admitted for management of abdominal pain. An abdominal radiograph shows significant stool burden, and she is started on a bowel cleanout. Her physical examination is notable for more than 10 warts surrounding the anus, with no other warts seen on examination. Which of the following should be pursued as part of the management of this patient?

    A. Endoscopy and colonoscopy to evaluate for inflammatory bowel disease
    B. Culture for human papillomavirus (HPV) infection
    C. Biopsy of the warts
    D. Confidential social history
    E. Thyroid testing

11. A 4-year-old female presents to the emergency department with difficulty breathing, stomach pain, abdominal swelling, and puffy eyes. Her laboratory tests are notable for proteinuria, a sodium of 129 mEq/L, normal complete blood count (CBC), and a serum albumin of 2.0 g/dL. Which of the following complications is the patient at risk for?

    A. Urinary tract infection
    B. Deep venous thrombosis
    C. Nephrolithiasis
    D. Hypotension
    E. Focal renal abscesses

12. A 4-year-old previously healthy male presents with 1 day of leg pain and limp. He recovered from an upper respiratory tract infection (URI) 2 weeks ago. Since then, he has been afebrile. Family history is significant for rheumatoid arthritis in the paternal grandmother. On examination, manipulation of the left hip results in pain. He has an antalgic gait and avoids putting weight on his left leg. There are no rashes. An ultrasound shows

a left hip effusion. The remaining workup includes the following:

White blood cell count	8000 cells/mm³
C-reactive protein	0.5 mg/dL
Erythrocyte sedimentation rate	21 mm/h
Joint aspirate analysis	30,000 white blood cells/mm³
Blood culture	Pending
Synovial fluid culture	Pending

The referring physician is requesting hospitalization for further management. Of the following, which is the next best step in management?

A. Surgical washout of hip
B. Magnetic resonance imaging of the hip and pelvis
C. Intravenous antibiotics
D. Nonsteroidal anti-inflammatory drug
E. Systemic steroids

13. A 5-year-old passenger in a motor vehicle accident presents to the emergency room for evaluation. After a thorough assessment by the trauma team, her only identified injury is a 3-cm wound on her right lower leg with moderate surrounding soft tissue damage and bone extruding. Which of the following antibiotic regimens would be appropriate for infection prophylaxis?

A. Intravenous (IV) cefazolin
B. IV vancomycin and oxacillin
C. IV cefazolin and gentamicin
D. IV penicillin and streptomycin
E. IV vancomycin

14. A 4-year-old previously healthy male is admitted for persistent fevers. He has had fevers up to 102°F for 12 days and left underarm swelling. There have been no known sick contacts, no recent travel, and the only animal exposures are to the family cat and dog. His examination is significant for an enlarged, tender lymph node in the left axilla. His initial results are shown as follows:

White blood cell	21 K/μL
Hemoglobin	12.5 g/dL
Platelets	220 K/μL
Neutrophils	40%
Lymphocytes	55%
Monocytes	4%
Eosinophils	1%

Basophils	0%
Erythrocyte sedimentation rate (ESR)	73 mm/h
C-reactive protein (CRP)	2.0 mg/dL
Blood culture	No growth at 24 hours

Which of the following is the first-line treatment for this patient's diagnosis?

A. Ceftriaxone
B. Azithromycin
C. Rifampin
D. Clindamycin
E. Amoxicillin

15. A 2-month-old male presents to the emergency department with jaundice and poor weight gain. His initial workup reveals a conjugated hyperbilirubinemia, and he undergoes an extensive workup. A liver biopsy reveals a paucity of interlobular bile ducts. Which of the following is most likely to be present in this patient?

A. Hypotonia
B. Congenital heart disease
C. Abdominal wall defects
D. Immunodeficiency
E. Polydactyly

16. You are the attending for a 15-year-old male with idiopathic scoliosis who is postoperative day 3 from a posterior spinal fusion. Overnight, the patient is noted to have increased swelling in his left lower extremity. A venous Doppler ultrasound confirms the presence of a nonoccluding thrombus in his left iliac vein. During rounds, a resident suggests starting the patient on a heparin infusion. Of the following, why would enoxaparin be a better choice than intravenous (IV) heparin?

A. Enoxaparin has a faster onset of action than heparin
B. Enoxaparin can be completely reversed by protamine if bleeding were to occur
C. Enoxaparin can be administered on an outpatient basis after discharge
D. Enoxaparin is more effective than heparin at treating venous thromboemboli
E. Enoxaparin does not require therapeutic laboratory monitoring after initiation

17. An 18-year-old male with a history of coarctation of the aorta repaired in the neonatal period is transferred from radiology to the emergency room with acute onset generalized urticaria, lip swelling, abdominal pain, facial flushing, and pruritus. He was receiving intravenous radiocontrast for magnetic resonance imaging of

the brain when the symptoms began. About an hour after presentation, he received intramuscular epinephrine of 0.01 mg/kg dose, and his symptoms improved. Three hours later, he began to have wheezing, tachypnea, and worsening abdominal pain. He has an oxygen saturation of 90%, a respiratory rate of 28 breaths per minute, a heart rate of 120 beats per minute, and a blood pressure of 80/50 mm Hg. What most likely led to the recurrence of his symptoms?

A. Multiple anaphylactic triggers
B. Adverse reaction to epinephrine
C. Delay in epinephrine administration
D. Rapid normal saline infusion
E. Lack of glucocorticoid administration

18. An 18-month-old female with a history of a resolved viral upper respiratory tract infection (URI) 2 weeks ago presents to the emergency department with fatigue and poor oral intake. Her temperature is 36.5°C, heart rate 165 beats per minute, respiratory rate 60 breaths per minute, blood pressure 90/65 mm Hg, and oxygen saturation 96%. Her examination is significant for crackles in bilateral lung fields, a II/VI systolic murmur with a gallop, a palpable liver edge 3 cm from the midcostal margin, and capillary refill time less than 2 seconds. Which of the following studies would be the most diagnostic?

A. Abdominal ultrasonogram with Doppler
B. Chest radiograph
C. Blood culture
D. Respiratory viral panel (RVP)
E. Echocardiogram

19. A 16-year-old male is brought into the emergency department after collapsing during a prolonged summer football practice. His temperature is 41°C, heart rate 123 beats per minute, blood pressure 103/72 mm Hg, respiratory rate 34 breaths per minute, and oxygen saturation 95%. He is disoriented, is slurring his speech, and appears flushed and diaphoretic. Which of the following is the next best step in management?

A. Start fluid resuscitation with isotonic fluid
B. Apply ice packs to the axillae, groin, and neck
C. Administer oral acetaminophen
D. Administer intravenous dantrolene
E. Start empiric intravenous ceftriaxone

20. A 4-month-old female presents to the emergency department with fevers, cough, congestion, and increased work of breathing. Her symptoms started 3 days ago and have continued to worsen. Her temperature is 39°C, respiratory rate 65 breaths per minute, heart rate 150 beats per minute, blood pressure 90/55 mm Hg, and oxygen

saturation 93% on room air. Her lung examination reveals multiple sounds, including rhonchi, crackles, and wheezing. Which of the following treatments may be considered for this patient during her inpatient stay?

A. Corticosteroids
B. Albuterol
C. Racemic epinephrine
D. Chest physiotherapy
E. Nebulized hypertonic saline

21. An 18-month-old male with mild developmental delay presents after two febrile seizures 10 hours apart. The episodes were brief, generalized, and tonic-clonic and lasted less than 5 minutes. For the past 2 days, he has had congestion, rhinorrhea, and fever with maximum temperatures of 38.4°C. His neurological examination is normal, and he is generally well appearing. Which of the following is the best counseling to provide to his parents?

A. He is not likely to have another seizure with future febrile illnesses
B. He does not require evaluation with an electroencephalogram (EEG)
C. He has a higher risk of epilepsy than the general population
D. Giving him acetaminophen with illnesses will prevent future seizures
E. A computerized tomographic (CT) scan of the head will likely find an underlying diagnosis

22. A 16-year-old female with no past medical history is currently admitted with dehydration and poor oral intake due to throat pain. On morning rounds, the patient reports that she has also had knee pain. On physical examination, she has bilateral tonsillar enlargement with erythema noted. On admission, she had a rapid strep test, extended viral panel, and monospot test, which were all negative. What is the next step in management?

A. Obtain neck and knee imaging
B. Continue symptomatic treatment
C. Send throat culture
D. Send Epstein-Barr virus (EBV) titers
E. Send gonorrhea testing

23. A 3-month-old, full-term female presents to the emergency department due to an episode of color change. The family reports a 15-second period when the infant appeared to stop breathing, her hands and feet turned blue, and she appeared unresponsive. The episode self-resolved, and she cried immediately on being picked up. She has never had any similar episodes. On arrival, her vital signs are a temperature of 37.2°C, heart rate of 120 beats per minute, respiratory rate of 25 breaths per minute, and

an oxygen saturation of 100% on room air. Her physical examination is within normal limits. Which of the following would be the most appropriate management?

A. No workup is necessary based on the history and examination, and the infant may be briefly observed on continuous pulse oximetry
B. A chest radiograph (CXR) should be obtained to rule out a pulmonary etiology of the episode
C. An echocardiogram should be obtained to rule out a cardiac etiology of the episode
D. A complete blood count (CBC) with differential should be obtained to rule out possible infections
E. The infant should be discharged with home cardiorespiratory monitoring and follow-up with their primary care provider within 24 hours

24. A 10-year-old boy is admitted with newly diagnosed diabetes. After a 3-week hospitalization, his blood glucose has normalized, and he is being discharged with close outpatient follow-up. His grandmother asks you if he has type 1 or type 2 diabetes. Which of the following would most suggest a diagnosis of type 2 diabetes in this patient?

A. Low C-peptide
B. Absence of anti-insulin antibodies
C. Absence of pancreatic islet autoantibodies
D. High body mass index (BMI)
E. Genetic testing for type 2 diabetes

25. A 9-year-old former preterm female is admitted for weight loss and malnutrition. Her mother reports that the patient is unable to swallow due to severe pain. She has had several admissions at local hospitals for similar complaints, with negative evaluation, including swallow study, computed tomography (CT) of the neck and chest, and endoscopy. She was able to demonstrate weight gain and adequate oral intake each time and was discharged home with recommendations for outpatient follow-up. Despite several multidisciplinary meetings, the mother insists the patient needs a gastrostomy tube (G-tube) to prevent dehydration and further admissions. Which of the following is the next best step in the management of this patient?

A. Repeat CT
B. pH probe
C. Chromosomal analysis
D. Report to Child Protective Services (CPS)
E. Gastrostomy tube placement

26. An 8-year-old female is admitted to the floor with acute onset of periorbital edema, abdominal pain, and abnormal urinalysis. While receiving supportive care, nephrology is consulted to discuss a renal biopsy. Which of the following would indicate a need for a kidney biopsy in this patient?

A. Steroid-resistant nephrotic syndrome
B. Age of patient
C. Periorbital edema
D. Transient proteinuria
E. Family history of renal disease

27. A 3-year-old girl presents with 4 days of lower extremity rash and abdominal pain. There are petechiae and palpable purpura on the buttocks, thighs, and calves bilaterally. The abdominal pain is crampy and "comes and goes." She is afebrile with no changes in oral intake, stooling, or urination. She has had some aches in her hips and knees. She is otherwise well appearing. Laboratory testing reveals normal blood cell counts, coagulation studies, and urine studies. Of the following, which is the next best step in treatment?

A. Intravenous immunoglobulin
B. Ceftriaxone
C. Methylprednisolone
D. Naproxen
E. Watchful waiting

28. A 7-year-old boy presents to the emergency department with fever, knee pain, and limp for 2 days. His physical examination is significant for swelling and warmth in the left knee, inability to flex the left knee due to pain, and inability to bear weight on the left side. The remainder of his physical examination is normal. His C-reactive protein level is elevated, erythrocyte sedimentation rate is 60 mm/h, and white blood cell count is 20×10^9/L. His synovial fluid was found to have 100×10^9/L with a differential of 90% polymorphonuclear leukocytes (PMNs). Which of the following is the most commonly cultured pathogen in this patient's diagnosis?

A. Gram-positive cocci in clusters
B. Gram-positive β-hemolytic cocci in chains
C. Gram-positive α-hemolytic diplococci
D. Gram-negative diplococci
E. Gram-negative coccobacilli

29. A 9-month-old boy is admitted for a left arm abscess requiring intravenous antibiotics after a failure of outpatient treatment with oral antibiotics. He was born at 38 weeks' gestational age with a normal birth weight of 2900 g and no complications during his nursery stay. Over the past 3 months, he has had two episodes of purulent otitis media and one episode of bacterial pneumonia. His mother says he has loose malodorous stools and has not been gaining weight for the past few months. His examination demonstrates an alert infant

with weight of 7.9 kg, hepatomegaly, and a 2-cm abscess on his left forearm with ecchymoses on his upper and lower extremities. His laboratory studies are significant for thrombocytopenia of $70 \times 103/\mu L$, hemoglobin of 9.5 g/dL, white blood cell count of $3000/\mu L$, alanine aminotransferase of 80 IU/L, and absolute neutrophil count of 1000 cells/μL. Due to his underlying congenital condition, what is he at risk for long term?

A. Diabetes mellitus
B. Long bone fractures
C. Leukemia
D. Bronchiectasis
E. Progressive myoclonic epilepsy

30. A recently adopted 2-month-old boy is brought to the emergency department for evaluation of his face turning blue when crying very hard. An echocardiogram confirms a diagnosis of tetralogy of Fallot with pulmonary stenosis, and he is admitted to the floor for preoperative optimization. Soon after his arrival on the floor, you are called to his bedside due to a sustained desaturation to 75% while he is crying. You attempt to soothe the patient and position him knees to chest. What are the next most reasonable steps in management?

A. Oxygen, fluid bolus, prostaglandin E_1
B. Oxygen, morphine, phenylephrine
C. Oxygen, morphine, prostaglandin E_1
D. Morphine, fluid bolus, prostaglandin E_1
E. Morphine, phenylephrine, prostaglandin E_1

31. A confused 16-year-old boy is dropped off at the emergency department by his friends about an hour after school ends. His temperature is 39.5°C, and his heart rate is 130 beats per minute. On examination, he has dilated pupils and dry mucous membranes. He is incoherent and seems to be grabbing at things that no one else sees. His parents are contacted and state that he was fine this morning when he left the house. Which of the following medications is the best treatment for his condition?

A. Dantrolene
B. N-Acetylcysteine
C. Physostigmine
D. Cefepime
E. Atropine

32. An 18-month-old male presents to the emergency department (ED) after swallowing a small, round object from the back of a singing toy. In the ED, his vital signs are as follows: temperature 37°C, respiratory rate 35 breaths per minute, heart rate 130 beats per minute, blood pressure 90/55 mm Hg, and oxygen saturation 99%. Chest radiography shows a small, round, radiopaque object with a radiolucent rim in the right mainstem bronchus. The patient has a cough with some intermittent stridor on examination but no other symptoms. The mother reports that since the patient is otherwise doing well, she will take him home for monitoring like she did previously when her daughter swallowed a piece of a toy. Which of the following is the best next step in management?

A. Discharge the patient home with clear instructions for the parents
B. Confirm location of the toy with computerized tomography (CT) of the chest
C. Admit for overnight monitoring with plans for bronchoscopy in the morning
D. Administer 10 mL of honey followed by charcoal
E. Arrange for the patient to be taken to the bronchoscopy suite for immediate object removal

33. An 8-year-old female is admitted with concerns for moderate dehydration and poor oral intake requiring intravenous fluids. She has a temperature of 39.8°C, heart rate of 146 beats per minute, respiratory rate of 24 breaths per minute, and a blood pressure of 105/62 mm Hg. On examination, she is noted to be uncomfortable and crying. There is nuchal rigidity and a positive Brudzinski sign. The remainder of her examination is unremarkable. As the admitting physician, you are concerned for bacterial meningitis. Which of the following is the best empiric antimicrobial treatment?

A. Ceftriaxone
B. Ceftriaxone and vancomycin
C. Ampicillin, ceftriaxone, and rifampin
D. Ampicillin and gentamicin
E. Meropenem and vancomycin

34. A 15-year-old female presents to the emergency room for worsening throat pain. Her parents report that she has had fevers to 38.8°C at home, with poor oral intake and fatigue for the past 3 days. She was previously at a sleepover at her friend's house, and two of the other people at the sleepover currently have similar symptoms. In the emergency room, vital signs are notable for temperature 39.3°C, respiratory rate 18 breaths per minute, blood pressure 110/72 mm Hg, heart rate 98 beats per minute, and oxygen saturation 98%. Her physical examination is significant for bilateral tonsillar enlargement with bilateral cervical lymphadenopathy and hepatosplenomegaly. The emergency department calls to admit the patient to the inpatient wards. Which of the following is associated with this patient's diagnosis?

A. Myocarditis
B. Soft tissue infections
C. Paronychial infections

D. Increased risk of fractures

E. Hyperglycemia

35. A 6-month-old female infant born at term is now admitted to the hospital for bronchiolitis. Her weight and length from birth and this visit are shown in the growth chart in Figure 1.1.

She is exclusively breastfed and has a small emesis after most feeds. Her stools are yellow, seedy, loose, and nonbloody. She feeds every 3 hours and

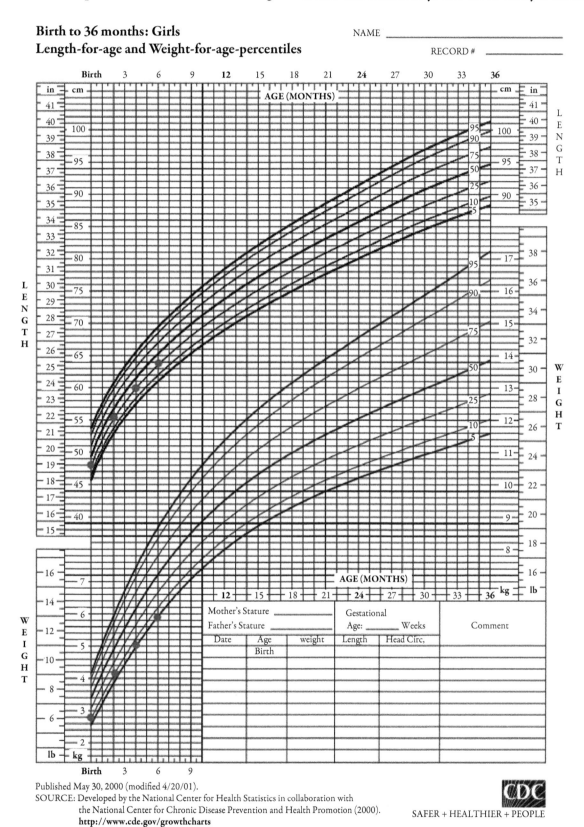

Birth to 36 months: Girls
Length-for-age and Weight-for-age-percentiles

NAME _____

RECORD # _____

Published May 30, 2000 (modified 4/20/01).

SOURCE: Developed by the National Center for Health Statistics in collaboration with
the National Center for Chronic Disease Prevention and Health Promotion (2000).
http://www.cde.gov/growthcharts

SAFER + HEALTHIER + PEOPLE

Figure 1.1

sleeps about 6 hours at night. What is the best next step?

- A. Supplement with formula after every feeding
- B. Initiate a proton pump inhibitor
- C. Provide reassurance
- D. Perform a 48-hour calorie count
- E. Laboratory evaluation with complete blood cell count and complete metabolic panel

36. A 5-year-old boy recently diagnosed with type 1 diabetes mellitus is admitted to the hospitalist service for management of a large abscess. His blood glucose is more than 300 mg/dL without acidosis. On review of his history, he has had multiple missed endocrinology clinic visits. The family reports that administering injections is against their religion, so they have not been giving insulin as prescribed. Instead, they have been giving him cinnamon supplements, which they read can help with diabetes. They expressed understanding that insulin is necessary to prevent life-threatening complications such as diabetic ketoacidosis, but they do not want their child to receive this treatment. What is the best next step?

- A. Advise the family to stop giving cinnamon since this is exacerbating his diabetes
- B. Accept the parents' refusal of diabetes treatment due to their religious freedoms
- C. Report the family to Child Protective Services for concern for medical neglect
- D. Formally evaluate the parents' competence for medical decision-making
- E. Treat the abscess but defer diabetes management and discussion to his outpatient endocrinologist

37. A 12-year-old female with no past medical history presents with vaginal bleeding for 4 weeks. The bleeding has been constant and is associated with abdominal pain. Menarche occurred 2 years ago. Her periods typically occur monthly and last 7–10 days with heavy bleeding. She denies any history of being sexually active. She takes no medications. Her vital signs are reassuring. A urine pregnancy test is negative. Which of the following tests is most likely to result in a diagnosis for this patient?

- A. von Willebrand factor antigen and activity assays
- B. Prothrombin time and activated partial thromboplastin time
- C. Bleeding time
- D. Platelet count
- E. Dilute Russell viper venom time

38. A 14-year-old girl is hospitalized with 4 weeks of fatigue, fever, and rash. During that time, she has had decreased energy, reduced appetite, muscle aches, and pains in multiple joints. Her fevers have occurred daily and are greater than 39°C. Three days ago, she developed a facial rash. On examination, she appears fatigued and pale. There is an erythematous rash of her bilateral cheeks with sparing of the nasolabial folds. She is tachycardic with a pericardial rub. Her lungs are clear bilaterally. Laboratory studies obtained prior to hospitalization include leukopenia, thrombocytopenia, anemia, elevated creatinine, hematuria, and nephrotic-range proteinuria. Of the following, which diagnostic test is most important to confirm her diagnosis?

- A. Rheumatoid factor (RF)
- B. Antinuclear antibodies (ANA) titer
- C. Antineutrophil cytoplasmic antibodies (ANCAs)
- D. Epstein-Barr virus (EBV) antibodies
- E. Antistreptolysin O antibodies (ASO)

39. A 3-year-old girl is hospitalized for workup of progressive arm pain for the last week. Her temperature 38.5°C, and the remaining vitals are normal. She has point tenderness without swelling of the mid upper arm on the right side. Laboratory tests demonstrate elevation in white blood cell count, C-reactive protein level, and erythrocyte sedimentation rate. Magnetic resonance imaging of her arm demonstrates bone focal marrow edema of the right humerus. The antibiogram for the region shows methicillin-resistant staphylococcus aureus (MRSA) prevalence of 3% of *Staphylococcus aureus* isolates. Which of the following is the best empiric antibiotic regimen for this patient?

- A. Cefepime
- B. Cefazolin
- C. Vancomycin
- D. Cephalexin
- E. Amoxicillin-clavulanate

40. A male infant is born at a gestational age of 39 weeks to a 29-year-old mother who is now gravida 3, para 3 (G3P3). His mother's prenatal laboratory testing is unremarkable. At the time of delivery, the infant is noted to have a rash consisting of nonerythematous 2- to 3-mm pustules that cover the infant's forehead, neck, chest, abdomen, and back as seen in Figure 1.2. The infant's physical examination is otherwise reassuring, and his vital signs are normal for age. What is the best next step in the management for this infant?

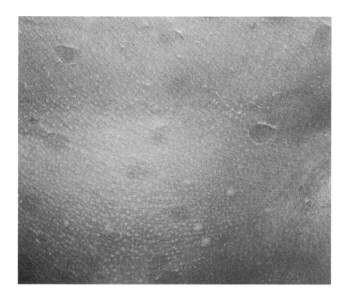

Figure 1.2

A. Blood, urine, and cerebrospinal fluid cultures
B. Viral swab of an unroofed lesion for polymerase chain reaction testing
C. Empiric broad-spectrum antibiotics
D. Maternal viral serologies
E. Reassurance

41. A 6-week-old female presents to the emergency department with 2 weeks of vomiting. The patient's birthweight was 3.31 kg, and she has been tracking along the 50th percentile for weight. Episodes of emesis occur five to six times per day, typically occurring 20 to 30 minutes after feeds. The emesis is not bloody or bilious, and the patient does not seem to be in pain during episodes. She is exclusively breastfed and has been having three or four yellow, seedy stools per day. Her parents deny any other symptoms, and her examination is unremarkable. What is the most appropriate test to confirm the patient's diagnosis?

A. Endoscopy
B. Upper gastrointestinal series with small bowel follow-through
C. Scintigraphy (milk scan)
D. Impedance probe
E. No diagnostic test necessary

42. A 3-year-old Asian male is hospitalized with community-acquired bacterial pneumonia. He was recently adopted, and his parents report that he was otherwise previously healthy. He is receiving 2 L/min of supplemental oxygen via nasal cannula, and his only medication is ampicillin. On hospital day 2, parents note dark-colored urine. His hemoglobin is 7.5 g/dL, down from 11.5 g/dL on admission. Peripheral smear demonstrates Heinz bodies. Which test would provide the definitive diagnosis?

A. Osmotic fragility
B. Ristocetin cofactor
C. Hemoglobin (Hb) electrophoresis
D. Glucose-6-phosphate dehydrogenase assay
E. Direct Coombs test

43. A patient requires a computed tomography (CT) scan of the abdomen with contrast but has a history of a reaction to an iodine-based contrast agent. You determine that completing the CT with contrast is necessary and that no other test will suffice. Which of the following reactions to contrast is *not* likely to be prevented by premedication with a corticosteroid?

A. Hypertension
B. Tachycardia
C. Diffuse urticaria and pruritus
D. Bronchospasm
E. Laryngeal edema

44. A neonate is noted to be cyanotic since his birth 1 hour ago. He is afebrile, and his respiratory rate is 60 breaths per minute. His oxygen saturation is 79% when calm, and it does not improve when placed on supplemental oxygen. On physical examination, there is no heart murmur, and his lungs are clear to auscultation. A chest radiograph demonstrates cardiomegaly, increased pulmonary vascular markings, and an egg-shaped cardiac silhouette. An echocardiogram is ordered. What is the best next step in management?

A. Knees to chest
B. Inotropic support
C. Diuretics
D. Antibiotics
E. Prostaglandin E_1 (PGE_1)

45. A 13-year-old boy presents to the emergency department complaining of diarrhea, vomiting, cough, and weakness after doing yardwork on a summer day. He notices his eyes have been watery, and he is drooling. His initial vitals are notable for a heart rate of 42 beats per minute. Which of the following mechanisms best explains his symptoms?

A. Inhibition of cholinesterase activity
B. Toxin-mediated activation of cytokine pathways
C. Inflammation resulting in peripheral nerve demyelination
D. Inhibition of acetylcholine activity

E. Decreased activity of an enzyme found on the intestinal brush border

C. Glaucoma
D. Skeletal deformities
E. Hypercalcemia

46. A 3-year-old female with no past medical history and normal growth and development is admitted for pneumonia. The father reports frustration that this is her sixth admission in the last year for pneumonia. On review of her history, the hospitalist notes that all of her previous pneumonias have been in the right middle lobe. She had computed tomography (CT) of the head and chest done at 6 months of age after a fall, which showed normal lung anatomy. This morning, her temperature is 37.2°C, respiratory rate is 35 breaths per minute, heart rate is 100 beats per minute, blood pressure is 93/60 mm Hg, and oxygen saturation is 99%. She has continued to improve throughout her admission and is noted to have no increased work of breathing on examination. What is the next step in management?

A. No further investigation is warranted
B. Extend antibiotic therapy to 3–4 weeks of treatment
C. Start prophylactic antibiotics to prevent future pneumonias
D. Repeat chest CT
E. Emergent bronchoscopy

47. A 1-day-old male is being evaluated in the newborn nursery due to concerns for a large erythematous patch involving the left forehead, eyelid, and cheek, as seen in Figure 1.3. The birth history is unremarkable, and there is no history of trauma during delivery. There are no other rashes noted on examination. In addition to seizures, what else is this child at increased risk for?

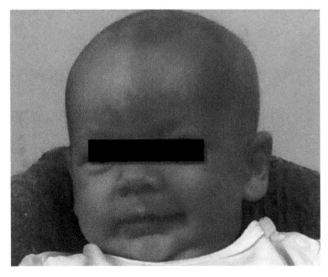

Figure 1.3

A. Plexiform neurofibromas
B. Cardiac rhabdomyomas

48. An 18-month-old male is admitted with bronchiolitis and is on day 3 of hospitalization. On morning rounds, the mother reports that his breathing is overall improved. His vital signs this morning are temperature 37°C, respiratory rate 30 breaths per minute, blood pressure 98/60 mm Hg, heart rate 98 beats per minute, and oxygen saturation 99% on room air. He has had improved oral intake and tolerated 8 ounces of milk this morning. The mother does report that she was concerned overnight that he is having throat pain. His throat examination reveals no tonsillar enlargement or exudate, and his uvula is midline. The overnight resident sent a rapid strep test, which was noted to be positive. What is the best next step in management?

A. Start a treatment course of oral amoxicillin
B. Start a treatment course of intravenous ampicillin
C. Monitor throat pain and start antibiotics tomorrow if throat pain is not improved
D. Monitor throat pain and start antibiotics if respiratory status worsens
E. Monitor throat pain; antibiotics are not indicated

49. A 14-year-old previously healthy female is being admitted to the hospital after presenting with severe muscle aches in her legs and dark urine after a track meet yesterday. Her laboratory work is are shown below, and electrocardiogram (ECG) results are shown in Figure 1.4. The emergency department physician has placed a peripheral intravenous catheter and given a normal saline bolus. What is the best next intervention?

Sodium	130 mmol/L
Potassium	7.2 mmol/L
Bicarbonate	17 mmol/L
Chloride	97 mmol/L
Blood urea nitrogen	50 mg/dL
Creatinine	2.8 mg/dL
Glucose	92 mg/dL
Calcium	10.7 mg/dL
Creatinine kinase	80,000 U/L

A. Intravenous furosemide
B. Subcutaneous insulin
C. Intravenous calcium gluconate
D. Oral Kayexalate
E. Intravenous calcium chloride

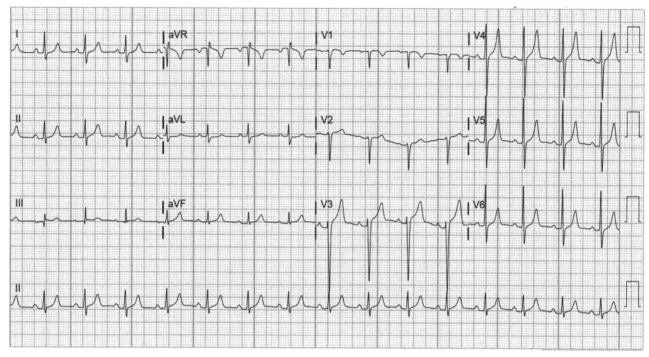

Figure 1.4

50. You are consulted in the emergency department (ED) to see a 12-year-old boy whose father reports that over the past 3 weeks the son has been drinking 3–4 L of water a day and urinating at least every 1–2 hours. He has wet his bed multiple times. His blood glucose is 101 mg/dL. Urine studies reveal a specific gravity of 1.003 and is otherwise unremarkable. What is the best next step in management?

A. Limiting his water intake
B. Fasting blood glucose and pancreatic antibodies
C. Oral glucose tolerance test
D. Early morning blood and urine testing with electrolytes
E. Treatment with desmopressin

51. A 7-year-old female presents to the emergency department for vaginal bleeding. On examination, a doughnut-shaped mass is seen protruding from the urethral opening, with significant erythema and a small amount of bleeding. What is the best next step?

A. Report concern for abuse to Child Protective Services
B. Sitz bath and estrogen cream
C. Steroid cream
D. Pelvic ultrasound
E. Vaginal irrigation

52. A 4-year-old male with an indwelling urinary catheter presents with fever and dysuria for 2 days. He takes cephalexin daily for urinary tract infection (UTI) prophylaxis. He has had multiple UTIs in the past but does not recall which antibiotics were used for treatment. Past urine culture results are not available. On the examination, he is tired appearing, is moderately dehydrated, and has tenderness to palpation in the suprapubic region. A urinalysis is positive for leukocyte esterase and has numerous white blood cells on microscopy; nitrites are negative. A urine Gram stain shows gram-positive cocci, and a urine culture is sent. He is admitted to the floor and started on intravenous fluids. Which of the following is the most appropriate empiric treatment for this patient while awaiting urine culture results?

A. Ceftriaxone
B. Trimethoprim-sulfamethoxazole
C. Ampicillin
D. Gentamicin
E. Nitrofurantoin

53. A 22-month-old boy presents with fever, right leg pain, and refusal to walk for 3 days. The pain occurs with rest and with activity. His vitals are normal, and he is well appearing. His right thigh is tender and mildly swollen without skin changes or fluctuance. He has a bug bite on his hand with excoriation but no swelling or redness. He has full passive range of motion at the knee and hips. He refuses to bear weight. Laboratory tests demonstrate a white blood cell count of 15×10^9/L, C-reactive protein level of 8 mg/L, and erythrocyte sedimentation rate of 75 mm/h. Blood cultures are

obtained. Which of the following imaging studies is the best next step in the workup of this patient?

   A. Magnetic resonance imaging (MRI) of the lower extremity
   B. Hip ultrasound
   C. Plain radiograph of the lower extremity
   D. Radionuclide scan using technetium Tc 99m
   E. Computed tomography (CT) of the lower extremity

54. A 16-year-old previously healthy male presents with rash. He first noticed a single "red spot" a few days ago, but it has since increased in size (see Figure 1.5). The patient reports that the rash is not itchy or painful. His vital signs are appropriate for age, and the rest of his physical examination is normal. There are no swollen joints or abnormal neurologic findings. There are no known sick contacts or recent illnesses. His only travel history is a camping trip in Wisconsin with friends 2 weeks ago. He has had no exposures to new foods or animals. Of the following, which is the best next step in management?

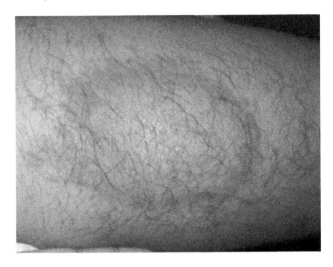

Figure 1.5

   A. Antibody testing
   B. Skin biopsy
   C. C-reactive protein and erythrocyte sedimentation rate
   D. Empiric antibiotic treatment
   E. Emollients and ongoing monitoring

55. A 6-month-old male presents to the emergency department with 1 day of bloody stools and intermittent inconsolability. He was born at full term and has been otherwise healthy. Between episodes, the patient is calm and slightly more sleepy than usual. He is breastfed, has incorporated several new foods over the past 2 months, and has been feeding well with normal urine output. He has not had any other symptoms and has been growing well along the 50th percentile for weight and length.

Which of the following is associated with the patient's most likely diagnosis?

   A. Breastfeeding
   B. Recent immunization
   C. Secondhand smoke exposure
   D. History of prematurity
   E. Recent episode of bacterial otitis media

56. A 10-year-old male with sickle cell disease presents with fever to 39°C and poor oral intake. His physical examination is consistent with mild dehydration but is otherwise normal. The patient is started on ceftriaxone and intravenous fluids and is admitted the hospital. Overnight, he develops hypoxemia, with oxygen saturations of 86% in room air. Supplemental oxygen is applied with improvement in saturations. A chest x-ray is obtained and demonstrates a right middle lobe infiltrate. What is the best addition to the antibiotic regimen for this patient?

   A. Clindamycin
   B. Vancomycin
   C. Ampicillin
   D. Azithromycin
   E. Penicillin

57. An 8-week-old boy born at full term with a history of delayed umbilical cord separation is admitted with recurrent omphalitis requiring intravenous antibiotics. On examination, he is a well-appearing infant with a dry, necrotic umbilical cord. The skin around the umbilicus is erythematous and tender to palpation. What infectious complications is this patient most at risk for in the future?

   A. Osteomyelitis
   B. Viral lower respiratory tract infections
   C. Fungemia
   D. Suppurative adenitis
   E. Recurrent bacterial lung and skin infections

58. A 6-week-old former full-term baby girl with a known large, unrepaired ventricular septal defect (VSD) is admitted due to poor weight gain. Her mother reports that over the last 2 days, she has been taking increasingly less feeds and seems to get tired and sweaty while feeding. She has a heart rate of 180 beats per minute, respiratory rate of 65 breaths per minute, and rales bilaterally. Which of the following represents the most likely ratio of pulmonary (Q_p) to systemic (Q_s) blood flow for this child?

   A. $Q_p{:}Q_s = 0.2$
   B. $Q_p{:}Q_s = 0.5$

C. $Q_p:Q_s = 0.7$
D. $Q_p:Q_s = 1.0$
E. $Q_p:Q_s = 2.5$

59. A 6-year-old boy is brought to the hospital after being bitten by a venomous snake in the left calf 2 hours ago. He complains of severe pain to the affected leg. He has not had any nausea, vomiting, difficulty breathing, or changes in his mental status. His vital signs show a temperature of 36.8°C, heart rate of 125 beats per minute, respiratory rate of 24 breaths per minute, blood pressure of 110/76 mm Hg, and oxygen saturation of 99%. Examination of his left calf shows two puncture wound marks with surrounding edema and ecchymosis and is tender to touch. The remainder of his examination is unremarkable. Laboratory evaluation, including electrolytes, coagulation panel, renal function, creatine kinase, and cardiac function are all within normal limits, except a platelet count of 110 platelets/μL. Which of the following is the most accurate assessment of his degree of envenomation?

A. None ("dry bite")
B. Mild
C. Moderate
D. Severe
E. Unable to determine with the information provided

60. The medical team is evaluating a 2-year-old male in the emergency department (ED) after presenting with concern about an aspiration event. His parents report that he was eating popcorn about an hour ago and was noted to have a choking event; they are concerned that he aspirated a piece of popcorn. Which of the following symptoms is consistent with aspiration?

A. Wheezing and decreased air movement
B. Increased work of breathing and crackles
C. Rhonchi and mediastinal crunch
D. Pleural friction rub and stridor
E. Transmitted upper airway sounds and rales

61. An 11-year-old female who was recently treated for sinusitis with amoxicillin now presents with fever, headache, left arm weakness, altered level of consciousness, and vomiting. Which of the following is the most appropriate empiric antibiotic choice?

A. Gentamicin, vancomycin, and cefazolin
B. Gentamicin and ceftriaxone
C. Ceftriaxone and metronidazole
D. Vancomycin and metronidazole
E. Tobramycin and nafcillin

62. You are caring for a 5-year-old patient admitted with a retropharyngeal abscess. The father reports that symptoms began 3 days prior to presentation and progressed to the point that the patient was no longer able to tolerate any oral intake. The patient has been on intravenous ampicillin/sulbactam and has been improving. Which of the following statements is true?

A. Peritonsillar abscesses are uncommon infections in the pediatric population
B. Retropharyngeal abscesses are commonly caused by a single organism
C. Peritonsillar abscesses most commonly occur in patients under 1 year of age
D. Retropharyngeal abscesses can spread to the chest as a complication
E. Retropharyngeal infections are more likely than peritonsillar abscesses to require surgical intervention

63. You receive a call from a community pediatrician about a 12-month-old patient that is in her office for a well check. She has seen the child for all her prior visits, but the family missed the 9-month well check. The pediatrician shares the growth chart in Figure 1.6.

This child's weight-for-height z score is 3 or less. Other than the missed well check, the pediatrician has no concerns about the family. By parental report the patient is taking adequate calories. The pediatrician is asking for your guidance on next steps. Which of the following would you recommend?

A. Order outpatient laboratory tests and have the patient return for a follow-up in 1 week
B. Begin oral supplementation with formula and have the patient return for follow-up in 1 week
C. Begin nasogastric tube (NGT) supplementation with formula and have the patient return for follow-up in 1 week
D. Request an urgent outpatient gastroenterology consultation for the patient
E. Admit the patient to the hospital for evaluation

64. You are rounding in the newborn nursery and see a 1-day-old with a bulbous nose and a cleft palate. You hear a murmur on examination and order an echocardiogram. Laboratory studies are significant for a serum calcium level of 6.3 mg/dL. What is the most likely cause of this patient's hypocalcemia?

A. Hypoparathyroidism
B. CHARGE association
C. Maternal vitamin D deficiency
D. Hypogammaglobulinemia
E. Inadequate intake

Birth to 36 months: Girls
Length-for-age and Weight-for-age-percentiles

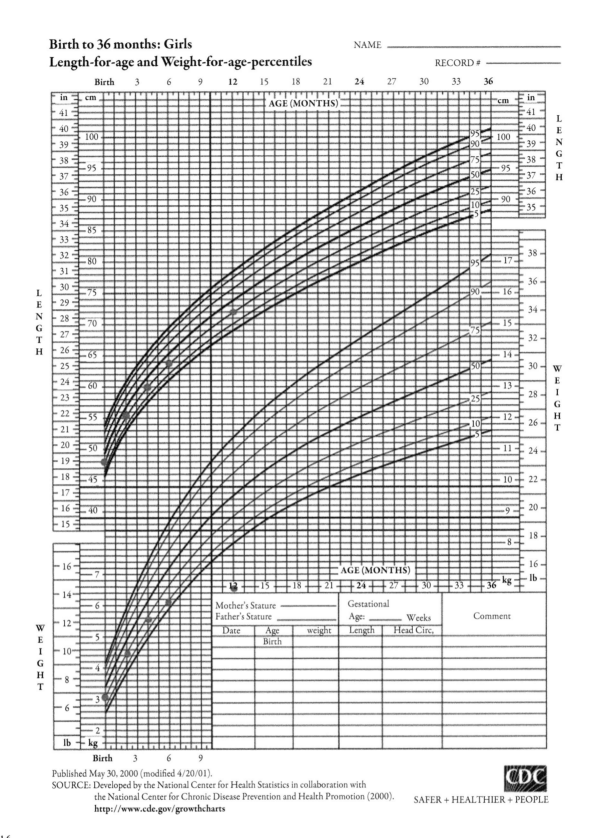

Published May 30, 2000 (modified 4/20/01).
SOURCE: Developed by the National Center for Health Statistics in collaboration with
the National Center for Chronic Disease Prevention and Health Promotion (2000).
http://www.cde.gov/growthcharts

SAFER + HEALTHIER + PEOPLE

Figure 1.6

65. A 5-month-old male presents to the hospital with fever and left arm shaking. The parents report no known ingestion or trauma preceding this change. On examination, the patient is fussy and inconsolable and has a witnessed episode concerning for left-sided focal seizure. Computed tomography (CT) of the head demonstrates a subdural and subarachnoid hemorrhage with mild focal mass effect on the right. His hemoglobin is 9.5 g/dL; platelets are 312,000/μL; aspartate aminotransferase (AST) is 38 U/L; lipase is less than 10 U/L; prothrombin time (PT) is 14.7 seconds; and partial thromboplastin time (PTT) is 101 seconds. A skeletal survey is normal. What is the best next step in management?

A. Lumbar puncture
B. Report to Child Protective Services (CPS)
C. Factor 8 infusion
D. Abdominal ultrasound
E. Brain magnetic resonance imaging (MRI)

66. A 2-year-old boy with no significant past medical history presents to the emergency room with fever and decreased urine output. He has not had a wet diaper for 2 days and appears tired today. One week ago, he had developed a dry cough and was diagnosed with a respiratory infection. His vital signs include a temperature of 101.5°F, a respiratory rate of 45 breaths per minute, an oxygen saturation of 88%, a heart rate of 135 beats per minute, and a blood pressure of 100/70 mm Hg. On examination he is ill appearing and alert, has right-sided lung crackles and diminished breath sounds, and has multiple sites of extensive petechiae. His clinical studies are significant for azotemia, elevated creatinine, normocytic anemia, thrombocytopenia, elevated white blood cell count, and a chest radiograph showing a right-sided effusion. The patient is admitted for sepsis and dehydration. Which of the following complications is this patient *not* at risk of developing during his hospitalization?

A. Coronary artery abnormalities
B. Anemia requiring red blood cell transfusion
C. Hyperkalemia
D. End -stage renal failure
E. Thrombosis

67. An 8-year-old previously healthy male is hospitalized with facial rash and weakness. The rash started a few weeks ago and was initially erythematous and localized to his upper eyelids. His primary care provider recommended starting an antihistamine. The rash has now spread to his bilateral cheeks and has a purplish hue. He also finds it more difficult to rise from a chair. Physical examination is notable for proximal muscle weakness with normal distal muscle strength and purplish-red discoloration of his bilateral upper eyelids. Of the following, which laboratory studies are most likely to support the diagnosis?

A. Complete blood cell count and differential
B. Creatine kinase (CK) and lactate dehydrogenase (LDH)
C. Lyme immunoglobulin (Ig) G and IgM
D. Anti–double-stranded DNA
E. C-reactive protein and erythrocyte sedimentation rate

68. A 4-year-old boy is hospitalized with 2 days of worsening rash. The rash started as a few red "spots and rings" that have persisted and spread. He has had fevers up to 104°F and complains of aches in his knees and ankles. He was diagnosed with otitis media 10 days ago and just completed a course of amoxicillin. He has been taking ibuprofen for discomfort. His mother has been applying scented lotion on his skin after baths. Your examination is significant for a diffuse blanching rash and mild facial and lower extremity edema (as seen in Figure 1.7). The rash also involves the lateral borders of the feet but spares the palms and soles. There is no mucosal involvement. Of the following, which is the most likely underlying trigger of the child's symptoms?

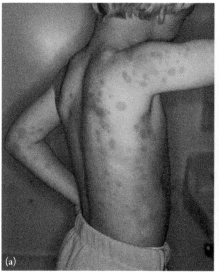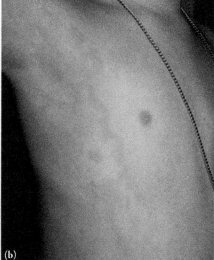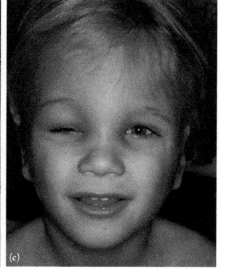

(a)   (b)   (c)

Figure 1.7

A. Amoxicillin
B. Ibuprofen
C. Parabens
D. Herpes simplex virus (HSV)
E. *Mycoplasma pneumoniae*

69. A 15-year-old female is admitted for management of severe epigastric abdominal pain and vomiting. Her symptoms have been present for 4 days and have worsened since onset. Her examination is significant for diffuse abdominal tenderness without rebound or guarding and no appreciable masses. Her serum amylase and lipase are significantly elevated. The patient has been admitted three times over the past year for similar episodes. Additionally, the patient's mother has similar episodes. Which of the following genes is associated with the patient's most likely underlying diagnosis?

A. *JAG1*
B. *NOTCH2*
C. *SPINK1*
D. *PRSS1*
E. *CFTR*

70. A 16-year-old obese female with a history of mild persistent asthma is admitted to the hospital with shortness of breath and chest pain. Her asthma is well controlled at baseline, and she has no other medical problems. Her medications are fluticasone, albuterol, and an oral contraceptive. On physical examination, she is afebrile; her heart rate is 120 beats/min, respiratory rate is 30 breaths/min, and oxygen saturation is 88% on room air. Her lungs are clear to auscultation bilaterally. A chest x-ray is normal. Of the following, which is the best next diagnostic study?

A. Echocardiogram
B. Ventilation/perfusion scintigraphy
C. Helical computed tomographic (CT) pulmonary angiography
D. D-dimer
E. Magnetic resonance pulmonary angiography

71. A 7-week-old female is admitted for acute diarrhea requiring intravenous hydration. Per her parents, her stools are occasionally bloody. She has been gaining weight appropriately. On review of systems, her parents deny fever, fussiness, vomiting, runny nose, cough, or other significant symptoms. Her examination is reassuring. Her basic metabolic panel, complete blood count, and abdominal x-ray are all within normal limits. She has a diet of breastmilk and cow milk–based

formula. What is the most likely cause of this patient's bloody loose stools?

A. Lactose intolerance
B. Food protein–induced proctitis/proctocolitis of infancy
C. Eosinophilic gastroenteritis
D. Necrotizing enterocolitis
E. Malrotation with volvulus

72. A 9-year-old boy with Duchene muscular dystrophy (DMD) is hospitalized with new fatigue and shortness of breath that worsens while lying in bed. A chest radiograph reveals an enlarged heart and prominent pulmonary vascular markings. His echocardiogram shows evidence of a cardiomyopathy that has progressed from a previous echocardiogram. Which of the following is the most likely form of cardiomyopathy in this patient?

A. Hypertrophic cardiomyopathy
B. Dilated cardiomyopathy
C. Restrictive cardiomyopathy
D. Arrhythmogenic cardiomyopathy
E. Noncompaction cardiomyopathy

73. A 3-year-old boy is seen in the emergency department after his parents witnessed him ingesting a coin. His x-ray demonstrates a coin located in the distal esophagus. He remains asymptomatic, denying pain, difficulty breathing, or trouble swallowing his secretions. Which of the following is the most appropriate next step?

A. Admit to the hospital and plan for emergent endoscopic removal within the next 2 hours
B. Admit to the hospital and plan for urgent endoscopic removal within the next 24 hours if the coin remains in the esophagus
C. Admit to the hospital and plan for observation until spontaneous passage
D. Discharge home, with plan to follow-up with an outpatient pediatrician within the next 24 hours
E. Discharge home, with plan to observe for passage of the coin in his stool

74. A 12-year-old female with a history of moderate persistent asthma presents to the emergency room with severe shortness of breath and wheezing. Vital signs are significant for a respiratory rate of 32 breaths per minute and oxygen saturation of 92% on ambient air. Arterial blood gas shows pH 7.37, $PaCO_2$ 32 mm Hg, PaO_2 65 mm Hg, and bicarbonate 19 mEq/L. She is given intravenous methylprednisolone, three nebulized albuterol and ipratropium treatments, and supplemental oxygen. Follow-up vital signs 1 hour later are notable for a respiratory rate of 18 breaths per minute and oxygen saturation of 95% on 3 lL/min of supplemental oxygen via nasal cannula. A repeat arterial blood gas is obtained and shows pH 7.25, $PaCO_2$ 49 mm Hg, PaO_2 75 mm Hg, and bicarbonate 20 mEq/L. What is the best next step in the management of this patient?

A. Begin continuous albuterol treatment
B. Prepare to obtain an advanced airway
C. Administer intravenous magnesium
D. Begin heliox therapy
E. Administer a second dose of intravenous steroids

75. A 17-year-old male with a history of sickle cell disease presents with acute onset of vertigo, dizziness, headache, and unsteadiness on his feet for the past 12 hours. He has been afebrile and has not had any other illness symptoms. What is the most appropriate next step in evaluation?

A. Computed tomography of the head
B. Quantitative vestibular testing
C. Magnetic resonance imaging (MRI) of the brain
D. Echocardiogram
E. Lumbar puncture

76. You are called to the emergency department (ED) for a 5-year-old female with unilateral facial swelling. Her parents report that her symptoms started 3 days prior to presentation and have continued to worsen. The area is erythematous and warm to the touch. Her family denies any trauma or insect bites to the area. She has had decreased oral intake over this time, with two voids in the past 24 hours. In the ED, she is afebrile, and her vital signs are stable. On physical examination, she has right-sided facial swelling that is very tender to palpation. You note that there is some pus visible at the Stenson duct. Which of the following is a potential complication of this condition?

A. Facial nerve palsy
B. Tonsillar swelling
C. Cyclic vomiting
D. Migraine headaches
E. Upper extremity paresthesia

77. A 9-month-old previously healthy female is admitted with lethargy, fevers, and decreased oral intake in septic shock. She undergoes a sepsis workup, including a urine and blood culture. She is started on intravenous ceftriaxone. Initial blood and urine cultures are growing *Escherichia coli* (*E. coli*). A repeat blood culture shows no growth, and the patient is back at her baseline, afebrile and well appearing. What is the best next step?

A. Obtain a voiding cystourethrography (VCUG)
B. Repeat a urine culture to document clearance
C. Obtain an echocardiogram
D. Provide a peripherally inserted central catheter (PICC) for prolonged intravenous antibiotic course
E. Transition to oral antibiotics based on sensitivities

78. You are asked to admit a 6-year-old boy from the emergency department (ED) for altered mental status. According to his parents, for the past several months he has been less active than usual and is now sleeping most of the day. He was previously healthy with normal development. A complete blood count, comprehensive metabolic profile, and infectious workup, including lumbar puncture, have not revealed a diagnosis. On physical examination, you note a diffusely enlarged thyroid gland. You admit the patient and send serum studies, which reveal the following:

Thyroid-stimulating hormone (TSH) 434 mIU/L (range 0.5–4.3 mIU/L)
Free thyroxine (T_4) 0.5 ng/dL (range 0.9–1.4 ng/dL)
Corticotropin (ACTH) 18 ng/L (range 9–57 ng/L)
Cortisol 9 μg/dL (range 2–13 μg/dL)

What is the appropriate next step in management?

A. Check thyroid antibodies
B. Obtain a thyroid scan
C. Start low-dose levothyroxine
D. Perform a thyroid biopsy
E. Obtain brain imaging

79. A 1-year-old male with a history of failure to thrive presents to the emergency department with right leg pain and inability to bear weight. His mother reports he fell from standing height and immediately began to cry. An x-ray of the affected extremity demonstrates a femur fracture with evidence of osteopenia. Which of the following is most likely to yield the diagnosis?

A. Head computed tomography (CT) scan
B. Social history
C. Skeletal survey
D. Peripheral blood smear
E. Serum and urine electrolytes

80. A 17-year-old female with no significant past medical history is admitted for severe abdominal pain. The pain has been present for 2 days across the lower

abdomen. She has also had nausea and nonbloody emesis and states that she has not been able to tolerate anything by mouth for 24 hours. Her temperature is 38.6°C, heart rate is 109 beats per minute, respiratory rate is 16 breaths per minute, and oxygen saturation is 99% on room air. On examination, she appears uncomfortable and has severe tenderness to palpation and rebound tenderness across the lower abdomen. A pelvic examination is notable for purulent discharge from the cervical os and bilateral adnexal tenderness. A urine pregnancy test is negative. Abdominal and pelvic ultrasounds and a computed tomographic scan of the abdomen are negative, showing a normal appendix and normal ovaries. Which of the following is the most appropriate treatment for this patient?

A. Clindamycin and gentamicin
B. Levofloxacin and metronidazole
C. Piperacillin-tazobactam
D. Ampicillin and doxycycline
E. Azithromycin and metronidazole

81. A 16-year-old previously healthy male is hospitalized after presenting to the emergency department with knee pain. Two days ago, his right knee became tender and swollen. He also notes that his left ankle has been "bothering him" for the past 4 days. He has been afebrile and denies recent illness, other joint pain, rash, oral lesions, abdominal pain, diarrhea, or urinary symptoms. He does well in school and enjoys playing basketball. He is sexually active with a single female partner. He denies drug or alcohol use. His vital signs are normal. On examination, his right knee is swollen but nonerythematous. Flexion of the right knee is limited due to pain. His posterior left ankle is swollen and tender to palpation without overlying skin changes. Palpation of his sacroiliac joints elicits mild tenderness. All other joints are normal. He has bilateral conjunctival injection. Laboratory studies are notable for erythrocyte sedimentation rate of 21 mm/h, C-reactive protein of 4 mg/L (normal < 1), and white blood cell count of 10,500 cells/mm³. Of the following, testing for which infectious pathogen is most likely to yield a positive result?

A. *Staphylococcus aureus*
B. Group A *Streptococcus*
C. *Chlamydia trachomatis*
D. *Campylobacter jejuni*
E. *Haemophilus influenzae*

82. A 5-year-old boy is referred by his primary care physician for hospital admission for management of severe eczema. He has widespread eczematous lesions over his face and extremities without evidence of superinfection.

He often cannot sleep due to itching. Emollients, topical steroids, and wet wraps have been trialed in the past, resulting in transient improvement, though adherence has not been consistent. His parents are upset that he has not improved and find his condition difficult to manage due to their work schedules and other child care obligations. You agree to hospitalize the child. Of the following, what is the best next step in management?

A. Intravenous nafcillin and topical hydrocortisone
B. Intravenous methylprednisolone
C. Wet wrap therapy (WWT) with topical triamcinolone
D. Calcineurin inhibitor therapy
E. Initiation of biologic therapy

83. A 3-week-old former full-term male presents to the emergency department with bilious emesis and abdominal distension. The patient's symptoms began 4 hours prior to presentation. He is otherwise asymptomatic and has been breastfeeding well with 4-5 yellow, seedy stools per day. On examination, the patient has notable abdominal distension with a rigid abdomen and hypoactive bowel sounds. He is hypotensive and has poor perfusion. After appropriate fluid resuscitation, what is the next most appropriate step in management?

A. Administration of systemic corticosteroids
B. Emergent surgical exploration
C. Gastric decompression
D. Administration of broad-spectrum antibiotics
E. Administration of packed red blood cells

84. A 2-year-old female is hospitalized with acute pyelonephritis. She demonstrates clinical improvement on intravenous antibiotics, and the medical team is preparing to discharge her home on oral antibiotics. On chart review, the hospitalist notes that the patient's most recent hemoglobin was 8.2 g/dL, hematocrit 24.6 g/dL, and mean corpuscular volume 65 fL. White blood cell count was elevated on admission but normalized, and platelet count is normal. The patient's skin color is pale. She is well perfused and has normal vital signs. Parents deny any history of bloody stools or other bleeding. The patient is described as a picky eater who dislikes meat. She drinks approximately 16 ounces of cow's milk per day. Of the following, what is the most appropriate next step?

A. Elimination of cow's milk from the diet
B. Initiation of oral iron supplementation and follow-up with primary care provider
C. Referral to a hematologist
D. Red blood cell transfusion
E. Initiation of vitamin B$_{12}$ supplementation

85. A fully vaccinated 5-year-old female with a history of obesity is admitted to the hospital. Ten days ago, she was diagnosed with an intergluteal abscess and is completing a 14-day course of trimethoprim-sulfamethoxazole. Five days ago, she developed a pruritic rash, which started in the groin and has spread to the back, arms, and legs. She has had intermittent fevers one or two times per day for 3 days, reaching a maximum of 38.4°C. On examination, you note diffuse urticarial lesions on the abdomen, back, and all four extremities. There are no lesions in the oropharyngeal, perianal, or vagina mucosa. She appears tired. Inflammatory markers are elevated. The skin lesions evolved slowly, with individual lesions lasting for more than a day. Some lesions now have central areas of clearing. Which of the following is the most appropriate next step?

A. Discontinue trimethoprim-sulfamethoxazole
B. Discontinue trimethoprim-sulfamethoxazole and start corticosteroids
C. Discontinue trimethoprim-sulfamethoxazole and start clindamycin
D. Nuclear medicine tagged white blood cell scan
E. Allergy skin testing with trimethoprim-sulfamethoxazole

86. A rapid response is called for tachycardia in a 9-month-old female who is hospitalized with bronchiolitis. She is afebrile with a heart rate of 230 beats per minute (beats/min) without variation. Her blood pressure and respiratory rate are normal. On examination, the patient is alert and well perfused. The nurse has informed you that the infant's heart rate was 140 beats/min a few minutes ago and suddenly rose to more than 200 beats/min prior to your arrival. The nurse put an ice-water bag over the infant's face for a few seconds, which failed to lower the heart rate. An electrocardiogram (ECG) rhythm strip is shown in Figure 1.8. What is the best next step in management?

A. Propranolol
B. Normal saline bolus
C. Adenosine
D. Verapamil
E. Synchronized cardioversion

87. A 2-year-old girl presents to the hospital after ingesting an unknown object from her mother's purse. She is asymptomatic. Which of the following objects, if found in the esophagus, would prompt emergent endoscopic removal?

A. Single magnet
B. Quarter
C. Bead
D. Watch battery
E. Safety pin

88. A 9-year-old male with a history of asthma presents to the emergency room with wheezing and difficulty

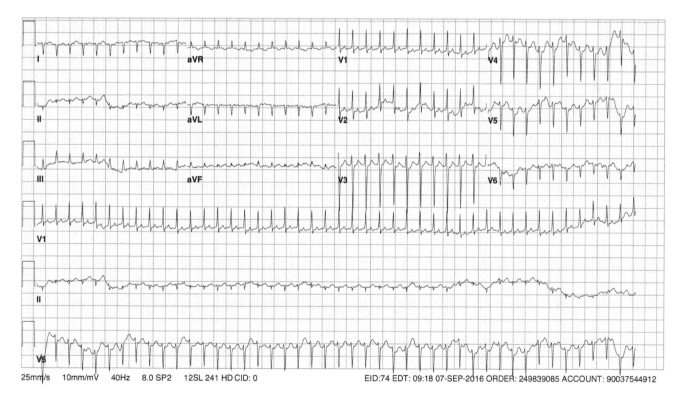

25mm/s   10mm/mV   40Hz   8.0 SP2   12SL 241 HD CID: 0   EID:74 EDT: 09:18 07-SEP-2016 ORDER: 249839085 ACCOUNT: 90037544912

Figure 1.8

breathing. His vital signs are notable for a respiratory rate of 36 breaths per minute, heart rate of 100 beats per minute, and oxygen saturation of 95%. His physical examination demonstrates moderately increased work of breathing and diffuse bilateral expiratory wheeze. He is started on nebulized albuterol and ipratropium bromide, to be given over the next hour. Thirty minutes into his treatment, the provider notices a change in oxygen saturation to 90%, with stable tachypnea and mildly increased tachycardia. What is the next step in management?

A. Obtain arterial blood gas
B. Prepare to obtain an advanced airway
C. Administer intravenous magnesium sulfate
D. Stop nebulized treatment and switch to albuterol and ipratropium bromide via metered dose inhaler (MDI)
E. Administer oxygen via nasal cannula

89. A 6-month-old female term infant is presenting with abnormal movements described by her mother as sudden arm and leg stiffening with her head bending forward. These episodes seem to happen most often when waking from sleep and have been increasing in frequency. On physical examination, you note hypomelanotic macules. Of the following, which do you expect to find on neuroimaging?

A. Lissencephaly
B. Subependymal nodules
C. Absent corpus collosum
D. Acute ischemic lesions
E. Pituitary hypoplasia

90. A 5-year-old female presents to the emergency department (ED) with unilateral facial swelling and redness. The patient's symptoms started 5 days prior to presentation. She has had blood work and computed tomography (CT) of the face, the results of which are currently pending. On physical examination, the patient has left-sided facial swelling with tenderness. On bimanual intraoral palpation, there is a hard entity along the Stenson duct. What is the best next step in management?

A. Obtain magnetic resonance imaging (MRI) of the face in addition to the CT
B. Administer a sialagogue
C. Perform gentle massage of the right side of the face
D. Perform a dental examination
E. Perform facial nerve electromyography

91. A 2-year-old male is being evaluated for fever. He has a history of necrotizing enterocolitis at birth resulting in short-gut syndrome and total parenteral nutrition (TPN) dependence requiring a central line. He has no other symptoms. His line site appears clear. What is the most appropriate initial step in his care?

A. Treat the fever with acetaminophen and discharge
B. Start treatment with antibiotics and admit
C. Obtain a peripheral blood culture
D. Obtain a central line culture and a peripheral blood culture
E. Remove the central line

92. An 11-year-old girl with a history of asthma is admitted with shortness of breath, chest pain, and increased use of her albuterol inhaler for the past 2 weeks. On physical examination, her blood pressure is 125/71 mm Hg, and her heart rate is 115 beats per minute. She appears anxious. You palpate a diffusely enlarged thyroid gland. Laboratory testing reveals the following:

Thyroid-stimulating hormone (TSH): less than 0.01 mIU/mL (range 0.4–5.0 mIU/mL)
Free thyroxine (T_4): 7.6 ng/dL (range 0.9–1.8 ng/dL)
Total triiodothyronine (T_3): more than 650 ng/dL (range 60–181 ng/dL)

What is the most appropriate next step in management?

A. Thyroidectomy
B. Thyroid biopsy
C. Start methimazole
D. Obtain thyroid-stimulating immunoglobulin (TSI) antibodies
E. Start propranolol

93. A 6-month-old female presents to the emergency department with irritability and rash. Her temperature is 38°C. She is inconsolable and has a diffuse erythematous rash with a sharp line of demarcation on the middle back that spares the buttocks. She has intact fluid-filled and ruptured blisters, as well as areas of peeling. She is admitted to the hospitalist team for hydration. What is the best next step in management?

A. Intravenous nafcillin
B. Bacterial culture from the ruptured blister
C. Thorough medication history
D. Skeletal survey
E. Skin biopsy

94. A 7-year-old male with no past medical history presents with left testicle pain and dysuria for the past several hours. He denies nausea, vomiting, or any history of trauma. He is afebrile. On examination, his

scrotum has mild swelling, and the left testicle is tender. Both testicles have normal lie, and his cremasteric reflex is intact. He is circumcised and has no skin lesions. A Doppler ultrasound of the scrotum indicates normal blood flow in both testicles. A urinalysis is normal, and a urine culture is sent. What is the most appropriate treatment for this patient?

    A. Ceftriaxone and azithromycin
    B. Cephalexin
    C. Ofloxacin
    D. Urology consultation
    E. Supportive care

95. A 17-year-old African American female presents to the emergency department with 1 month of fatigue and cough and 5 days of shortness of breath. She has been seen several times by medical providers and been treated with albuterol and a course of azithromycin for atypical pneumonia without improvement. She has no past medical history and has not had similar illnesses in the past. She denies any fevers, vomiting, weight loss, diarrhea, rashes, or joint pain. She has not traveled recently and does not have any risk factors for tuberculosis. She denies tobacco or e-cigarette use. On examination, she is well nourished with mild tachypnea and frequent coughing. She has normal oxygen saturations. There is no nasal congestion or focal lung findings on auscultation. Computed tomography of the chest shows bilateral hilar lymphadenopathy and diffuse pulmonary nodules. An angiotensin-converting enzyme (ACE) level obtained by her primary care provider is elevated. Based on her most likely diagnosis, what is the most important laboratory study to obtain next?

    A. Serum calcium level
    B. Serum sodium level
    C. Antineutrophil cytoplasmic antibodies
    D. Complement levels
    E. Complete blood cell count with differential

96. A 10-year-old boy is referred by his primary care provider for hospitalization after 2 months of bloody diarrhea, abdominal pain, and an 8-pound weight loss. He stools three to six times daily, including overnight. The abdominal pain is crampy and intermittent. The pain does not prevent him from going to school. He also endorses fatigue and intermittent mild joint pains. He denies fever, recent travel, and exposure to animals or undercooked foods. His mother has hypothyroidism and his maternal grandmother has rheumatoid arthritis. His primary care provider sent stool for infectious studies, which have returned negative. On examination, he is thin and pale with diffuse mild tenderness to palpation of his abdomen. There are

several tender erythematous nodules on his bilateral anterior legs. Which of the following best describes his dermatologic condition?

    A. Erythema infectiosum
    B. Erythema migrans
    C. Erythema multiforme
    D. Erythema nodosum
    E. Erythema toxicum

97. A 4-year-old male is admitted for management of constipation. This is his fifth admission in the last 2 years for similar episodes, all of which have been treated with a bowel clean-out. The patient was placed on a bowel regimen after his first admission, and his primary pediatrician has been increasing the regimen with each admission. The patient is compliant with all medications. Of note, the patient first passed meconium at 30 hours of life. The patient has occasional abdominal pain but no other notable symptoms. He is growing well along the 50th percentile for weight and height. What finding is most likely to be seen on intestinal biopsy?

    A. Intraepithelial lymphocytosis
    B. Villous atrophy
    C. Absence of rectal ganglion cells
    D. Granuloma formation
    E. No abnormalities

98. A 3-year-old male undergoing chemotherapy for acute myelogenous leukemia is admitted to the hospital with fever and neutropenia. He has no localizing signs of infection. The patient is placed on empiric cefepime. On hospital day 4, the patient remains febrile and neutropenic. Aerobic blood cultures, anaerobic blood cultures, and urine culture show no growth of bacteria. Of the following, which is the most appropriate next step?

    A. Change cefepime to aztreonam
    B. Perform a lumbar puncture
    C. Obtain a stool culture
    D. Repeat a urine culture
    E. Start micafungin

99. A 3-year-old male is admitted for respiratory distress due to pneumonia and is started on 4 L/min oxygen by nasal cannula. He has a history of recurrent otitis media and sinusitis. This is his third admission for pneumonia. On examination, he is underweight, febrile, and nontoxic appearing, and you note that he does not have tonsils. What immunology laboratory test would confirm the most likely diagnosis?

    A. Natural killer cell enumeration
    B. Serum immunoglobulin (Ig) A levels

C. Flow cytometry for Bruton tyrosine kinase (BTK) protein expression
D. Dihydrorhodamine assay
E. Lymphocyte enumeration panel

100. A 9-day-old male presents with emesis. He was born at full term with no complications. On examination, he is lethargic and severely dehydrated, and you note hyperpigmentation of his scrotum. The sodium level is 122 mEq/L. Which of the following laboratory results would be consistent with this patient's diagnosis?

A. Metabolic alkalosis
B. Hyperglycemia
C. Hyperkalemia
D. Decreased plasma renin
E. Increased aldosterone

101. An 8-week-old male is referred to the emergency department by his pediatrician for failure to thrive. His parents report fussiness and a lack of interest in feeding. On examination, the patient appears well hydrated but irritable. He has a small laceration of the frenulum, which parents state they had not noticed before. What is the best next test to evaluate this patient?

A. Computed tomography (CT) of the head without contrast
B. Coagulation studies
C. Serum electrolytes
D. Complete blood count
E. Chest and abdomen radiograph

102. A 9-year-old male presents to the emergency department with swelling intermittently over the past few weeks. It is most prominent in the morning. He has had no recent illness and denies blood in his urine. He has otherwise been in his usual state of health. In the emergency department, his blood pressure is 148/99 mm Hg with a heart rate of 97 beats per minute. On physical examination, you note prominent periorbital edema and mild pitting edema of his lower extremities. The rest of his examination is normal. His laboratory test values are as follows:

Urinalysis: 3+ protein, 1+ blood
Urine protein: 350 mg/dL
Urine creatinine: 82 mg/dL
Serum creatinine: 0.4 mg/dL
Triglycerides: 220 mg/dL
C3: normal
C4: normal
Albumin: 2.2 g/dL

Which of the following factors is an indication for renal biopsy for this patient?

A. Elevated triglycerides
B. Microscopic hematuria
C. Hypertension
D. The patient's age
E. Edema

103. An 8-year-old male is admitted in respiratory distress with concern for bacterial pneumonia. He has a history of obliterative bronchiolitis, bronchiectasis, allergic rhinitis, and chronic diarrhea. He is on inhaled glucocorticoids, albuterol, and antihistamines and has been on several courses of antibiotics. On examination, he is underweight and tired and has sinus tenderness, purulent rhinorrhea, dry cough, shallow breathing, and bilateral crackles and wheezing on lung auscultation. What laboratory study would be helpful in diagnosing the most likely underlying disease in this patient?

A. Serum immunoglobulin panel
B. Complete blood count (CBC) with differential
C. Lymphocyte proliferation studies
D. Dihydrorhodamine assay
E. Bacterial blood culture

104. A 2-week-old neonate admitted to your service is found to have a heart rate of 75 beats per minute but is otherwise well appearing. His mother had been on steroids for a "disease flare" during pregnancy. His electrolytes, including potassium, calcium, and magnesium, are normal. His echocardiogram does not demonstrate structural abnormalities of the heart. What is the rhythm on his electrocardiogram (ECG), pictured in Figure 1.9?

A. Sinus arrhythmia
B. Second-degree atrioventricular (AV) block
C. Sinus bradycardia
D. Third-degree AV block
E. Premature ventricular complex (PVC)

105. A 4-year-old boy is brought to the emergency department immediately after ingesting lighter fluid at a family barbeque. He has a mild cough but is stable on room air. He is made nil per os (nothing by mouth) and is admitted to the floor for continued observation. About 15 hours after admission, you are called for desaturations to 87% and a temperature of 38.2°C. On examination, you hear crackles in the right lower lung fields, but the patient is breathing comfortably and is alert. He responds well to supplemental oxygen. What is the appropriate next step?

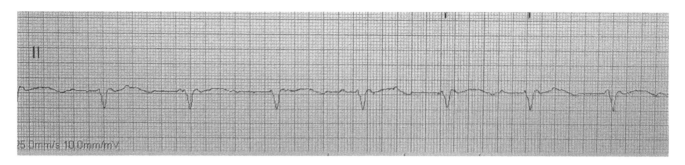

Figure 1.9

A. Administer azithromycin
B. Administer ceftriaxone
C. Intubate and transfer to the intensive care unit for closer monitoring
D. Continue to monitor with no additional intervention
E. Administer prednisone

106. A 12-year-old girl is hospitalized due to an asthma exacerbation. She receives twice-daily prednisolone, albuterol every 2 hours, and continuous intravenous fluids during her stay. On hospital day 3, she develops a new oxygen requirement of 3 L/min via nasal cannula to maintain oxygen saturation of 92% or greater. Her other vital signs are significant for a temperature of 37.2°C, heart rate of 115 beats per minute, and blood pressure of 100/67 mm Hg. Her lung examination reveals bilateral crackles and a moderate expiratory wheeze. What is the most appropriate next step in management?

A. Start broad-spectrum antibiotics
B. Stop albuterol and start levalbuterol
C. Start heliox (80/20 helium/oxygen blend)
D. Increase frequency of corticosteroids
E. Administer a diuretic

107. A 4-month-old male is admitted to the hospitalist service with difficulty feeding over the last 48–72 hours. The mother reports the child has started having increasing difficulty latching on to the bottle. His urine output has remained normal, but his stools have recently decreased and become more solid. The family has recently started introducing solid food into the patient's diet but deny giving the patient any honey or home-canned food products. On examination, the patient has generalized weakness with poor head control. When placed in a supine position, the patient's hips fall to an abducted position. He has a sluggish pupillary response and a weak suck reflex. The remainder of the physical examination, including vital signs, is normal. There is no family history of neuromuscular or genetic disorders. What is the underlying mechanism of this condition?

A. Inhibition of acetylcholine release from the presynaptic membrane
B. Abnormal mutation in *SMN1* gene
C. Maternal antibodies against acetylcholine receptors in the postsynaptic membrane
D. Genetic mutation in mitochondrial DNA
E. Antibodies against gangliosides (immunoglobulin [Ig] G anti–GQ1b antibody)

108. A healthy 5-year-old boy presents with a 6-day history of rhinorrhea and left neck swelling that is enlarging despite amoxicillin/clavulanate use for 2 days. He has had a fever to 101°F and fatigue. On examination, you note limited neck range of motion, tender left anterior cervical lymphadenopathy with overlying erythema, and a 1-cm area of central fluctuance. Contrast-enhanced computed tomography (CT) shows a 1.5 by 1.8 cm abscess. What is the best initial management of this patient?

A. Oral trimethoprim/sulfamethoxazole
B. Intravenous (IV) clindamycin or vancomycin
C. Intravenous vancomycin and ceftriaxone
D. Fine-needle aspiration
E. Surgical drainage

109. A 2-year-old male with short-gut syndrome and total parenteral nutrition (TPN) dependence is admitted for fever. Blood cultures have been obtained and broad-spectrum empiric antibiotics are started. His central line site appears clear. On hospital day 1, he is well appearing and afebrile. His mother asks if the central line will need to be removed and replaced. Which of the following is an indication for central line removal?

A. The central line culture is positive for a *Candida* species
B. The central line and peripheral cultures are positive for a gram-negative species
C. The central line and peripheral cultures are positive for gram-positive cocci
D. The central line and peripheral cultures are growing an organism at less than 24 hours

E. The central line has been in place for more than 1 year

110. You admit a 2-week-old baby whose newborn screen is concerning for an elevated thyroid-stimulating hormone (TSH) level. The newborn is well appearing. Which of the following is most likely to cause a false-positive screen?

A. Prematurity
B. Low birth weight
C. An elevated maternal TSH level
D. A newborn screen obtained after 24 hours of life
E. A maternal history of Graves' disease

111. A 4-year-old girl is brought to the emergency department by her mother due to complaints of genital pain. She attends day care but denies any sexual abuse. On examination, she has two ulcerative, erythematous lesions on her vulva. What is the next step in the evaluation and treatment of this patient?

A. Swab the lesions for herpes simplex virus (HSV) by polymerase chain reaction (PCR)
B. Obtain serum HSV serology
C. Prescribe empiric acyclovir
D. Report to Child Protective Services
E. Conduct a forensic genital examination

112. A 14-year-old male with a history of migraines presents with watery diarrhea for 5 days. Several household members have similar symptoms. He denies abdominal pain. He has had persistent headaches during this time and has been taking ibuprofen every 6 hours without relief. He has urinated very little today. He has been afebrile. Laboratory and imaging results are as follows:

Serum sodium: 140 mEq/L
Serum creatinine: 1.4 mg/dL
Urinalysis: specific gravity 1.010, epithelial cell casts, no red blood cells, trace protein, 1+ ketones
Urine osmolarity: 300 mOsm/kg
Urine sodium: 75 mEq/L
Urine creatinine: 25 mg/dL
Renal ultrasound: normal

Which of the following best describes this patient's renal function?

A. Prerenal acute kidney injury (AKI)
B. Intrinsic AKI
C. Postrenal AKI
D. Chronic kidney disease (CKD)
E. Normal renal function for age

113. A 7-year-old girl presents with right knee swelling and limp. She started sporadically limping 2 months ago, but her parents attributed it to overuse during soccer season. There was no trauma to the knee at the time of symptom onset. Over the past 6 weeks, her knee has become more swollen. She now complains that her knee "won't bend well" when she first wakes up in the morning, but this improves throughout the day. She denies fevers, rashes, weight loss, and diarrhea. They have not tried any treatments, as she seems to be functioning well and attending school with no issues. Her vital signs are normal. Her physical examination is notable for edema, warmth, and mildly decreased range of motion of the right knee without tenderness or erythema. All other joints are normal. The rest of the physical examination is unremarkable. Complete blood count, erythrocyte sedimentation rate, C-reactive protein, and lactate dehydrogenase are normal. Lyme antibodies and tuberculosis testing are negative. A radiograph of the affected knee shows a small joint effusion without bony changes. Of the following, what is the most appropriate initial treatment?

A. Therapeutic arthrocentesis
B. Nonsteroidal anti-inflammatory drug (NSAID)
C. Empiric antibiotic therapy
D. Methotrexate
E. Oral prednisone

114. A previously healthy 14-year-old girl presents to the emergency department with a worsening skin lesion of her left thigh. The lesion initially looked "like a pimple." Over the past 2 days, the skin around the lesion has become tender and red. She denies fevers, other skin lesions or rashes, and decreased fluid intake. Neither she nor her close contacts have a history of similar lesions. She denies any known insect bites or trauma.

On evaluation, her vital signs are normal. Her skin examination is notable for a 3 by 3 cm mildly erythematous lesion that is tender, warm, and fluctuant with a central pustule. Her examination is otherwise normal. An ultrasound of the lesion is done and shows a 2.8 by 2.3 cm fluid collection within the cutaneous tissues. A complete blood cell count was without leukocytosis. A blood culture was obtained. The emergency department physician calls you to discuss admission for intravenous antibiotics. Which of the following is the most appropriate treatment?

A. Warm compresses
B. Incision and drainage
C. Incision and drainage and oral antibiotic therapy
D. Oral antibiotic therapy
E. Intravenous antibiotic therapy

115. A 4-year-old female presents with 2 days of periumbilical pain, fever, and diarrhea. She had vomiting on the first day of illness. She eats a regular diet, has tried no new foods, and has not traveled. Your physical examination findings are significant for fever to 39.2°C, a pulse of 115 beats per minute, and pain on palpation with guarding in the right lower quadrant. What is the most likely cause of her diarrhea?

A. Viral gastroenteritis causing secretory losses
B. An inflamed appendix causing irritation of the colon
C. Deficiency of the lactase enzyme
D. Urinary tract infection
E. *Escherichia coli* infection leading to loss of surface area for absorption

116. The hospital pediatrics service is asked to consult on a 9-year-old male who develops prolonged bleeding following oral surgery. On further history, the patient has always bruised easily and has frequent nosebleeds. He has no prior surgical history. His mother has a history of prolonged bleeding following childbirth. Complete blood cell counts and peripheral smear are normal. Of the following, which is the most likely diagnosis?

A. Von Willebrand disease
B. Hemophilia A
C. Hemophilia B
D. Bernard-Soulier syndrome
E. Wiskott-Aldrich syndrome

117. A 4-year-old female with chronic eczema is admitted for cellulitis. Her examination is notable for coarse facial features, poor growth, scoliosis, multiple patches of dry skin, and lichenification and excoriations along her upper extremities. There is an area of skin breakdown in the left antecubital fossa associated with erythema and soft tissue swelling with several blisters. She is started on intravenous vancomycin and acyclovir to cover for possible herpes simplex virus or *Staphylococcus aureus* infection. Her history is concerning for recurrent sinusitis and chronic upper airway infections and multiple family members with similar medical problems. Clinical studies reveal normal complete blood count. The most likely underlying immunodeficiency in this patient is associated with which of the following?

A. Aphthous ulcers
B. Facial tetany
C. Delay in shedding of primary teeth
D. Thrombocytopenia
E. Peripheral neuropathy

118. An 11-year-old boy is admitted due to chest pain and shortness of breath that started while he was playing soccer. Initial workup is remarkable for elevated troponin and C-reactive protein. Parents report that about 2 weeks ago he recovered from an acute diarrheal illness, but he is otherwise a healthy child with no cardiac history. Which of the following tests is the gold standard to confirm the diagnosis?

A. Chest x-ray
B. Electrocardiogram (ECG)
C. Echocardiogram
D. Cardiac magnetic resonance imaging (MRI)
E. Endomyocardial biopsy

119. A 3-year-old girl presents to the emergency department after her parents noticed that she was difficult to arouse. There is no family history of medical problems except for chronic pain in the mother. On examination, the patient is sleepy with pinpoint pupils and shallow breathing at a rate of 12 breaths per minute. Her heart rate is 72 beats per minute, and her blood pressure is 78/42 mm Hg. Her urine drug screen is negative, including opioids. Which of the following is the best next step?

A. Flumazenil
B. Naloxone
C. Gastric lavage
D. Atropine
E. Naltrexone

120. A 2-year-old male presents to the emergency room with respiratory distress. According to his mother, the patient has a history of constipation and frequent bouts of coughing. On this occasion, he has had fever and cough for 3 days, with worsening difficulty breathing over the last 12 hours. Vital signs are significant for fever, tachypnea, tachycardia, and oxygen saturation of 91%. His growth curve indicates weight below the first percentile. Examination reveals diminished breath sounds on the left side and scattered crackles throughout. A chest radiograph shows near-complete opacification of the left lung. He is started on intravenous antibiotics, supplemental oxygen, and chest physiotherapy. A follow-up chest radiograph in 2 days is normal, and his symptoms have begun to improve. What should your discharge plan for this patient include?

A. Refer for a chloride sweat test as an outpatient
B. Obtain newborn screening test
C. Obtain a computed tomographic (CT) scan of the chest prior to discharge
D. Obtain a blood test for immunoglobulin G (IgG) prior to discharge
E. Refer to Child Protective Services

121. A pediatric hospitalist is called by the emergency department to evaluate a patient with new-onset hallucinations. The parents report the patient, a 15-year-old female, has been endorsing auditory hallucinations for several days and has had increasingly aggressive behavior. The patient has had a gradual cognitive decline over the last 8 weeks. Normally a very bright and cheerful adolescent, she has recently been less interactive, with fluctuating periods of responsiveness. On examination, the patient is alert but appears confused with disorganized speech. A basic urine drug screen and head computed tomography are negative. Which is the most likely cause of this patient's presentation?

A. Human immunodeficiency virus (HIV) encephalitis
B. Synthetic cathinone ("bath salt") intoxication
C. Anti–N-methyl-D-aspartate (NMDA) encephalitis
D. Cerebrovascular accident
E. Arbovirus encephalitis

122. A 3-year-old healthy female presents with a 6-week history of intermittent fever and facial swelling. Her parents deny recent upper respiratory infection, mouth pain, trauma, or tick or animal exposures. Physical examination reveals a normal oropharynx with submandibular nontender lymphadenopathy (LAD) with overlying induration and violaceous discoloration of the skin. What is the most appropriate next step in evaluation?

A. Culture of tissue from incision and drainage
B. Acid-fast bacillus stain of tissue from fine-needle aspiration
C. Computed tomography (CT) of the neck, chest, abdomen, and pelvis
D. Panoramic radiographs of the face
E. Purified protein derivative (PPD) skin test

123. A 2-year-old, healthy male presents for persistent fevers. His symptoms started 14 days ago with fevers, nasal congestion, and cough. They resolved for 1–2 days but then returned. The remainder of the review of systems is negative. He attends day care. His examination is unremarkable. What is the best next step?

A. Obtain an echocardiogram
B. Provide reassurance without further workup or treatment
C. Administer empiric ceftriaxone
D. Consult rheumatology for further evaluation
E. Obtain a C-reactive protein (CRP) and erythrocyte sedimentation rate (ESR)

124. A 5-year-old previously healthy girl is brought to the emergency department (ED) with lethargy and vomiting. According to her mother, she was tired the previous evening and went to bed without eating dinner. She woke up this morning not feeling well and within 30 minutes started vomiting. A blood glucose in the ED is 45 mg/dL. A critical sample is collected, and she is given an intravenous dextrose bolus. This has happened three times over the past several months. Each episode has occurred in the morning, typically preceded by a very active day during which she didn't eat much. Based on the most likely diagnosis, which of the following would you expect to see on this patient's critical sample?

A. Low free fatty acids
B. Low growth hormone
C. Low cortisol
D. Low insulin
E. Low ketones

125. A 2-year-old boy with a history of developmental delay and multiple food allergies is admitted for evaluation of 8 weeks of persistent bloody stools. The mother shows you a series of photos of soiled diapers that appear to be full of blood. The child's hemoglobin is normal, and he has been gaining weight normally. He has a normal-appearing stool during your examination, and a fecal occult blood test is negative. What is the best next step in management?

A. Colonoscopy
B. Allergy testing
C. Fecal calprotectin
D. Stool culture
E. Observation of additional stools

126. A 14-year-old girl with no past medical history presents with abdominal fullness for 2 weeks. Ultrasound of the abdomen shows a large multicystic mass with a small solid component extending from the right ovary. The right ovary appears to be much larger than the left ovary. Computed tomographic (CT) scan demonstrates that the mass is well circumscribed, does not appear to be invading the surrounding tissues, and has three small focal areas of calcification within the solid component. Which of the following is least likely to be a complication of her condition?

A. Malignant transformation
B. Hypotension and fever
C. Anti–N-methyl-D-aspartate (NMDA) receptor encephalitis

D. Ovarian torsion

E. Addison disease

127. An 8-year-old boy with systemic juvenile idiopathic arthritis (sJIA) is hospitalized with daily fevers to 40.5°C for the past 4 days. On the day of admission, he developed worsening headache, joint pains, fatigue, and decreased oral intake, prompting evaluation in the emergency department. He has no sick contacts or recent travel. Vital signs include temperature 40°C, heart rate 150 beats per minute, respiratory rate 28 breaths per minute, blood pressure 86/50 mm Hg, and oxygen saturation 97% on room air. He is ill appearing and lethargic with diffuse lymphadenopathy and hepatosplenomegaly but no meningismus. Initial laboratory testing shows a white blood cell count of 10,000 cells/mm³, anemia, thrombocytopenia, elevated ferritin (15,000 ng/mL), elevated triglycerides (300 mg/dL), and low fibrinogen (150 mg/dL), with additional laboratory test results pending. Compared to baseline laboratory testing obtained 2 weeks ago, which of the following is most likely to be decreased?

A. Erythrocyte sedimentation rate (ESR)

B. C-reactive protein (CRP)

C. Aspartate aminotransferase (AST)

D. Creatinine

E. Lactate dehydrogenase (LDH)

128. A previously healthy 2-year-old boy presents to the emergency department with rash and fever. His mother reports that he first felt warm a few days ago but was still active and eating normally. His mother then noticed several small red spots that turned into blisters on his hands, which have since spread to his diaper region as well as the soles of both feet. Over the past 24 hours, he has started to refuse any oral intake and has only had one wet diaper. Vital signs are significant for fever to 39.0°C and tachycardia. He is normotensive. His physical examination is notable for flat erythematous papules and vesicles present on the palmar and plantar surfaces of the hands and feet and diaper region. There are numerous small vesicles and ulcers on the palate and posterior oropharynx. His capillary refill is 3 seconds with dry oral mucosa. A bolus of intravenous normal saline is administered. You agree to hospitalize the patient. Of the following, what is the best next step in management?

A. Swab lesions for herpes simplex virus polymerase chain reaction testing and start intravenous acyclovir

B. Draw a blood culture and start intravenous clindamycin

C. Obtain complete blood count, C-reactive protein, and erythrocyte sedimentation rate

D. Administer intravenous hydration and acetaminophen

E. Consult dermatology for skin biopsy

129. A 3-year-old male presents with 6 days of abdominal pain, vomiting, bloody diarrhea, decreased urine output, and fatigue. He is found to have a hemoglobin of 6.3 g/dL, platelets of 34 × 10⁹ cells/L, and a creatinine of 1.2 mg/dL. Which of the following is likely present in his stool culture?

A. *Salmonella*

B. *Campylobacter*

C. *Escherichia coli*

D. *Clostridium difficile*

E. *Yersinia*

130. A 3-year-old female presents with acute onset of petechiae and bruising. Her parents report that last week the patient had a fever and upper respiratory symptoms that self-resolved. Complete blood cell counts are remarkable for platelets of 9,000/mm³. The physician suspects immune thrombocytopenic purpura (ITP) and plans to begin corticosteroid therapy. Of the following, what is the most important laboratory test to obtain before starting treatment?

A. Prothrombin time and partial thromboplastin time

B. Indirect Coombs test

C. Peripheral smear

D. Rh blood group typing

E. Fibrinogen level

131. A 6-week-old female is brought to the emergency department for fever to 100.9°F. Her father states that she has been feeding normally and has good urine output. Her rectal temperature on arrival is 100.5°F; her heart rate is 130 beats per minute, respirations are 25 breaths per minute, and oxygen saturation is 99%. Her physical examination demonstrates a well-appearing infant with clear lungs bilaterally and capillary refill time less than 2 seconds. Which of the following is a recommended part of this patient's workup?

A. Urinalysis

B. Respiratory pathogen panel

C. Erythrocyte sedimentation rate (ESR)

D. Lumbar puncture (LP)

E. Chest radiograph

132. A 16-year-old previously healthy girl presents with worsening chest pain and fever for 2 days. Her chest pain is described as stabbing over her midchest, is worse with deep breaths, and is improved by sitting upright and leaning forward. She reports that about a week ago she had a runny nose, sore throat, and cough. On echocardiogram, a moderate-size pericardial effusion is noted, with no evidence of tamponade or myocardial involvement. What is the next most appropriate step in management?

A. High-dose nonsteroidal anti-inflammatory (NSAID)
B. Colchicine
C. Pericardiocentesis
D. Corticosteroid
E. Ceftriaxone and vancomycin

133. A 5-year-old girl presents to the emergency department with altered mental status after being found in the garage with a bottle of antifreeze. Which of the following laboratory findings would you expect for this patient?

A. Ethanol 30 mg/dL
B. Partial pressure of carbon dioxide ($PaCO_2$) 52 mm Hg
C. Alanine aminotransferase 70 U/L
D. Bicarbonate 14 mEq/L
E. Creatinine 1.8 mg/dL

134. During morning rounds, the medical student is presenting a 2-year-old patient admitted for increased work of breathing as a transfer from an outside emergency room. The patient's symptoms started 4 days ago with cough, cold, and congestion after his older brother had the same symptoms. At the outside hospital, he had received oral prednisone, two albuterol nebulizer treatments, one hypertonic saline nebulization treatment, and chest physiotherapy. The chest radiograph demonstrated bilateral air space disease but no evidence of pneumonia. This morning, the patient's vital signs show a temperature of 37°C, respiratory rate 35 breaths per minute, heart rate 110 beats per minute, blood pressure 94/52 mm Hg, and oxygen saturation 99% monitored on a continuous pulse oximeter on room air. On lung auscultation, he is noted to have course breath sounds with scattered rhonchi and wheezes. The medical student asks about the current recommendations related to this diagnosis. Which of the following is correct?

A. Oral corticosteroids are recommended
B. Chest radiography is an important diagnostic tool
C. Inhaled short-acting β-agonists should be part of initial routine care
D. Chest physiotherapy can be helpful in clearing secretions

E. Continuous pulse oximetry is not recommended routinely

135. A 15-year-old female is being admitted with an intractable bifrontal headache associated with repeated episodes of nausea and vomiting and sensitivity to light and sound. She has taken a few doses of acetaminophen with caffeine at home for the past day with limited improvement. Her family history is notable for migraine headaches. Of the following, the best treatment option is:

A. Acetaminophen and ibuprofen
B. Oxycodone and intravenous promethazine
C. Intravenous fluids and oral topiramate
D. Intravenous ketorolac and intravenous prochlorperazine
E. Intravenous ketorolac and oral amitriptyline

136. A 3-year-old unvaccinated male presents to the emergency room with abrupt onset of difficulty breathing. His mother reports the patient was in his normal state of health this morning, but over the course of the day developed increased work of breathing and significant drooling. He is now refusing to drink liquids. His mother has not noticed any runny nose or cough. On examination, the patient appears anxious. He is sitting upright with his nose pointed up and mouth held open, with notable pooling secretions. He has inspiratory stridor and tachypnea, but otherwise clear lung sounds. He becomes distressed when the physician attempts to examine his oropharynx. Vital signs are notable for fever, tachycardia, and oxygen saturation 96% on ambient air. What is the next step in the management of this patient?

A. Obtain neck radiographs
B. Intubate the patient in the emergency room
C. Administer intravenous vancomycin
D. Move patient emergently to the operating room with otolaryngology
E. Administer intravenous corticosteroids

137. A 10-year-old previously healthy female is admitted to the hospital for prolonged fevers. She reports nightly fevers up to 103°F for the last 3 weeks; these fevers are often accompanied by a salmon-colored, maculopapular rash. She is more fatigued but continues to attend school and participate in sports. She recently complained of bilateral knee pain, but her parents have attributed this to "growing pains." The family history is significant for hypothyroidism in her mother. Her physical examination is significant for bilateral axillary lymphadenopathy. Her primary care provider obtained laboratory tests and imaging 1 week ago:

White blood cells	18 K/μL
Hemoglobin	10.5 g/dL
Hematocrit	30%
Platelets	300 K/μL
Neutrophils	59%
Lymphocytes	36%
Monocytes	4%
Eosinophils	3%
Basophils	0%
Erythrocyte sedimentation rate (ESR)	73 mm/h
C-reactive protein (CRP)	2.0 mg/dL
Blood culture	Negative
Rapid strep	Negative
Knee x-ray	Normal

What is the best next step in management?

A. Monitor fever trend
B. Obtain magnetic resonance imaging (MRI) of the lower extremities
C. Obtain *Bartonella* serology
D. Consult rheumatology
E. Obtain peripheral blood smear

138. You are consulted by the emergency department for a 12-year-old male with poorly controlled ulcerative colitis (UC) who is presenting with bloody stools and altered mental status. His blood pressure is 145/81 mm Hg. On physical examination, he has a round face, supraclavicular fat pads, and abdominal striae. He has been taking steroids since his UC diagnosis last year. You are considering Cushing syndrome as a possible comorbidity for this patient. Which of the following tests, if abnormal, would confirm the diagnosis?

A. Serum cortisol
B. Corticotropin (ACTH) stimulation test
C. Early morning salivary cortisol
D. Overnight dexamethasone suppression test
E. 24-hour urinary free cortisol and late-night salivary cortisol

139. A 14-year-old male presents with a sore throat, fever, and red-brown urine for the past 2 days. He has no associated rhinorrhea, sneezing, or cough. To the surprise of his parents, he has occasionally had red-brown urine in the past when he had similar cold-like symptoms. He has had no pain. There is no family history of hematuria. Blood pressure is normal for age and

height. A physical examination is notable for swollen, erythematous tonsils bilaterally with palatal petechiae. A pharyngeal bacterial culture swab is sent. Urinalysis demonstrates 17 red blood cells per high-power field but no white blood cells. Which of the following is most likely to represent this patient's laboratory results?

A. Normal C3, normal C4
B. Low C3, normal C4
C. Normal C3, low C4
D. Low C3, low C4
E. Low C3, elevated C4

140. A previously healthy 16-year-old girl presents with left knee pain and swelling for 1 week. On review of systems, she reports four episodes of loose, nonbloody stools each day and crampy abdominal pain for the past month. She has had no fevers. On review of her growth chart, you see that she weighs 55 kg today, which is down from 60 kg at her well-child check 4 months ago. She denies intentional weight loss. On evaluation, she is mildly tachycardic, but all other vital signs are normal. She has cutaneous and conjunctival pallor. Three aphthous ulcers are noted in her posterior oropharynx. Her left knee is swollen, warm, and tender and has limited flexion. Her other joints are normal. Her abdomen is diffusely tender to palpation. Of the following, which of these is most likely to yield a definitive diagnosis?

A. Arthrocentesis
B. Knee radiograph
C. Stool culture
D. Vaginal swab for gonococcal and chlamydial testing
E. Esophagogastroduodenoscopy and colonoscopy

141. A 14-day-old female presents to clinic for evaluation of multiple skin lesions. On examination, she has a hemangioma involving the scalp, forehead, and left eyelid that measures 7 cm in diameter. There are smaller hemangiomas on the back and right leg as well as a midline sternal pit. A murmur was noted in the nursery, with echocardiogram revealing a small ventriculoseptal defect (VSD). She was born by spontaneous vaginal delivery without complications with an unremarkable prenatal history. You agree to hospitalize her for evaluation and monitoring while starting appropriate medical therapy. What anticipatory guidance regarding medical therapy is most appropriate to provide for parents at discharge?

A. Check a blood pressure prior to each dose
B. Check a blood sugar prior to each dose
C. Obtain a pulse oximeter to monitor the heart rate
D. Avoid periods of fasting for longer than 4 hours

E. Avoid administration of the medication in the evening

142. A 13-year-old female with a history of systemic lupus erythematosus (SLE) presents with fever, right upper quadrant (RUQ) pain and anorexia for the last 8 hours. She has some nausea but no vomiting or diarrhea. Her physical examination is significant for a temperature of 38.9°C, mild dehydration, and RUQ tenderness on palpation. Her skin examination is normal. Her initial workup is significant for a leukocytosis and a very mild elevation in alkaline phosphatase, aspartate aminotransferase (AST), and alanine aminotransferase (ALT). Her bilirubin is normal. What is the most likely diagnosis for this patient?

A. Primary sclerosing cholangitis
B. Fitz-Hugh-Curtis syndrome
C. Acute acalculous cholecystitis
D. Acute cholangitis
E. Hepatitis A

143. A 15-year-old male with sickle cell disease (hemoglobin SS) is hospitalized for an acute vaso-occlusive crisis. His pain control is improving on intravenous morphine and intravenous fluids. Overnight the hospitalist is called to his bedside for the patient's altered mental status. On physical examination, the patient has left hemiparesis and left hemisensory loss. Of the following, which test is most likely to provide a definitive diagnosis?

A. Brain magnetic resonance imaging (MRI) with diffusion and T2-weighted images
B. Head computed tomography (CT)
C. Head and neck CT angiography
D. Lumbar puncture
E. Transcranial Doppler ultrasound

144. A 2-week-old girl presents with decreased oral intake and increased sleepiness for a day. On examination she is noted to be afebrile with a respiratory rate of 85 breaths per minute, heart rate of 200 beats per minute, II/VI systolic ejection murmur, absent femoral pulses, and delayed capillary refill time. Her lungs are clear and symmetric on auscultation. What is the most likely pathophysiologic mechanism of her decreased cardiac output and cardiogenic shock?

A. Left outflow tract obstruction
B. Right outflow tract obstruction
C. Left-to-right shunting leading to preferential flow to pulmonary bed
D. Decreased myocardial contractility
E. Decreased diastolic filling of the heart

145. A 14-year-old boy is admitted after falling off his skateboard unhelmeted. You are paged 6 hours after admission because the patient is less arousable. You notice that his systolic blood pressure has increased 15 mm Hg to 130 mm Hg, and his heart rate has decreased to 45 beats per minute. Which of the following is the most appropriate next diagnostic test?

A. Electrocardiogram
B. Magnetic resonance imaging (MRI) of his head with contrast
C. Computed tomography (CT) of his head without contrast
D. Sodium level
E. Echocardiogram

146. You are caring for a late preterm infant in the transitional care nursery who has been admitted for over 6 weeks. During the first 2 days of life, she had hypothermia requiring the warmer. She had hypoglycemia after birth and required dextrose-containing fluids for a total of 3 days. She also required a nasogastric tube for feeding, but for the past 2 weeks has been feeding well by mouth and is voiding five or six times per day. The patient's mom reports that she is very concerned about her daughter's lungs given her prematurity and had heard about a vaccine to protect against respiratory syncytial virus (RSV). In discussion with the family, why would this patient be ineligible for this vaccine?

A. Degree of prematurity
B. History of feeding difficulty
C. History of hypoglycemia
D. History of temperature instability
E. Prolonged length of stay in the hospital

147. A 5-year-old female presents with acute ataxia and left-sided arm weakness associated with irritability and fatigue. The patient complains of headache and has hyperreflexia on examination. One week ago, she had an upper respiratory infection but has been afebrile. Magnetic resonance imaging (MRI) of the brain and spine demonstrates large multifocal, asymmetric, poorly defined white matter lesions. Lumbar puncture with cerebrospinal fluid (CSF) analysis demonstrates a negative Gram stain, and the culture is pending. Which of the following is the best treatment for this patient?

A. Broad-spectrum antibiotics
B. High-dose corticosteroids
C. Antithrombotic therapy
D. Intravenous fluids
E. Intravenous levetiracetam

148. A 2-year-old male arrives with his father to the emergency department with noisy breathing and cough. The father states the patient has had a runny nose and low-grade fever for the past 2 days. This morning the patient developed a cough, and the father noted a rattling noise with deep inhalation. He has had decreased intake of solids but continues to drink fluids. In the emergency department, vital signs are notable for a temperature of 37.2°C, respiratory rate 27 breaths per minute, heart rate 132 beats per minute, and oxygen saturation 97% on ambient air. Physical examination reveals an erythematous oropharynx, inspiratory stridor, clear lung sounds, and mild abdominal retractions. An occasional "barking" cough is noted. Which of the following is the most common cause of this patient's illness?

A. Influenza virus
B. Respiratory syncytial virus (RSV)
C. Rhinovirus
D. Parainfluenza virus
E. Adenovirus

149. A 12-year-old female is admitted for headache unresponsive to oral acetaminophen and ibuprofen. She reports weekly headaches for the last year, exacerbated by stress at school. She denies changes in vision, syncope, nausea, or vomiting and has never been woken up by the headache. She is a straight A student but has increasingly missed more days of school due to her headaches. She received intravenous ketorolac with resolution of her acute headache, but her mom would like to discuss treatment options for her recurrent headaches prior to discharge. Which of the following do you recommend?

A. Continued use of acetaminophen and ibuprofen as needed
B. Relaxation training with biobehavioral feedback
C. Oxycodone as needed
D. Acupuncture
E. Propranolol daily as a preventive medication

150. A previously healthy 18-month-old male is admitted for viral bronchiolitis and found to have a blood glucose of 56 mg/dL. Serum sodium is 129 mEq/dL, and potassium is 5.2 mEq/dL. He is tired appearing but arousable. His mother says he is often difficult to wake up in the mornings, but then "perks up" later in the day. His work of breathing has improved on 1 L/min of oxygen, and the rest of his examination is reassuring. Which of the following would help confirm the cause of this patient's hypoglycemia?

A. Dexamethasone suppression test
B. Low plasma renin

C. Corticotropin (ACTH) stimulation test
D. Low serum ketones
E. Low plasma corticotropin

151. A 13-year-old female with a history of recurrent urinary tract infections presents with fever, intermittent sharp left-sided flank pain, red-tinged urine, vomiting, and an inability to tolerate fluids by mouth. She is hemodynamically stable. A urinalysis is positive for leukocyte esterase and nitrites, the urine pH is 8.5, and microscopy reveals red blood cells, white blood cells, and crystals. A urine culture is sent. The patient is started on intravenous fluids, ketorolac, tamsulosin, and ceftriaxone. An abdominal ultrasound is pending. Which of the following types of nephrolithiasis is least likely to respond to medical therapy alone?

A. Calcium oxalate
B. Cysteine
C. Struvite (magnesium ammonium phosphate)
D. Urate (uric acid)
E. Citrate

152. A 17-year-old previously healthy male presents with dehydration due to painful oral lesions. In the past he has had both oral and genital lesions, sometimes associated with fever. He reports difficulty seeing items on the projector screen at school and denies headaches, vomiting, joint pain, sexual activity, or any recent travel history. He has a heart rate of 110 beats per minute but otherwise his vitals are normal. His physical examination demonstrates multiple ulcers with a white-gray base and erythematous halo on the tongue, cheeks, palate, and lips. There are also several ulcerated lesions present on the scrotum, some of which have healed into scars. In addition to intravenous (IV) fluids and pain control, what is the best next step in management?

A. Herpes simplex virus polymerase chain reaction test and IV acyclovir
B. Rapid plasmin reagin and IV penicillin
C. Bacterial culture and IV clindamycin
D. Colchicine
E. Topical high-potency corticosteroids

153. A 4-year-old boy was admitted from the emergency department due to a suspected infection of his scalp. For the past several weeks, he had some itching, scaling, and hair loss of his right posterior scalp. Over the past 2 weeks, the area has become swollen, red, and boggy with occasional bloody and purulent drainage. His mother endorses tactile fevers but has not used a thermometer at home. His vitals are appropriate for age. On examination, a scalp lesion is noted (see Figure 1.10). There is

localized alopecia over the lesion. He has a few enlarged and tender right-side occipital lymph nodes. He is otherwise well appearing without other skin lesions. The emergency department sent fluid from the lesions for bacterial culture. Of the following, what is the most appropriate initial treatment?

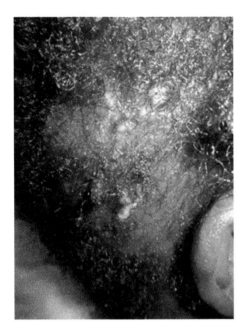

Figure 1.10

A. Intravenous micafungin
B. Intravenous vancomycin
C. Oral clindamycin
D. Oral terbinafine
E. Topical triamcinolone

154. A 14-day-old, full-term male presents to the emergency department with jaundice. The patient spent 3 days in the neonatal intensive care unit after birth, receiving phototherapy for hyperbilirubinemia, but has otherwise been doing well. He has been taking 2–3 ounces of formula every 3 hours and is waking appropriately overnight for feeds. He is having eight wet diapers and two greenish-brown stools per day. On examination, the patient is well appearing with jaundice to the level of the abdomen and notable scleral icterus. Laboratory evaluation reveals no evidence of hemolysis and an unconjugated bilirubin level of 16 mg/dL. All other liver function measures are normal. Which therapy is most likely to treat this patient's underlying condition?

A. Increasing feed volumes
B. Levothyroxine
C. Exclusion of galactose from diet
D. Phenobarbital
E. Periodic packed red blood cell transfusions

155. A 2-year-old female with sickle cell disease presents with severe fatigue and pallor. On physical examination, her temperature is 37.5°C, heart rate is 160 beats/min, respiratory rate is 45 breaths/min, and oxygen saturation is 96%. She has abdominal distension, and the spleen tip is palpable in the right lower quadrant. Her hemoglobin is 5.8 g/dL, compared to her baseline of 8 g/dL. Of the following, which is the most appropriate next step in management?

A. Exchange transfusion
B. Intravenous morphine
C. Intravenous crystalloid
D. Surgical consultation
E. Intravenous ceftriaxone

156. A 6-year-old boy with meningitis is admitted to a rural community hospital without an intensive care unit. On examination, he has a temperature of 39.2°F, heart rate of 150 beats per minute, respiratory rate of 40 breaths per minute, and blood pressure of 95/65 mm Hg. He appears sleepy and has cool extremities but has intact peripheral pulses. His capillary refill time is 3 seconds. His white blood cell count is 20 × 10⁹/L. In addition to starting broad-spectrum antibiotics, which of the following would be the best next step in management?

A. Normal saline 20 mL/kg bolus
B. Maintenance intravenous fluids
C. Dextrose 10% 2.5 mL/kg
D. Epinephrine infusion
E. Hydrocortisone stress dose

157. You are consulted in the emergency department to evaluate a 2-year-old girl with altered mental status. She is unresponsive and breathing slowly. The remainder of her vitals are within normal limits. Her pupils are equal and reactive, and she has normoactive bowel sounds. You recommend a urine drug screen. For which of the following substances will this child most likely test positive?

A. Opiates
B. Cannabis
C. Phencyclidine (PCP)
D. Cocaine
E. Amphetamines

158. A 12-month-old female born at 27 weeks' gestation is being admitted for increased work of breathing and respiratory distress. Her parents report that starting 3 days prior to presentation, she developed nasal congestion and cough. Her brother, who is in day care,

has the same symptoms. Her parents noted that over the past few days, her respiratory symptoms have been worsening, and she has been increasingly tachypneic. On presentation, her vital signs show a temperature of 38°C, respiratory rate of 45 breaths per minute, heart rate of 140 beats per minute, blood pressure of 110/50 mm Hg, and oxygen saturation of 94%. Her physical examination is notable for some mild nasal flaring with intermittent grunting and moderate substernal retractions. What is the best next step in this patient's management?

A. Swab for respiratory syncytial virus (RSV)
B. Start antihypertensive medication
C. Start oxygen therapy
D. Administer acetaminophen
E. Give normal saline 20 mL/kg bolus

159. A 3-year-old male is admitted for difficulty walking. The patient was in his normal state of health when he woke up from a nap this afternoon with an abnormal gait. His father describes the gait as "staggered" and "swaying from side to side." The family denies any recent fevers, weight loss, or head trauma. His father does report the patient had a "cold" 2 weeks ago that gradually resolved with only supportive care. On examination, you note the patient seems unsteady when sitting on the table and has a stumbling, wide-based gait when attempting to walk. Brain magnetic resonance imaging is normal, and a urine drug screen is negative. Based on this patient's presentation, what is the most likely diagnosis?

A. Posterior fossa tumor
B. Polyethylene glycol intoxication
C. Guillain-Barré syndrome
D. Meningitis
E. Acute cerebellar ataxia

160. You are evaluating a healthy 3-year-old male with a 5-day history of fever and right-sided neck swelling. His parents state that his illness began with rhinorrhea and redness of both eyes, which have now resolved. On physical examination, he is irritable and refuses to move his neck. He has a 2 by 3 cm right lateral tender neck mass without fluctuance or overlying erythema. He is admitted for intravenous antibiotics. After 48 hours, you note no improvement in his neck swelling, but a new diffuse erythematous maculopapular rash has developed. Which of the following diagnostic tests would be most helpful to establish the diagnosis?

A. Alanine aminotransferase (ALT) and albumin
B. Cerebrospinal fluid (CSF) white blood cell count and protein

C. Neck ultrasound
D. Epstein-Barr virus (EBV) serology
E. Consultation with a pediatric dermatologist

161. A 12-year-old, previously healthy female is admitted for severe pain of her right lower extremity. She suffered a mild ankle sprain playing soccer 4 months ago and since then has had worsening lower extremity pain. She reports constant pain, sensitivity to touch, and intermittent mottling and coolness to the extremity. The physical examination is significantly limited by hyperalgesia but no noted deformity or skin changes. Complete blood count, C-reactive protein, erythrocyte sedimentation rate, and creatinine kinase are all within normal limits. Magnetic resonance imaging of the right lower extremity is normal. Which of the following is the best treatment option for this patient?

A. Physical therapy
B. Ketamine infusion
C. Sympathetic nerve block
D. Gabapentin
E. Amitriptyline

162. A 10-year-old patient with dilated cardiomyopathy initially admitted in heart failure is being transferred out of the intensive care unit (ICU) to your service. In the ICU, the following thyroid function tests were ordered as part of her cardiac workup:

Thyroid-stimulating hormone (TSH): 0.1 mIU/mL (0.5–4.3)
Free thyroxine (T_4): 0.8 ng/dL (0.9–1.4)

Which of the following laboratory findings would be expected in this patient?

A. Low thyroxine-binding globulin (TBG)
B. Low reverse T_3
C. High transthyretin (TTR)
D. Elevated free T_4 index
E. Elevated thyroid-stimulating immunoglobulin (TSI) antibodies

163. A 15-year-old obese female presents with severe right-side lower abdominal pain, nausea, vomiting, and a low-grade fever. The abdominal pain started suddenly a few hours ago following exercise. She is writhing on the examination bed in pain, and her abdomen is tender to palpation, particularly in the right lower quadrant. A urine pregnancy test is negative. Abdominal and pelvic ultrasounds show a normal appendix as well as a large, edematous right ovary. The left ovary is normal in appearance. On Doppler, the right ovary has normal

blood flow that is similar to that of the left ovary. Which of the following is the most significant risk factor for this patient's condition?

A. Pelvic inflammatory disease
B. Ovarian mass
C. Prior abdominal surgery
D. Endometriosis
E. Intrauterine device

164. A 3-year-old girl was hospitalized for dehydration after 5 days of fever, sore throat, and mouth sores. Her mother denies conjunctival injection, extremity swelling, arthritis, rash, vomiting, or diarrhea. Her physical examination demonstrates cervical lymphadenopathy and oropharyngeal aphthous ulcers. Laboratory workup demonstrates normal complete blood cell count with differential, lactate dehydrogenase, uric acid, complete metabolic panel, and erythrocyte sedimentation rate. C-reactive protein is mildly elevated. Testing for respiratory viruses and herpes simplex is negative. She is currently well appearing and drinking adequately. Her mother reports that the patient regularly has similar episodes of self-resolving fever, mouth sores, and "swollen glands." They have occurred every 4 weeks for the past 3 months. She is asymptomatic between episodes. Of the following, what instructions should be given to family at discharge?

A. Schedule antipyretics to prevent fevers
B. Urgent referral to otolaryngology for tonsillectomy is indicated if fevers persist
C. Keep a fever and symptom diary and follow closely with the primary care provider
D. Seek immediate evaluation for antibiotic prescription if she has fevers above 38.5°C
E. No ongoing monitoring is needed as fevers are common in the pediatric population

165. An 11-month-old boy is admitted after experiencing self-limited episodes of brisk flexion of his arms and extension of his neck over the past week. These episodes have occurred multiple times per day. He does not have any loss of consciousness. He has otherwise been well. His primary care provider identified mild fine motor and language delays, but elicited no other significant past medical history. On examination, he is well appearing with hypopigmented macules noted on his back (see Figure 1.11). Electroencephalography (EEG) is performed and demonstrates random high-amplitude slow waves with frequent multifocal spikes. Of the following, which is the most appropriate next step in evaluation?

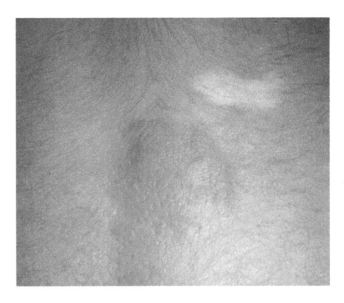

Figure 1.11

A. Skin biopsy
B. Focused genetic testing
C. Brain magnetic resonance imaging (MRI), echocardiogram, and renal ultrasound
D. Brain, spine, and cardiac MRI
E. Lumbar puncture, echocardiogram, and abdominal ultrasound

166. A 3-year-old male presents to the emergency room after swallowing four magnetic beads. The patient does not have any respiratory distress, abdominal pain, or dysphagia and is otherwise well appearing on examination. An abdominal radiograph is obtained and shows multiple radioopaque objects in the stomach. Which of the following is the most appropriate intervention for this patient?

A. Serial radiographs to monitor progression of foreign bodies
B. Initiation of total bowel clean-out
C. Endoscopy for removal of foreign bodies
D. Reassurance and discharge home
E. Administer sucralfate

167. An 8-year-old male presents with fatigue and shortness of breath. In the past 24 hours, his parents have noted that he appears pale and has yellow discoloration of his eyes. He reports painless dark urination. The patient recently completed a course of azithromycin for pneumonia. His physical examination is notable for sinus tachycardia, a systolic murmur, and scleral icterus. His hemoglobin is 6.5 g/dL, and cold agglutinin titers are elevated. Which of the following additional laboratory findings would be expected in this patient?

A. Low plasma free hemoglobin
B. Red blood cells on urine microscopy

C. High alanine and aspartate aminotransferase
D. Low leukocyte count
E. Positive direct antiglobulin test

168. The pediatric surgical service consults you for hypertension in a 7-year-old girl who is postoperative day 2 from an appendectomy. During hospitalization, the patient's blood pressure has been consistently 12–15 mm Hg above the 95th percentile for her height and age using a manual, appropriate size cuff. The patient is well hydrated, pain is well controlled, and she is tolerating a normal diet. She denies headache, blurry vision, shortness of breath, swelling, and chest pain. Discussion with her primary pediatrician reveals a similar blood pressure at a recent visit. Which classification is most accurate?

A. Elevated blood pressure
B. Stage 1 hypertension
C. Stage 2 hypertension
D. Hypertensive urgency
E. Hypertensive emergency

169. A 16-year-old boy is admitted to your service after being stabilized following a drug overdose. During your social history, he admits that he recreationally uses inhalants, but insists that he only does this occasionally. As part of your anticipatory guidance, which of the following risks should be emphasized for this occasional user?

A. Peripheral neuropathy
B. Subacute combined degeneration syndrome
C. Sudden death from cardiac arrest
D. Megaloblastic anemia
E. Toxic leukoencephalopathy

170. A 3-year-old male with a history of hypoxic ischemic encephalopathy, chronic respiratory failure with ventilator dependence, and chronic enteral feeds via gastrostomy tube is admitted to the hospital for a malfunctioning gastrostomy tube. On his third day of admission, he develops a fever of 38.4°C and mild hypoxemia requiring an increase in his fraction of inspired oxygen (FiO_2) from 21% to 35%. His nurse describes an increase in secretions from his tracheostomy tube, which have also become slightly green-tinged in color, over the last 12 hours. His current vital signs are heart rate 124 beats per minute, blood pressure 101/56 mm Hg, respiratory rate 24 breaths per minute, and oxygen saturation 94% on 35% FiO_2. On examination, you note the patient to have purulent secretions at the opening of his tracheostomy and transmitted upper airway noise on auscultation. A chest radiograph shows a properly placed

tracheostomy tube and no lung infiltrates. What is the best next step in management?

A. Start broad-spectrum antibiotics with vancomycin and ceftriaxone
B. Obtain tracheal aspirate for Gram stain and culture
C. Consult the pulmonologist for direct visualization of the tracheostomy
D. Perform chest physiotherapy
E. Start glycopyrrolate

171. A 2-month-old male is being evaluated in the emergency department for poor weight gain. His mother reports the patient has had feeding difficulties since birth, especially when attempting to latch. The pregnancy was only notable for polyhydramnios. There is no family history of neuromuscular disorders. On examination, the infant has moderate head lag and a poor suck reflex but is able to lift his extremities against gravity. Deep tendon reflexes are present. His testes are undescended bilaterally. Of the following, which is the most likely diagnosis?

A. Prader-Willi syndrome
B. Trisomy 21
C. Spinal muscular atrophy type 1
D. Infantile botulism
E. Congenital myotonic dystrophy

172. You are admitting a 9-year-old male with a history of bilateral sensorineural hearing loss for presumed peritonsillar abscess. When he developed left lateral neck swelling, his parents brought him to the emergency department because he has required intravenous antibiotics in the past for similar symptoms. A contrast-enhanced computed tomographic (CT) scan shows a left-side abscess just below the angle of the mandible, with an enhancing tract toward an enlarged left palatine tonsil. In addition to surgical evaluation, what diagnostic test is indicated?

A. Serum thyroid function testing (TFTs)
B. Contrast-enhanced magnetic resonance imaging (MRI) of the head and neck
C. Immunoglobulin panel
D. Renal ultrasound
E. Serum uric acid and lactate dehydrogenase (LDH)

173. A 6-week-old male presents with forceful, projectile vomiting for 7 days. He is diagnosed with idiopathic hypertrophic pyloric stenosis. On examination, he is moderately to severely dehydrated. What is the most likely laboratory finding you may see in this patient?

A. Hypokalemic hypochloremic metabolic acidosis
B. Hypokalemic hypochloremic metabolic alkalosis

C. Hyperkalemic hyperchloremic metabolic acidosis

D. Hyperkalemic hyperchloremic metabolic alkalosis

E. Hyperkalemic hypochloremic metabolic alkalosis

174. You admit a 16-year-old with type 1 diabetes (T1D) for ongoing fatigue, persistent gastrointestinal pain, and weight loss. His diabetes has been well controlled with an insulin pump, and his total daily dose of insulin has been steadily decreasing over the past year. His examination is unremarkable. His heart rate is 87 beats per minute, respiratory rate is 18 breaths per minute, and his blood pressure is 99/65 mm Hg. Which of the following laboratory tests are most important to perform in this patient?

A. HLA-B27 typing

B. Thyroid-stimulating hormone (TSH), free thyroxine (T_4)

C. Tissue transglutaminase immunoglobulin (Ig) A

D. Rheumatoid factor (RF), antinuclear antibody (ANA), anti–double-stranded DNA (anti-dsDNA) antibody

E. Basic metabolic panel, corticotropin (ACTH), cortisol, plasma renin activity

175. A 13-year-old female with a history of migraines with vision changes presents with vaginal bleeding for 5 weeks. She becomes dizzy on standing and has been increasingly fatigued in the last week. The bleeding has been waxing and waning and is associated with crampy abdominal pain. Menarche occurred 18 months ago, and previously her periods had occurred monthly, lasting for 5 days with moderate bleeding. She denies ever having been sexually active. She takes no medications. She appears pale. Her vital signs are reassuring, although her heart rate is elevated to 117 beats per minute. A urine pregnancy test is negative. Her hemoglobin level is 6.2 g/dL. She is admitted to the pediatric ward, and a packed red blood cell transfusion is ordered. Which of the following is the most appropriate initial treatment for this patient?

A. Combination oral contraceptive

B. Intravenous estrogen infusion

C. Tranexamic acid

D. Progestin-only oral contraceptive

E. Intravenous iron infusion

176. You are called to the nursery to see a 1-day-old boy for rash. He was born to a 17-year-old mother by vaginal delivery. Her prenatal care was minimal, with only her rubella immune status being documented. Gestational age of the infant is unknown. Group B *Streptococcus* status was unknown, but the mother received appropriate antibiotic prophylaxis. The infant is well appearing, with diffuse rash (see Figure 1.12). He has an irregular heart rhythm on examination, so an electrocardiogram is obtained and shows a type II second-degree heart block. While updating the mother, you note she has prominent parotid and submandibular glands. On additional history, she reports having chronic dry eyes and mouth, joint aches, fatigue, and "swollen glands." While they are bothersome, she has never sought medical care for these symptoms. Of the following, a positive result of which of the following maternal tests would support the most likely diagnosis?

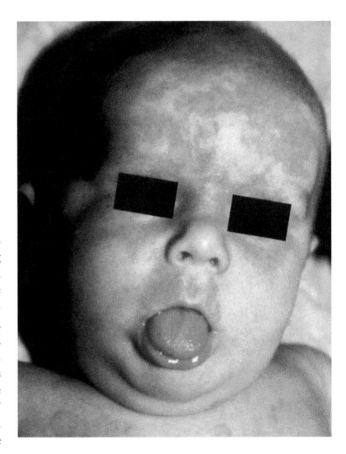

Figure 1.12

A. Antinuclear antibody (ANA)

B. Anti-Ro and anti-La antibodies

C. Antimyeloperoxidase and antiproteinase 3 antibodies

D. Cytomegalovirus polymerase chain reaction

E. *Toxoplasma gondii* antibodies

177. A 14-month-old girl with a history of a febrile seizure with right upper extremity Todd's paralysis is hospitalized following a 1-minute episode of bilateral arm and leg shaking with upward eye deviation. After the episode spontaneously resolved, the patient seemed to be sleepy. On history you discover that her development was normal until her 12-month well-child visit, when her pediatrician noted mild speech and fine

motor delay. Her vital signs at the time of admission are normal. Except for weakness in the right upper extremity, her neurological examination is normal. She has a flat, erythematous birthmark on her left forehead and right upper eyelid. Given her presentation, evaluation by which of the following specialists would be most appropriate?

A. Cardiology
B. Nephrology
C. Ophthalmology
D. Otolaryngology
E. Pulmonology

178. A 4-year-old male presents to the emergency department with new-onset bloody stools for 2 days. Per his parents, the patient has not had any other symptoms, including vomiting, diarrhea, abdominal pain, or fever. His stools appear homogeneous in consistency and are dark red in color. He stools once per day with soft consistency and has not had any history of constipation. He has been eating normally and is gaining weight appropriately. The parents report no changes to his diet, and he has not recently consumed any pigmented foods. On examination, the patient has normal vital signs. His abdomen is soft and nontender with no organomegaly. No anal fissures or hemorrhoids are noted. Which diagnostic test is most likely to reveal the etiology of the patient's symptoms?

A. Colonoscopy
B. Stool culture
C. *Helicobacter pylori* stool antigen
D. Abdominal ultrasound
E. Technetium Tc 99m scan

179. A 2-year-old male with hemophilia A presents with swelling and pain following trauma to his right calf. On physical examination, the right calf is tender to palpation and has overlying ecchymoses. The right knee and ankle joints are normal with good range of motion. The distal right lower extremity is pink with brisk capillary refill and normal pulses. Of the following, which is the appropriate therapy for this patient?

A. Desmopressin acetate
B. Factor VIII concentrate
C. Factor IX concentrate
D. Tranexamic acid
E. Fasciotomy of the right lower leg

180. A 13-year-old previously healthy boy is seen in the emergency department for headaches and blurry vision. His blood pressure is 181/115 mm Hg and remains elevated on two additional checks using a manual, appropriate size cuff. His physical examination confirms visual changes. A workup for secondary causes of hypertension is initiated. Of the following, which is the most appropriate next step in management?

A. Do not initiate antihypertensives until all workup is complete
B. Initiate a short-acting antihypertensive with the goal of rapidly decreasing his blood pressure to the 90th percentile
C. Initiate a short-acting antihypertensive with the goal of gradually decreasing his blood pressure to the 90th percentile
D. Initiate a short-acting antihypertensive with the goal of rapidly decreasing his blood pressure to the 95th percentile
E. Initiate a short-acting antihypertensive with the goal of gradually decreasing his blood pressure to the 95th percentile

181. You are paged to a pediatric trauma in the emergency department. An adolescent female is wheeled in from a motor vehicle accident, and you notice she is making unintelligible sounds, her eyes are opening only to pain, and she is posturing with abnormal flexion. What is the appropriate immediate next step?

A. Computed tomography (CT) of the head
B. Type and screen
C. Central venous catheter placement
D. Urine pregnancy test
E. Intubation

182. A 7-month-old male born at 28 weeks' gestation who requires enteral feeds via gastrostomy tube and 2 L/min oxygen via nasal cannula at home presents to the hospital with grunting and hypoxemia. His clinical examination and chest radiograph are concerning for pneumonia. He is admitted for intravenous (IV) antibiotics, IV fluids, and increased oxygen support. He continues to tolerate full enteral feeds. He initially improves, but on hospital day 3 he is noted to have increased work of breathing and diffuse wheezing. His oxygen saturation is 95% on 3 L/min oxygen, and his other vital signs are within normal limits. A trial of nebulized albuterol is not effective. A repeat chest radiograph shows new bilateral interstitial lung markings and perihilar fullness. What is the best next step in the management of this patient?

A. Administer nebulized ipratropium-albuterol
B. Increase the oxygen flow rate
C. Start inhaled budesonide
D. Administer furosemide

E. Broaden antibiotic coverage

183. A 16-year-old female presents to the emergency department with severe headache for the past 2 days. She describes the headache as a constant, pulsatile pain. In addition, she has noted transient episodes of blurry vision. She was recently started on minocycline to treat acne. Her vital signs are normal for age. Her body mass index is at the 97th percentile for age. On examination, the patient is sitting in a dark room in obvious discomfort. Pupillary reflexes and extraocular movements are intact. Funduscopic examination reveals bilateral papilledema. The remainder of her examination is within normal limits. Computed tomography (CT) of the head reveals no focal findings with normal-size ventricles. A lumbar puncture is obtained with an opening pressure of 38. Cerebrospinal fluid (CSF) analysis demonstrates glucose 55 mg/dL, protein 32 mg/dL, red blood cell 1, and white blood cells 0. Pregnancy testing is negative. Based on this patient's most likely diagnosis, what is the best initial treatment for this condition?

A. Topiramate
B. Intravenous ceftriaxone and vancomycin
C. Lumboperitoneal shunt
D. Acetazolamide
E. Furosemide

184. A 2-year-old male is admitted for dehydration, fever, and irritability. He has a 3-week history of intermittent fever and upper respiratory symptoms. Physical examination is notable for a moderately erythematous left tympanic membrane, along with erythema and tenderness over the left mastoid process. Peripheral white blood cell (WBC) count is 26×10^9/L, and C-reactive protein (CRP) is 81 mg/L. Cerebrospinal fluid analysis (CSF) shows a WBC count of 10/mm^3 and protein of 50 mg/dL. He is receiving vancomycin and ceftriaxone, while cultures are pending for presumed bacterial mastoiditis. On hospital day 2, he has new-onset vomiting and worsening irritability. The best next step in this patient's care is to

A. Obtain head computed tomography with venography
B. Obtain an electroencephalogram (EEG)
C. Check serum creatinine and random vancomycin level
D. Start a proton pump inhibitor
E. Obtain renal ultrasound with Dopplers

185. You are preparing to discharge a patient who is frequently admitted to the hospitalist service for acute episodes of pain. You last discharged him 5 months earlier. He requires a new prescription for a controlled opioid medication today. According to the Centers for Disease Control and Prevention (CDC), when should you check your state's Prescription Drug Monitoring Program (PDMP) for this patient?

A. Before writing a new prescription for a controlled substance if you have not checked the PDMP in the last 3 months
B. Before writing a new prescription for a controlled substance if you have not checked the PDMP in the last 30 days
C. Only when you have suspicion for opioid abuse
D. When requested by pharmacy
E. When requested by a family member

186. You admit a 13-year-old boy with type 1 diabetes (T1D) and a blood glucose of 485 mg/dL. His venous blood gas shows a pH of 7.22. A serum bicarbonate level is 10 mmol/L, and his anion gap is 28. His grandfather says the patient is adherent to his insulin regimen and that the patient was recently diagnosed with another autoimmune disease. Of the following, what is the most likely cause of this patient's presentation?

A. Coexisting celiac disease
B. Insulin nonadherence
C. Coexisting primary adrenal insufficiency
D. Increased insulin requirement in puberty
E. Viral upper respiratory illness (URI)

187. A 10-year-old boy presents to the emergency department with left-side scrotal pain that began 3 hours ago. On physical examination, he is writhing in pain and unable to respond to your questions. His right testis is normal in appearance; his left testis is exquisitely tender to the touch, and you note a small blue mass through the scrotal skin. Your suspected diagnosis is confirmed by a scrotal ultrasound. Of the following, what is the most appropriate treatment for this patient?

A. Manual detorsion
B. Reassurance and discharge
C. Surgical detorsion and fixation
D. Warm compress and ibuprofen
E. Antibiotics

188. A 9-year-old girl presents to her primary care physician with 1 day of dark brown urine. For the past 1–2 months she has had intermittent fevers, vague joint pains, fatigue, and decreased appetite. She has developed a worsening rash within the past 2 weeks, which started as raised purple spots and now has the appearance seen in Figure 1.13. She is fatigued and, except for the rash, otherwise well appearing on examination. Her blood pressure is 120/80, but the rest of her vital signs

are normal. Laboratory studies show an elevated creatinine, C-reactive protein, and erythrocyte sedimentation rate as well as mild anemia, hematuria, and proteinuria.

Of the following, what is the best next step in management?

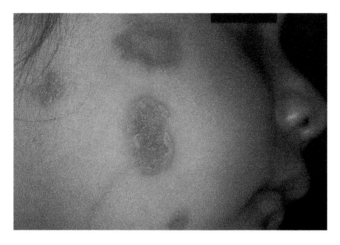

Figure 1.13

A. In-office biopsy of lesions
B. Systemic prednisone with close outpatient follow-up
C. Urgent outpatient dermatology and nephrology referrals
D. Referral to the nearest emergency department
E. Hospitalization for multidisciplinary evaluation and treatment

189. A 4-year-old previously healthy boy presents to the emergency department with fussiness and rash. Yesterday, he developed a bright red rash on his torso, which has since spread to all four extremities. His mother is worried that he is having oral pain, as he will no longer eat or drink. Five days ago, he was prescribed trimethoprim/sulfamethoxazole for an ear infection at urgent care. Vital signs are notable for tachycardia and otherwise are age appropriate. Physical examination demonstrates a diffuse erythematous rash with areas of blistering and skin sloughing, as well as oral, anal, and urethral mucositis. Of the following, which is the best next step in management?

A. Dermatology consultation for urgent biopsy
B. Swab of skin lesions for culture and discharge home with topical mupirocin
C. Discharge home with topical emollients
D. Hospitalize for supportive care with intravenous fluids, wound care, and pain control
E. Hospitalize for intravenous antistaphylococcal antibiotics

190. A 10-year-old otherwise healthy female presents to the emergency department with concerns for dehydration. The patient was in her normal state of health until 1 week prior to presentation, when she began having vomiting, diarrhea, and generalized abdominal pain. For the past 2 days, she has been having fevers as high as 38.7°C, three or four episodes of nonbloody, nonbilious emesis, and two nonbloody stools each day. She has not recently traveled. There is no family history of autoimmune disease. On examination, the patient is febrile to 38.1°C, is tachycardic to 115 beats per minute, and is generally ill appearing. She has notable scleral icterus, and her mucous membranes are dry. Her abdominal examination is notable for hepatomegaly and generalized tenderness with no rigidity or guarding. Her white blood cell count is 15,000 with a normal hematocrit and normal platelets. Her aspartate aminotransferase (AST) and alanine aminotransferase (ALT) are elevated at 850 and 1130, respectively. Her bilirubin is elevated at 10.2 mg/dL, primarily conjugated. A right upper quadrant ultrasound is unremarkable. The most likely diagnosis for this patient is

A. Autoimmune hepatitis
B. Hepatitis A infection
C. Hepatitis B infection
D. Cholelithiasis
E. Primary sclerosing cholangitis

191. A 12-year-old medically complex female is hospitalized with hematogenous osteomyelitis. Vascular access has been difficult, and a peripherally inserted central catheter (PICC) is placed in the right upper extremity for antibiotic administration. Several days into the hospitalization, the patient develops right upper extremity swelling. Ultrasonography with Doppler confirms a deep venous thrombosis. Of the following, which factor is associated with increased risk for catheter-related thrombosis?

A. Single- rather than double-lumen catheter
B. Small catheter diameter
C. Factor V Leiden mutation
D. Glanzmann thrombasthenia
E. Central rather than peripheral catheter insertion

192. A 10-year-old girl presents to the emergency department after a witnessed fainting event at school. She was playing basketball with her friends when she fell to the ground and was unresponsive for 10 seconds. There were no abnormal movements or incontinence during the episode. She returned to her baseline within several minutes. She does not remember feeling palpitations, shortness of breath, or lightheaded prior to the fall. She is currently asymptomatic, and her physical examination is normal. Which of the following is most likely to yield a diagnosis?

A. Electroencephalography (EEG)
B. Electrocardiography (ECG)
C. Expanded social history
D. Orthostatic vital signs
E. Basic metabolic panel

193. A 9-year-old previously healthy boy is admitted to your service after operative repair of a left tibial fracture with cast placement. He is now complaining of acutely increasing levels of pain that were previously responsive to acetaminophen. His toes are warm and well perfused. Which of the following is the most important next step?

A. Measure compartment pressures
B. Increase his pain medication
C. Obtain left leg x-rays
D. Start an anxiolytic
E. Reassure the patient

194. A healthy, fully immunized 5-year-old boy is admitted for respiratory distress. He has a history of 8 days of rhinorrhea, wet cough, and subjective fevers. His symptoms worsened 24 hours ago, prompting his pediatrician to start a course of amoxicillin for presumed bacterial pneumonia. On physical examination, he is febrile to 39°C, has a respiratory rate of 32 breaths per minute, and has an oxygen saturation of 95% on 2 L/min of 100% oxygen. He has moderate intercostal retractions and crackles over the left upper lung field. A chest radiograph shows left upper lobe consolidation. Influenza viral testing is negative. What is the most appropriate next step in the management of his condition?

A. Start ceftriaxone
B. Start ampicillin
C. Consult pulmonologist for bronchoalveolar lavage (BAL)
D. Continue amoxicillin and start azithromycin
E. Obtain urinary antigen testing

195. A 3-year-old boy is admitted to your pediatric hospital medicine service due to concerns for progressive weakness over the last few months. His mother reports the patient did not start walking until 20 months of age. He was adopted at birth, so the biological family history is unknown. While in the room, you observe the boy playing on the floor and using his hands to push himself up into a standing position. You suspect the patient has an inherited neuromuscular disorder. What is the most common mode of inheritance for this disease process?

A. X-linked recessive
B. Autosomal dominant
C. Autosomal recessive

D. Mitochondrial
E. X-linked dominant

196. A 5-year-old healthy male presents with 2 days of right eye redness and pain. He has also had 5 days of rhinorrhea, cough, and subjective fever. Physical examination is remarkable for right periorbital edema and erythema with photophobia and pain with movement of extraocular muscles. He has mild right proptosis and moderate midface tenderness. Contrast-enhanced computed tomography demonstrates a 10-mm by 15-mm medial subperiosteal abscess of the right orbital wall. Regarding the most likely diagnosis, which of the following statements is true?

A. The most likely predisposing factor is frontal sinusitis
B. Blood cultures are likely to be positive
C. Elevated white blood cell count (WBC) and C-reactive protein (CRP) levels are not predictive
D. Systemic corticosteroids have not been found to be beneficial
E. Conservative management with antibiotics alone is appropriate

197. A 16-year-old patient weighing 75 kg is admitted to the hospitalist service for acute worsening of her chronic pain. She normally takes extended-release oxycodone 10 mg orally twice daily. How many morphine milligram equivalents (MMEs) is this patient taking per day currently?

A. 10
B. 30
C. 50
D. 100
E. 120

198. A 7-year-old male with a history of type 1 diabetes mellitus presents to the emergency department with nausea, vomiting, and abdominal pain. He is afebrile, his heart rate is 145 beats per minute, respiratory rate is 35 breaths per minute, and oxygen saturation is 99%. His arterial blood gas demonstrates a pH of 7.15, and his basic metabolic panel is as follows: sodium 128 mmol/L, potassium 5.9 mmol/L, chloride 105 mmol/L, and bicarbonate 8 mmol/L. His blood glucose is 485 mg/dL, and his urine dip demonstrates 3+ ketones. The patient is awake and alert; his abdomen is mildly tender on palpation without guarding or rebound. Which of the following is the best next step in management?

A. Order computed tomography of the head
B. Administer sodium bicarbonate
C. Administer calcium gluconate

D. Give 10 mL/kg of intravenous (IV) normal saline

E. Start an IV insulin infusion at 1 unit/kg/h

199. A 16-year-old male presents to the emergency department with gross hematuria and severe flank pain. Which of the following is the most sensitive imaging modality to detect the likely diagnosis?

A. Computed tomography (CT) with contrast

B. CT without contrast

C. Ultrasound

D. Plain radiography

E. Magnetic resonance imaging (MRI)

200. An 18-month-old male is admitted with fever for the past 5 days, as well as conjunctival injection, swollen hands and feet, red and cracked lips, and a maculopapular rash. An echocardiogram is performed, which is normal. He is diagnosed with Kawasaki disease (KD) and started on aspirin; he is also given intravenous immunoglobulin (IVIG) at 2 g/kg delivered over 10 hours. Twenty-four hours after completion of the IVIG, the patient develops a fever to 38.5°C. What is the best next step in management?

A. Administer a second dose of IVIG

B. Initiate corticosteroids

C. Give acetaminophen

D. Give infliximab

E. Repeat echocardiogram

201. A 15-year-old previously healthy boy presents to the emergency department (ED) with redness, warmth, and pain of the right thigh. Five days ago, he scratched the area on a wooden fence. Initially, there was redness directly around the lesion, but the redness has since spread. He was seen in urgent care 3 days ago and given oral cephalexin, which he has taken as prescribed. He was brought to the ED after he developed a fever at home. Vital signs include a temperature of 39.1°C and a heart rate of 120 beats per minute. His other vitals are within normal parameters. There is a 5-cm superficial laceration of the right thigh without drainage or fluctuance, as well as a 10 by 14 cm surrounding area of confluent erythema and mild edema. There is tenderness directly over the laceration. He has full range of motion in the right lower extremity with good distal pulses. His white blood cell count is 16,000 cells/mm³ with 85% neutrophils. Blood cultures are pending. Of the following, which are the best next steps in management?

A. Discharge and continue oral cephalexin

B. Discharge with oral clindamycin

C. Admission and intravenous (IV) oxacillin

D. Admission and IV vancomycin

E. Urgent surgical evaluation

202. A 17-year-old male with ulcerative colitis (UC) presents to the emergency department with fatigue and pruritis. His symptoms began 2 weeks prior to presentation and have been getting progressively worse during that time period. He denies any fevers, abdominal pain, vomiting, or diarrhea. He reports that his UC has been well controlled on a daily regimen of mesalamine and that he has not had any flares in the last year. On examination, he has hepatomegaly and mild scleral icterus. His alkaline phosphatase is elevated at 315 U/L with aspartate aminotransferase (AST) and alanine aminotransferase (ALT) values of 75 and 90 mmol/L, respectively. What results would be expected on liver biopsy?

A. Fibrous obliteration of small bile ducts

B. Steatosis with portal inflammation

C. Portal mononuclear cell infiltrate surrounding the portal triad

D. Proliferation of hyperplastic hepatocytes surrounding a central stellate scar

E. Lobular inflammation with focal necrosis

203. A 15-year-old boy is being evaluated in the emergency department due to an episode of blacking out on a family trip to a water park on a very hot day. His father said that he was standing in line for a water slide when he swayed and started to fall backward. His father caught him and said he woke up within 20–30 seconds. The patient recalls feeling lightheaded, his vision fading to black, and then waking up in his father's arms. Before the event, he ate all of his lunch and was drinking water throughout the day. His physical examination is normal. Which of the following is the most likely cause of his syncopal episode?

A. An atrioventricular (AV) conduction abnormality with inability to increase stroke volume

B. Increased parasympathetic activity and vasodilation

C. A focal area of abnormal brain activity

D. A disorder in which emotions manifest through physical symptoms

E. Intravascular volume depletion resulting in decreased blood pressure while in an upright position

204. A 10-year-old girl is brought to the emergency department following a bite wound from a raccoon. You are consulted for prophylaxis recommendations. Her father states that she last received immunizations at 4 years of age. Which of the following regimens do you recommend?

A. Tetanus toxoid–containing vaccine, human tetanus immune globulin, rabies vaccine, and rabies immune globulin

B. Tetanus toxoid–containing vaccine, rabies vaccine, and rabies immune globulin only
C. Rabies vaccine and rabies immune globulin only
D. Tetanus toxoid–containing vaccine and rabies vaccine only
E. Tetanus toxoid–containing vaccine, human tetanus immune globulin, and rabies vaccine only

205. A 12-year-old male with hypoxic-ischemic encephalopathy and epilepsy has been hospitalized for 7 days for evaluation of poor weight gain. He was hospitalized 2 months ago for a wound infection following spinal fusion surgery. During this admission, gastric tube feeds were initiated, and he was started on omeprazole and cyproheptadine. He has developed tachypnea and hypoxia over the past 12 hours as well as focal crackles over the left lower lobe on auscultation. He has required chest physiotherapy and airway suctioning every 3 hours. A chest radiograph shows a left lower lobe opacification with volume loss. Which of the following is an established risk factor for the development of his condition?

A. Scoliosis
B. Homelessness
C. Use of proton pump inhibitors (PPIs)
D. Recent travel
E. Use of gastric feeding tubes

206. An 11-year-old previously healthy female presents following a first-time seizure at home. In the emergency department, computed tomography of the brain without contrast, complete blood count, and complete metabolic panel are normal. She is admitted for observation and further workup due to not returning to neurologic baseline. While on the floor, she begins having another generalized tonic-clonic seizure. On your assessment, her vital signs are as follows: heart rate 133 beats per minute, respiratory rate 14 breaths per minute, blood pressure 133/88 mm Hg, oxygen saturation 89%, temperature 37.6°C. Which of the following is the best next step in management?

A. Administer oral levetiracetam
B. Administer intravenous (IV) lorazepam
C. Administer IV diazepam
D. Provide supplemental oxygen
E. Obtain additional head imaging

207. A 12-year-old male with a history of chronic seasonal allergies and wheezing presents in spring with 7 days of nasal congestion, green rhinorrhea, and eye swelling. Today, he began complaining of frontal headache, and his mother noticed left forehead swelling. On physical examination, he is febrile to 102.8°F and has difficulty answering questions due to headache. He has moderate left periorbital and forehead edema with fluctuance and severe tenderness. His white blood cell count is 24 × 10⁹/L, and C-reactive protein is 20.1 mg/dL. What is the best next step in evaluation?

A. Brain magnetic resonance imaging (MRI) with gadolinium
B. Maxillofacial, thin-cut, contrast-enhanced computed tomography (CT) and axial imaging
C. Lumbar puncture
D. Electroencephalography (EEG)
E. Pediatric neurosurgery consultation

208. A 7-day-old male who was born at home presents with lethargy. Parents deny fever. There are no sick contacts. On examination, the infant is listless and has delayed capillary refill time. A basic metabolic panel shows sodium 130 mmol/L, potassium 6.5 mmol/L, chloride 105 mmol/L, bicarbonate 12 mmol/L, and glucose 40 mg/dL. A complete blood count and cerebrospinal fluid studies are reassuring. Following fluid resuscitation with normal saline, which of the following will best treat the underlying diagnosis?

A. Empiric antibiotics
B. Corticosteroids
C. Sodium bicarbonate injection
D. Breastmilk or formula
E. Dextrose-containing intravenous fluids

209. A 4-year-old female is admitted to the hospital in respiratory distress and is diagnosed with community-acquired pneumonia. She is started on ampicillin and 15 L/min of oxygen via high-flow nasal cannula. On hospital day 3, her oxygen requirement has improved to 0.5 L/min via simple nasal cannula. She remains on maintenance intravenous fluids due to poor oral intake. Her physical examination demonstrates a comfortable, alert, and responsive child with decreased breath sounds over the left lower lung fields and moist mucous membranes. A basic metabolic panel from this morning demonstrates a sodium of 130 mmol/L. Her serum osmolality is 260 mOsm/kg (normal is 275 to 290 mOsm/kg). Her urine osmolality is 140 mOsm/kg, and her urine sodium is 45 mEq/L. What is the recommended treatment for her hyponatremia?

A. Administer 10 mL/kg of 3% hypertonic saline
B. Administer 20 mL/kg of 0.9% normal saline
C. Give intranasal desmopressin
D. Change antibiotic from ampicillin to clindamycin
E. Restrict fluids to two-thirds of maintenance rate

210. A 7-month-old previously healthy male is admitted for management of pyelonephritis. He remains febrile despite 48 hours of ceftriaxone. Which of the following is the best next step?

A. Technetium-labeled dimercaptosuccinic acid (Tc 99m DMSA) scan
B. Renal and bladder ultrasound (RBUS)
C. Computed tomography (CT) of the abdomen
D. Blood culture
E. Voiding cystourethrography (VCUG)

211. A 3-week-old previously full-term female presents to the emergency department with vomiting. Her parents report 8–10 episodes of projectile vomiting over the 5 days prior to presentation. She had been feeding well until today but has been less interested over the last 12 hours. Her parents note the patient has had five wet diapers over the past 24 hours. They deny fevers, diarrhea, recent sick contacts, or other symptoms. On examination, the patient is afebrile with a pulse of 170 beats per minute. Her mucous membranes are moist with capillary refill time of less than 2 seconds. Her central pulses are strong. Her abdomen is soft, nondistended, with no organomegaly and no other appreciable masses. What is the most likely laboratory finding for this patient?

A. Hyperchloremia
B. Hypokalemia
C. Leukocytosis
D. Elevated conjugated bilirubin
E. Low bicarbonate

212. A 3-year-old previously healthy boy presents to the emergency room unresponsive and pulseless after ingesting several of his grandmother's potassium chloride supplements. Compressions and bag-mask ventilation are immediately initiated. The cardiorespiratory monitor confirms ventricular fibrillation. What is the immediate next step in management?

A. Intravenous calcium gluconate
B. Intravenous insulin
C. Intravenous epinephrine
D. 2 J/kg shock
E. 4 J/kg shock

213. An 18-month-old male is admitted for evaluation of failure to thrive. A thorough history has not yielded any concerning symptoms or social history, and the physical examination demonstrates a small-for-age child who is otherwise well appearing. Serum electrolyte studies are as follows: sodium 135 mmol/L; potassium 4.1 mmol/L; chloride 112 mmol/L; and bicarbonate 15 mmol/L. Which of the following diagnoses should be suspected?

A. Diabetes mellitus
B. Renal tubular acidosis (RTA)
C. Organic acidemia
D. Hyperaldosteronism
E. Mitochondrial disorder

214. A 10-year-old girl is brought to the emergency department following a deep bite to her ankle from her adult cat. You are consulted for antibiotic prophylaxis recommendations. Which of the following agents do you recommend?

A. Cephalexin
B. Clindamycin
C. Trimethoprim-sulfamethoxazole
D. Amoxicillin-clavulanate
E. Azithromycin

215. A 4-year-old girl with cerebral palsy and gastrostomy tube dependence is admitted with respiratory distress, hypoxemia, and increased secretions. This is her third admission in the past year for respiratory infection. On chest radiography, she has a right middle lobe consolidation. She is scheduled to undergo diagnostic bronchoalveolar lavage (BAL). What is the most likely finding from bronchoscopy and BAL fluid analysis?

A. Lipid-laden macrophages
B. Positive fungal staining
C. Foreign body
D. Bronchiectasis
E. Extrinsic airway compression

216. A 14-year-old male is admitted with concerns for recent changes in behavior. His family reports over the last 2 days he has been increasingly anxious and confused. He denies any headaches, trouble swallowing, changes in vision, abdominal pain, or diarrhea. He does endorse a recent cough for which he has been taking an over-the-counter cough medication for the last 48 hours. His medical history includes depression, for which he was started on fluoxetine 1 week ago. The family is not aware of any illicit drug use. Vital signs are temperature 100.6°F, heart rate 120 beats per minute, respiratory rate 10 breaths per minute, and blood pressure 138/82 mm Hg. On examination, he is able to correctly state his name but cannot identify his location or the current month. He appears agitated, is diaphoretic, and will intermittently stand up to pace back and forth but is able to follow commands. Strength testing is 5/5 throughout

with normal ambulation. His deep tendon reflexes are biceps 2+ and patellar 3+ with inducible ankle clonus bilaterally. Which of the following most likely explains this patient's symptoms?

A. Lysergic acid diethylamide (LSD) intoxication
B. Infectious meningitis
C. Serotonin syndrome
D. Neuroleptic malignant syndrome
E. Malignant hyperthermia

217. A 4-year-old female presents with acute onset of difficulty breathing. Her mother reports the patient developed symptoms over the course of a few hours, including drooling, muffled speech, and noisy breathing. On arrival to the emergency room, she appears anxious as she sits at the edge of the bedside with her nose pointed up. After an examination reveals significant drooling, stridor, tachypnea, and hypotension, she is intubated urgently and stabilized. What is the best choice in antimicrobial therapy for this patient?

A. Clindamycin
B. Cefotaxime
C. Vancomycin and ceftriaxone
D. Metronidazole and ceftriaxone
E. Piperacillin-tazobactam

218. You are admitting a 6-year-old boy with a history of juvenile dermatomyositis for fever. His white blood cell count is 1200 cells/mL with an absolute neutrophil count (ANC) of 302 cells/mL. The patient's medication list includes methotrexate, folate, and omeprazole. He had previously been on steroids, which were discontinued 3 months ago. You have ordered blood cultures and a 20-mL/kg normal saline bolus. Of the following, what is the most appropriate next step?

A. Granulocyte colony-stimulating factor (G-CSF)
B. Cefepime
C. Amphotericin
D. Ampicillin
E. High-dose methylprednisolone

219. A 14-year-old female presents to the emergency department with abdominal pain, tinnitus, vertigo, and nonbilious, nonbloody emesis. She reports taking half of a bottle of aspirin after her boyfriend broke up with her. What is the most likely electrolyte finding you may see in this patient's laboratory results?

A. Primary gap metabolic acidosis and a primary respiratory alkalosis
B. Primary gap metabolic acidosis and a secondary respiratory alkalosis

C. Primary respiratory alkalosis and a secondary gap metabolic acidosis
D. Primary nongap metabolic acidosis and a primary respiratory alkalosis
E. Primary nongap metabolic acidosis and a secondary respiratory alkalosis

220. A 3-day-old infant comes to the emergency department with lethargy, hypoglycemia, and hepatomegaly. She is found to have a urinalysis positive for ketones and reducing substances. What is this patient at increased risk for?

A. *Escherichia coli* sepsis
B. Neutropenia
C. Arrhythmias
D. Acute renal failure
E. Hearing loss

221. A 5-year-old girl presents to the emergency department with tea-colored urine and edema and is found to have a blood pressure of 132/84 mm Hg. Which of the following laboratory results would be consistent with the most common cause of this patient's presentation?

A. Low serum C3, low serum C4
B. Positive anti-DNase B
C. Stool culture positive for *Escherichia coli* O157:H7
D. Elevated urine calcium-to-creatinine ratio
E. Elevated anti–double-stranded DNA (dsDNA) titers

222. A 17-year-old previously healthy female presents to the emergency room with abdominal pain, nausea, and vomiting. Her symptoms began approximately 1 month ago and have progressively worsened. Her pain is located in the epigastric region, is worse after meals, and improves when she is lying prone. She has had daily nonbloody emesis over the last week, and today had two episodes of bilious emesis. She denies diarrhea or fevers. She reports that she has intentionally lost approximately 40 pounds over the last 2 months. On examination, she is afebrile with a pulse of 110 beats per minute and a blood pressure of 110/75 mm Hg. She is cachectic with a mildly distended abdomen and high-pitched bowel sounds. Her laboratory testing is remarkable for a normal lipase, normal electrolytes, and normal aspartate aminotransferase (AST), alanine aminotransferase (ALT), alkaline phosphatase, and bilirubin. Which study is most likely to reveal the patient's diagnosis?

A. Abdominal radiograph
B. Abdominal ultrasound
C. Magnetic resonance arteriography (MRA)
D. Upper endoscopy

E. Magnetic resonance cholangiopancreatography (MRCP)

223. A 10-year-old male athlete collapses on the rink during an ice hockey match on a Saturday and is found to be in pulseless arrest. Two bystanders immediately initiate cardiopulmonary resuscitation (CPR), and a third locates an automated external defibrillator (AED). A shock is delivered by the AED, and the boy has return of circulation prior to transport to the hospital. Which of the following factors is associated with successful outcomes for this patient?

A. Out-of-hospital arrest
B. Age
C. Shockable rhythm
D. Cold rink temperature
E. Weekend event

224. You are paged to a pediatric trauma in the emergency department. A 16-year-old boy is brought in by paramedics after being pulled from a lake. He is bradycardic, hypotensive, and unresponsive with a slow respiratory rate. The team has been unable to obtain an accurate core temperature. Which of the following interventions do you recommend next?

A. Administer fluids warmed to 42°C
B. Administer naloxone
C. Apply heat packs to his extremities
D. Administer dantrolene
E. Administer fluids warmed to 37°C

225. A previously healthy 8-year-old girl is being admitted with acute-onset fever, respiratory distress, and worsening cough after an influenza infection 2 weeks ago. On physical examination, she is ill appearing with temperature 39°C, respiratory rate 34 breaths per minute, and oxygen saturation 83% on room air. On auscultation, she has significantly decreased aeration and diffuse crackles on the right side. Chest radiography (CXR) shows blunting of the left costophrenic angle and a rim of fluid ascending the lateral chest wall. In regard to this child's condition, which of the following statements is correct?

A. Antibiotic treatment alone is typically insufficient
B. Empiric antibiotic coverage should include both gram-positive and gram-negative organisms
C. Chest computed tomography (CT) has higher sensitivity and specificity for evaluating the pleural space than ultrasound (US)
D. The prevalence of bacteremia is lower than in uncomplicated community-acquired pneumonia (CAP)

E. The need for surgical intervention is based on disease extent and severity

226. As a member of your institution's rapid response team, you are called to the bedside of a 6-year-old female due to concerns for new-onset seizure activity. She has a history of medulloblastoma and has recently undergone hematopoietic stem cell transplantation (HSCT). On your arrival, it is reported the patient's seizure activity ceased after 2 minutes without any pharmacological intervention. She has no prior history of seizures. The primary medical team reports the patient has had gradually worsening hypertension over the last 48 hours. She had been complaining of headache throughout the day, which was treated with acetaminophen. Based on this clinical history, which of the following is the best next step in management?

A. Lumbar puncture
B. Neurosurgery consult
C. Electrocardiogram (ECG)
D. Brain magnetic resonance image (MRI)
E. Intravenous fosphenytoin

227. You are called to evaluate an 18-month-old female who has presented to the emergency department with 3 days of runny nose, tactile fever, and occasional cough. Today, she developed worsening of her cough along with loud, noisy breathing while playing with her toys. Her appetite has decreased but she is drinking fluids regularly. Your examination reveals inspiratory stridor and a barky, nonproductive cough. The patient is given racemic epinephrine with moderate improvement of her symptoms. How would you describe the pathophysiology of this patient's condition?

A. Inflammation of the epiglottis and adjacent supraglottic structures due to bacteria
B. Inflammation of the larynx and subglottic airway due to a virus
C. Tracheal swelling and sloughing due to bacterial infection
D. Bronchoconstriction triggered by a viral infection
E. Alveolar filling of fluid, white blood cells, and debris, triggered by bacterial invasion of the lower respiratory tract

228. A 2-week-old, full-term boy presents to the emergency department (ED) with fever. He is ill appearing with no focal findings on examination. His mother had prolonged rupture of membranes and unknown prenatal care, but the delivery was unremarkable. The ED physician completes a full sepsis workup and initiates empiric antibiotics and acyclovir. Soon after admission, the cerebrospinal fluid (CSF) herpes simplex virus

(HSV) polymerase chain reaction (PCR) results return as positive. Which of the following is the most appropriate course of acyclovir for this patient?

A. Intravenous (IV) for 21 days followed by oral suppression for 3 months
B. IV for 14 days followed by oral suppression for 6 months
C. IV for 28 days followed by oral suppression for 3 months
D. IV for 21 days followed by oral suppression for 6 months
E. IV for 14 days followed by oral suppression for 3 months

229. A 4-year-old male with methylmalonic acidemia (MMA) presents to the emergency department (ED) with emesis and altered mental status. He appears listless on examination and has a capillary refill time of greater than 3 seconds. A point-of-care glucose is 58 mg/dL. A peripheral intravenous (IV) line is placed and blood for laboratory tests is drawn. What would be the best next step for this patient?

A. IV carnitine
B. 25% dextrose bolus
C. 10% dextrose with electrolytes
D. Normal saline bolus
E. Sodium phenylacetate–sodium benzoate

230. A 3-year-old girl with intermittent asthma and atopic dermatitis presents with a worsening facial rash. Over the past 3 days, the atopic dermatitis on her face became painful, and she developed punched-out erosions with hemorrhagic crusts. The rash has worsened despite application of 1% hydrocortisone cream and topical mupirocin ointment. Today, she developed a fever to 38.5°C and poor oral intake, prompting evaluation. What is the best next step in management?

A. Bacterial culture of lesion, start amoxicillin/clavulanate
B. Bacterial culture of lesion, await results to determine treatment
C. Viral polymerase chain reaction (PCR) of lesion, start acyclovir
D. Viral PCR of lesion, await results to determine treatment
E. Dermatology consultation, start topical triamcinolone

231. A 2-week-old, former full-term female presents to the emergency room with emesis. Over the past 4 hours she has had three episodes of nonbloody, bilious emesis.

Her parents deny any change in stooling patterns. She has been breastfeeding well and gaining weight appropriately with three soft, yellow stools per day. She has had no fevers. On examination, she is fussy but nontoxic appearing. She has mild abdominal distension with hypoactive bowel sounds with an otherwise soft abdomen and no appreciable masses. Her vital signs are within normal parameters. What is the most appropriate imaging study for this patient?

A. Hepatic iminodiacetic acid (HIDA) scan
B. Computed tomography (CT) of the abdomen
C. Barium enema
D. Upper gastrointestinal (GI) series
E. Magnetic resonance imaging (MRI) of the abdomen

232. A 3-year-old boy is admitted for evaluation of 6 days of fever, chills, and malaise. On examination, his temperature is 39.1°C, and he has nontender nodules on his palms. Three blood cultures that were performed on separate occasions reveal *Haemophilus parainfluenzae*. A urinalysis is significant for red cell casts and proteinuria. A transthoracic echocardiogram is normal. How many major and minor modified Duke criteria does this patient meet?

A. 0 major + 4 minor
B. 1 major + 3 minor
C. 2 major + 2 minor
D. 3 major + 1 minor
E. 4 major + 0 minor

233. A 3-year-old boy is brought to the emergency department by paramedics after being pulled from a lake in winter. He was submerged for approximately 8 minutes and required 15 minutes of resuscitation before being admitted for postresuscitation care. His initial blood gas had a pH of 7.18. Which of the following factors is most predictive of significant morbidity?

A. Water temperature
B. Initial blood gas
C. Resuscitation time
D. Patient age
E. Submersion duration

234. A 6-month-old girl presents with respiratory distress. Her parents report 2 days of rhinorrhea, cough, and fussiness. Today, she developed fast breathing and worsening cough. She is febrile to 38°C with a respiratory rate of 65 breaths per minute and heart rate 170 beats per minute. On physical examination, she is irritable, grunting, nasal flaring, and retracting with diffuse crackles and wheezing. Which of the following

arterial blood gas (ABG) results is most consistent with her underlying disorder?

A. pH 7.47, PaO$_2$ 55 mm Hg, PaCO$_2$ 28 mm Hg, bicarbonate 21 mEq/L
B. pH 7.25, PaO$_2$ 95 mm Hg, PaCO$_2$ 38 mm Hg, bicarbonate 25 mEq/L
C. pH 7.35, PaO$_2$ 50 mm Hg, PaCO$_2$ 42 mm Hg, bicarbonate 21 mEq/L
D. pH 7.39, PaO$_2$ 85 mm Hg, PaCO$_2$ 55 mm Hg, bicarbonate 33 mEq/L
E. pH 7.32, PaO$_2$ 90 mm Hg, PaCO$_2$ 90 mm Hg, bicarbonate 28 mEq/L

235. A 12-year-old is hospitalized for worsening weakness over the past 2 weeks. On physical examination, he has hyporeflexia and symmetrical 3+/5 strength in his bilateral lower extremities. Magnetic resonance imaging of the spine shows enhancement of the anterior spinal nerve roots. His cerebrospinal fluid was notable for 1 white blood cell, 1 red blood cell, glucose 57 mg/dL, and protein 183 mg/dL. Four weeks ago, he and his family had febrile gastroenteritis, which self-resolved with hydration and supportive care. Of the following, which is the most likely cause of his condition?

A. Molecular mimicry
B. Autoantibodies against acetylcholine receptors
C. Genetic mutation
D. Viral infection of the central nervous system
E. Tick salivary neurotoxin

236. A 17-year-old healthy female presents to the emergency department with severe tooth pain and fever. She is found to have a periapical abscess. Given the systemic symptoms, the on-call oral-maxillofacial surgeon recommends admission for parenteral antibiotics after incision and drainage of the abscess. Which of the following organisms is important to consider when formulating your treatment plan?

A. *Staphylococcus*
B. *Enterobacter*
C. *Bacteroides*
D. *Klebsiella*
E. *Proteus*

237. A 22-day-old full-term, previously healthy female is being admitted for fever. On examination, she is well appearing, and her mother's prenatal care and delivery were unremarkable. The patient's significant initial results are shown below. Blood, urine, and cerebrospinal fluid (CSF) cultures were collected. What empiric antibiotics would you recommend?

Blood:

White blood cells (WBCs)	16 K/μL
Bands	6%
Procalcitonin	12 ng/mL
Comprehensive metabolic panel	Within normal limits

Urinalysis:

Leukocyte esterase (LE)	3+
WBCs	10–50/high-power field

CSF:

Protein	110 mg/dL
Glucose	25 mg/dL
WBC	1100 cells/mm^3
Red blood cells	300 cells/mm^3
Neutrophils	72%

A. Ampicillin and gentamicin
B. Vancomycin and gentamicin
C. Vancomycin
D. Ceftriaxone
E. Ampicillin and ceftazidime

238. You are reviewing the medication list of a newborn's mother, which includes levothyroxine 150 mg taken during the pregnancy. Based on this finding, what additional question should be asked of the mother?

A. Do you plan to breastfeed?
B. Do you have a history of hyperthyroidism?
C. Was this medication also taken in the first trimester?
D. Were you counseled that your baby would need to be weaned off the medication due to the high dosage?
E. Did you have a fetal echocardiogram during the pregnancy?

239. A 9-year-old boy presents with worsening epigastric abdominal pain, emesis, and 3 pounds of weight loss in the past month. He has been stooling regularly and has had no fevers. He has always been a slow eater and feels like food gets "stuck" when he tries to swallow. His family history is only notable for atopy. What is the most appropriate study to obtain?

A. Upper gastrointestinal (GI) series with small bowel follow-through
B. Endoscopy
C. Abdominal ultrasound
D. Urea breath test
E. Allergy testing

240. A 2-year-old boy presents to the emergency department with complaints of fever, rash, and decreased oral intake. His mother reports daily fever for the past 6 days despite use of antipyretic medications. On physical examination, he is irritable and has dry mucous membranes, bright red lips, bilateral conjunctival injection without eye discharge, swelling of his hands, and a diffuse erythematous macular rash. Which of the following treatments is necessary to reduce the risk of long-term complications of this condition?

A. Aspirin
B. Corticosteroids
C. Normal saline
D. Intravenous immunoglobulin (IVIG)
E. Ibuprofen

241. A 14-year girl is admitted for workup of chest pain and exertional shortness of breath. She reports that she recently joined the track team and has noted these symptoms after running. On examination she has a mid-to-late systolic click with a high-pitched late systolic murmur. What is her most likely diagnosis?

A. Mitral valve prolapse
B. Hypertrophic cardiomyopathy
C. Atrial stenosis
D. Pulmonary stenosis
E. Myocarditis

242. You are called to admit a 3-year-old girl brought to the emergency department after a house fire. Her pulse oximetry reads 97%, but she is sleepy and vomiting with tachycardia, hypertension, and tachypnea. Which of the following should be included in her treatment regimen?

A. Hydroxocobalamin
B. Methylene blue
C. Naloxone
D. Sodium nitroprusside
E. Physostigmine

243. A 13-year-old girl with myotonic dystrophy and epilepsy is admitted for a 2-day history of somnolence. At baseline, she requires bilevel positive airway pressure when asleep and frequent chest physiotherapy. Aside from requiring an increase of her dose of valproic acid 2 weeks ago for increased seizure activity, she has been well without fever or symptoms of infection. On admission, she appeared fatigued but easily arousable, with a Glasgow Coma Scale (GCS) score of 13. She was placed on supplemental oxygen for tachypnea without retractions. Twelve hours later, she has developed agitation, headache, and tachycardia, with a GCS of 11. She has shallow respirations and nasal flaring, but

no retractions and clear lung fields. Which of the following arterial blood gas (ABG) analysis results is most consistent with her underlying disorder?

A. pH 7.47, PaO_2 55 mm Hg, $PaCO_2$ 28 mm Hg, bicarbonate 21 mEq/L
B. pH 7.25, PaO_2 95 mm Hg, $PaCO_2$ 38 mm Hg, bicarbonate 25 mEq/L
C. pH 7.35, PaO_2 50 mm Hg, $PaCO_2$ 42 mm Hg, bicarbonate 21 mEq/L
D. pH 7.39, PaO_2 85 mm Hg, $PaCO_2$ 55 mm Hg, bicarbonate 33 mEq/L
E. pH 7.31, PaO_2 95 mm Hg, $PaCO_2$ 90 mm Hg, bicarbonate 28 mEq/L

244. A 17-year-old male is hospitalized for evaluation and management of suspected acute psychosis. During his admission, the patient becomes progressively agitated and aggressive. He was given haloperidol intramuscularly for behavioral management. Following de-escalation, the patient was noted to have repetitive tongue protrusion, eye blinking, and head jerking. His vitals are as follows: heart rate 75 beats per minute, respiratory rate 14 breaths per minute, temperature 37°C, blood pressure 115/76 mm Hg, and oxygen saturation 100%. He appears distressed but follows commands, is oriented to self, and has an otherwise normal neurologic examination. Of the following, what is the best next step in treatment?

A. Human tetanus immune globulin
B. Lorazepam
C. Fosphenytoin
D. Benztropine
E. Dantrolene

245. A teenager with anorexia and severe malnutrition is admitted to your hospitalist service for initiation of a feeding protocol with nasogastric tube (NGT) feeds. What are the most critical electrolyte disturbances that may occur?

A. Hyperkalemia, hypophosphatemia, hypomagnesemia
B. Hypokalemia, hypophosphatemia, hypoglycemia
C. Hyperkalemia, hypophosphatemia, hyponatremia
D. Hypokalemia, hypophosphatemia, hypomagnesemia
E. Hyponatremia, hypophosphatemia, hypomagnesemia

246. A 2-day-old male is brought to the emergency department (ED) for poor feeding and lethargy. He had an uneventful newborn nursery course and was latching well prior to discharge earlier today. On examination, he is lethargic, afebrile, and tachypneic. His laboratory testing is as follows: sodium 136 mmol/L; potassium 3.9 mmol/

L; chloride 101 mmol/L; bicarbonate 25 mmol/L; glucose 95 mg/dL; and ammonia 815 mmol/L. Which of the following is the most likely diagnosis?

A. Mitochondrial disorder
B. Ornithine transcarbamylase (OTC) deficiency
C. Propionic acidemia
D. Fructosemia
E. Medium-chain acyl-CoA dehydrogenase deficiency (MCADD)

247. A 7-year-old female with a history of steroid-responsive nephrotic syndrome is admitted with a relapse. On day 2 of her admission, she acutely develops fever, decreased appetite, and diffuse abdominal pain. She has no dysuria or urinary urgency. The physical examination is notable for tachycardia, fever to 39.6°C, diffuse abdominal tenderness, a fluid wave, and ill appearance. Which of the following diagnoses is most likely?

A. Pneumonia
B. Urinary tract infection
C. Bacterial peritonitis
D. Myocarditis
E. Thromboembolism

248. A previously healthy 16-year-old competitive long-distance runner is admitted for observation following increasingly frequent episodes of lightheadedness, generalized weakness, fatigue, palpitations, and fainting. These episodes began shortly after she suffered a concussion during track and field practice about 6 months ago. She has since been unable to run and has spent most of her time outside of school in bed with recurrent headaches. Episodes occur most frequently in the morning when she gets out of bed. A complete metabolic profile, complete blood count, thyroid function testing, and electrocardiogram obtained at time of admission are all normal. While she is lying comfortably in her hospital bed, she has a heart rate of 80 beats per minute and a blood pressure of 116/76 mm Hg. Repeat vitals obtained 3 minutes after she stands up demonstrate a heart rate of 120 beats per minute and a blood pressure of 103/70 mm Hg. Her physical examination is reassuring. She is complaining of her typical morning headache. What is the most likely diagnosis?

A. Inappropriate sinus tachycardia
B. Postconcussive syndrome
C. Dehydration
D. Postural orthostatic tachycardia syndrome
E. Orthostatic hypotension

249. A 12-kg 2-year-old girl is brought to the emergency department from a house fire. She has suffered severe burns to her back and the back of her head with superficial burns on her posterior arms and legs. She is kept nil per os (nothing by mouth). Approximately how much fluid should she receive intravenously (IV) during the first 8 hours?

A. 350 mL
B. 1650 mL
C. 1000 mL
D. 1300 mL
E. 650 mL

250. An 8-year-old male with status asthmaticus is becoming more tachypneic with increasing accessory muscle use despite 24 hours of continuous albuterol use at 20 mg/h. His mental status is normal, and he is able to speak in complete sentences. His most recent arterial blood gas (ABG) analysis on 15 liters per minute of 100% oxygen via nonrebreather face mask shows pH 7.45, PaO$_2$ 65 mm Hg, and PaCO$_2$ 42 mm Hg. What is the best next step in managing this patient?

A. Continue current management
B. Increase oxygen flow rate
C. Initiate high-flow nasal cannula oxygen
D. Initiate mechanical ventilation
E. Increase continuous albuterol dose

251. A 10-month-old female is admitted to the hospitalist service for failure to thrive. You determine the likely cause is undernutrition. The infant's weight is 8 kg. Her ideal body weight (IBW) is 10 kg. What is the recommended dietary intake for this child to enable catch-up weight gain?

A. 40 kcal/kg/d
B. 60 kcal/kg/d
C. 100 kcal/kg/d
D. 140 kcal/kg/d
E. 180 kcal/kg/d

252. A 3-year-old male presents to the emergency department with 2 days of low-grade fever, vomiting, and diarrhea. He has been unable to tolerate fluids at home for the last 12 hours and has only urinated twice. His vital signs are notable for a temperature of 38.5°C, pulse of 122 beats per minute, and a normal blood pressure. He is awake, with slightly dry mucous membranes and a capillary refill of 2 seconds. His abdominal examination is benign. His volume depletion is thought to be mild to moderate, and you discuss treatment options with his family. Based on current guidelines, which of the following is recommended?

A. Intravenous bolus with normal saline
B. Maintenance fluids with 5% dextrose and normal saline

C. Discharge to home with oral replacement therapy
D. Oral replacement therapy of 50–100 mL/kg over 4 hours
E. Oral replacement therapy with 5 mL every 15 minutes

253. A healthy 4-year-old boy is brought into the emergency department following a submersion event in a backyard pool. His parents report that he was "under water" less than 1 minute and did not appear to lose consciousness. His examination reveals normal vital signs with oxygen saturation of 97% on room air. He is breathing comfortably with normal mentation. Which of the following is the most appropriate disposition for this patient?

A. Discharge home with strict return precautions
B. Continue to observe for 4–8 hours in the emergency department
C. Admit to inpatient pediatric unit due to the risk of developing complications
D. Admit to intensive care unit due to the risk of developing complications
E. Disposition is to be determined based on the results of his workup, including blood gas, complete metabolic panel, complete blood count, chest x-ray, and toxicology analysis

254. A 15-year-old male with Crohn's disease is admitted for abdominal pain and diarrhea. He is receiving total parenteral nutrition and corticosteroids through a peripherally inserted central catheter. On hospital day 3, he develops shortness of breath, cough, and generalized chest pain. His temperature is 38.7°C, blood pressure 138/84 mm Hg, respiratory rate 38 breaths per minute, heart rate 122 beats per minute, and oxygen saturation (SpO_2) of 84% on room air. His SpO_2 improves to 93% on 3 liters per minute of 100% oxygen. Arterial blood gas (ABG) analysis shows pH 7.48, PaO_2 55 mm Hg, and $PaCO_2$ 25 mm Hg. Chest radiography (CXR) demonstrates right lower lobe atelectasis. An electrocardiogram (ECG) shows sinus tachycardia with right axis deviation and right bundle branch block. What is the predominant pathophysiologic mechanism underlying this patient's hypoxemia?

A. Ventilation-perfusion (V/Q) mismatch
B. Right-to-left shunting
C. Diffusion impairment
D. Reduced fraction of inspired oxygen
E. Hypoventilation

255. You have a 23-month-old admitted to your hospitalist service for failure to thrive. Her growth chart is shown in Figure 1.14. Which of the following is closest to this child's estimated ideal body weight (IBW) in kilograms, using the growth chart in the figure?

A. 10.5 kg
B. 11.5 kg
C. 12.5 kg
D. 13.5 kg
E. 14.5 kg

256. A 16-month-old male with biliary atresia and a history of a hepatoportoenterostomy at 2 months of age presents to the emergency department with fever for 1 day. His temperature is 39.2°C, heart rate is 115 beats per minute, respirations are 20 breaths per minute, and blood pressure is 100/75 mm Hg. On physical examination, he has mild bilateral scleral icterus, lungs are clear to auscultation bilaterally with normal work of breathing, abdomen is tender in the right upper quadrant, and capillary refill time is less than 2 seconds. Laboratory workup demonstrates a direct bilirubin of 5.8 mg/dL. What is the best antibiotic regimen for this patient?

A. Ceftriaxone and vancomycin
B. Piperacillin/tazobactam
C. Trimethoprim/sulfamethoxazole (TMP/SMX)
D. Linezolid and meropenem
E. Cefepime

257. A previously healthy 18-month-old girl is admitted following a dog bite to the back of her head. Computed tomography demonstrates a small skull fracture. In addition to confirming her tetanus vaccination status, which of the following is the most appropriate next step in management while awaiting surgical consultation?

A. Observe for development of signs of infection
B. Initiate oral amoxicillin-clavulanic acid
C. Initiate oral cephalexin
D. Initiate parenteral ampicillin-sulbactam
E. Initiate parenteral ceftriaxone and metronidazole

258. A 17-year-old male with a history of congenital myopathy with mild proximal muscle weakness is admitted to the hospital with shortness of breath. He endorses significant dyspnea and fatigue with minor activities and is unable to lay flat due to difficulty breathing. His outpatient doctor has given him a course of levofloxacin, dexamethasone, and furosemide without improvement. On admission, his physical examination is notable for diminished but clear breath sounds throughout all lung fields. His oxygen saturation is 96% on 2 liters per minute via nasal cannula. A venous blood gas reveals pH

Birth to 36 months: Girls
Length-for-age and Weight-for-age-percentiles

NAME _____

RECORD # _____

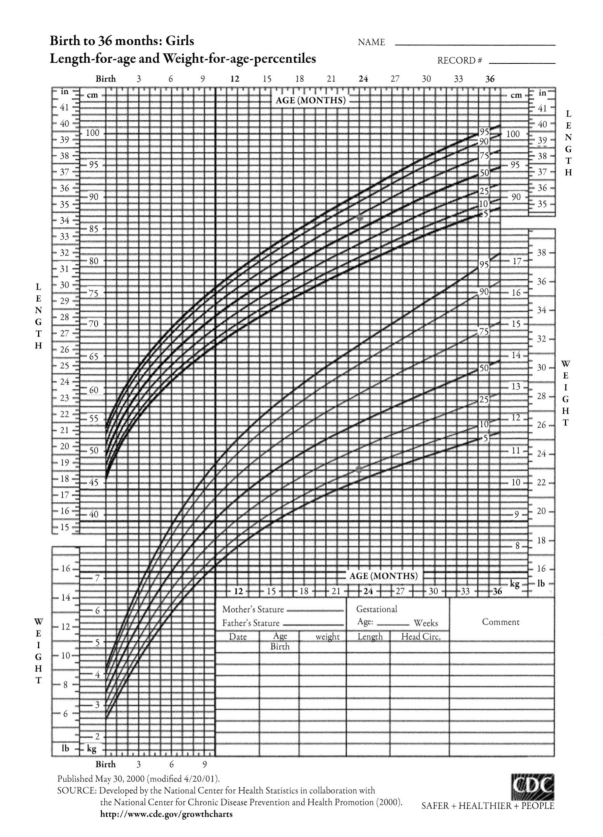

Published May 30, 2000 (modified 4/20/01).
SOURCE: Developed by the National Center for Health Statistics in collaboration with
the National Center for Chronic Disease Prevention and Health Promotion (2000).
http://www.cde.gov/growthcharts

SAFER + HEALTHIER + PEOPLE

Figure 1.14

7.31, PvCO$_2$ 79 mm Hg, PvO$_2$ 37 mm Hg, and bicarbonate 39 mEq/L. His chest radiograph shows low lung volumes and atelectasis. What is most likely to help this patient's symptoms?

A. Intravenous (IV) fluids
B. Increased oxygen via high-flow nasal cannula
C. IV immunoglobulin (IVIG)
D. Noninvasive positive pressure ventilation (NIPPV)
E. Inhaled corticosteroids

259. A 3-month-old, full-term male is admitted to the hospital due to an episode where he appeared to have perioral cyanosis, stopped breathing, and was unresponsive for 30 seconds. The episode resolved with light stimulation. He has no other associated symptoms, but several family members have a cough. His vital signs and physical examination are within normal limits. Based on the current guidelines for a brief resolved unexplained event (BRUE), what would be an appropriate workup?

    A. Chest radiograph (CXR)
    B. Pertussis testing
    C. Electroencephalogram (EEG)
    D. Echocardiogram
    E. Respiratory viral testing

260. A 3-year-old presents to the emergency department (ED) with irritability and decreased appetite that has gradually worsened over the past several days. She refused dinner last night and breakfast this morning, prompting her parents to bring her to the ED. Her abdomen is severely distended, so the ED physician orders an abdominal radiograph that shows a significant stool burden. Her mother reports that the patient has stooled once weekly for the past 2 months, and that the stools are large in diameter and painful to pass, occasionally obstructing the toilet. You admit her for a bowel clean-out. What part of this patient's presentation is concerning for an underlying disease as the cause of her constipation?

    A. Painful stool passage
    B. Patient age
    C. Once-weekly stooling pattern
    D. Severe abdominal distension
    E. Decreased appetite

261. A 3-year-old girl is brought to the emergency department complaining of severe arm pain. Her parents report seeing a black spider with red markings on its abdomen that may have bit her while she was playing in the garage. She is irritable and diaphoretic, with a heart rate of 160 beats per minute and blood pressure of 130/80 mm Hg. Her left arm shows a faint, erythematous targetoid lesion at the site of the bite, but is without swelling or induration. She has intermittent muscle tremors in her arm and complains of significant pain and tenderness to palpation. Which of the following is the most appropriate next step in treatment?

    A. Ice and elevation of the affected extremity
    B. Parenteral antibiotics
    C. Benzodiazepines
    D. Antivenom
    E. Opioid analgesics

262. A 13-year-old male with a history of severe persistent asthma is transferred out of the pediatric intensive care unit to the floor on day 4 of hospitalization for asthma exacerbation. He initially required continuous albuterol, heliox, and intravenous steroids, but is now on intermittent albuterol every 4 hours and oral corticosteroids. This is his 6th hospitalization for asthma in the last 12 months and his 10th course of corticosteroids. His home medications include high-dose beclomethasone metered dose inhaler (MDI), salmeterol MDI, albuterol MDI, and montelukast. Prior workup of his asthma included confirmatory spirometry and elevated immunoglobulin (Ig) E levels. What should your discharge planning for this patient include?

    A. Stop beclomethasone and salmeterol and start combination inhaled budesonide-formoterol
    B. Change MDI medications to nebulized formulations
    C. Refer for immunomodulator therapy
    D. Obtain pulmonary function tests prior to discharge
    E. Prescribe prolonged steroid taper

263. A 9-year-old male is referred for admission from his primary care provider (PCP) due to chronic pain of the lower extremities. The patient is a former 28-week infant with mild cerebral palsy. He underwent tendon release surgery at 6 years of age and again 8 months ago to improve his mobility. He is now able to ambulate with a walker. His parents report he has complained of bilateral lower extremity pain since his last surgery despite physical therapy three times per week and trials of nonsteroidal anti-inflammatory medications. There has been no known trauma since the surgery and no swelling or erythema of any of his joints. Which of the following symptoms support the diagnosis of neuropathic pain?

    A. Sharp, shooting, stabbing pain with distal radiation
    B. Throbbing, aching, pressure-like pain with proximal radiation
    C. Exacerbation of pain only with activity
    D. Absence of temperature and/or color change of the affected extremity
    E. Pain relief with opiates

264. A 6-year-old boy with muscular dystrophy is admitted following spinal surgery. He is nonambulatory and uses a wheelchair at home. A review of his laboratory tests shows the following:

Serum calcium 12.5 mg/dL (8.8–10.3)
Serum phosphorus 3.8 mg/dL (2.4–4.9)

Serum albumin 3.9 g/dL (3.1–4.8)
Parathyroid hormone (PTH) 9 ng/L (12–65)
25-hydroxy vitamin D 17 ng/mL (20–50 ng/mL)

Which of the following is the most likely cause of his high calcium?

A. Primary hypoparathyroidism
B. Vitamin D deficiency
C. Prolonged immobilization
D. Solid tumor
E. Secondary hyperparathyroidism

265. A 4-year-old girl is brought in to the emergency department by her grandmother, who reports that she found the patient with an empty bottle of "heart pills" and suspects she may have ingested several pills. Her vital signs reveal a heart rate of 47 beats per minute, blood pressure of 75/40 mm Hg, respiratory rate of 20 breaths per minute, and oxygen saturation of 99%. On examination, the patient is in no acute distress and has strong pulses. Laboratory evaluation reveals a normal basic metabolic panel with a glucose of 70. Which of the following intravenous medications should be administered next?

A. Normal saline bolus and atropine
B. Normal saline bolus and glucagon
C. Atropine and glucagon
D. Atropine and dextrose
E. Glucagon and epinephrine

266. A 7-year-old male with cystic fibrosis (CF) is admitted with worsening cough and increased sputum production. His prior bronchial cultures have grown *Pseudomonas aeruginosa* and methicillin-sensitive *Staphylococcus aureus*. He is started on intravenous (IV) piperacillin-tazobactam and IV ciprofloxacin, and new sputum cultures and a chest radiograph are obtained. His airway clearance therapy includes increased frequency of nebulized albuterol and the addition of nebulized hypertonic saline, along with his home chest physiotherapy regimen. On hospital day 3, the patient develops moderate hemoptysis that self-resolves after a few hours. His vital signs have not changed, and his laboratory tests show a stable hemoglobin since admission. A chest radiograph shows persistent bilateral infiltrates without interval change. His sputum culture demonstrates the same organisms as prior cultures. What is the next step in the management of this patient?

A. Start IV vancomycin
B. Stop IV ciprofloxacin

C. Stop nebulized hypertonic saline
D. Start inhaled dornase alfa
E. Obtain computed tomography (CT) of the chest with contrast

267. A 16-year-old female is admitted to the hospital with gradually worsening chronic fatigue, joint pains, and abdominal pain and now with dysuria and hematuria. She is noted to have findings on her laboratory tests as follows. What is the most likely diagnosis?

Serum calcium (Ca)	13 mg/dL
Serum creatinine	1.0 mg/dL
Serum albumin	3.6 g/dL
Serum phosphorus	1.2 mg/dL
Vitamin D, 25-OH, total (25(OH)D)	32 ng/mL
Parathyroid hormone (PTH)	375 pg/mL (range 18–80 pg/mL)
Urine calcium	30 mg/dL
Urine creatinine	120 mg/dL

A. Pseudohypercalcemia
B. Malignancy
C. Familial hypocalciuric hypercalcemia (FHH)
D. Disuse osteoporosis
E. Parathyroid adenoma

268. A 14-year-old male presents to the emergency department with altered mental status after attending a party. Which of the following ingestions would benefit most from immediate administration of activated charcoal?

A. Iron
B. Lithium
C. Alcohol
D. Aspirin
E. Bleach

269. A 10-year-old male with history of epilepsy is admitted with convulsions and is found to be hyponatremic to 124 mEq/L. His mother reports he has been tolerating his gastric tube feeds with no recent changes in his feeding regimen and no recent illness or exposures. His neurologist added an antiepileptic medication in the last couple months, but no other recent medication changes have been made. On examination, vital signs are within normal ranges, and he is well perfused with moist mucous membranes and no edema. Given the following laboratory test values, what is the classification of his hyponatremia?

Serum sodium (Na)	124 mEq/L
Serum potassium (K)	3.5 mEq/L
Serum chloride (Cl)	93 mEq/L
Serum blood urea nitrogen (BUN)	25 mg/dL
Serum creatinine	0.9 mg/dL
Serum glucose	80 mg/dL
Urine sodium (UNa)	30 mEq/L

A. Pseudohyponatremia
B. Hypertonic hyponatremia
C. Euvolemic hyponatremia
D. Hypovolemic hyponatremia
E. Hypervolemic hyponatremia

270. A 5-year-old female with a history of asthma presents to the hospital with shortness of breath. Her symptoms have worsened despite using her albuterol inhaler appropriately at home. On physical examination, she is tachypneic with substernal retractions and significant expiratory wheezing. Oxygen saturation is 93% on room air. She is given oral dexamethasone and three combined albuterol-ipratropium nebulizer treatments with mild improvement. Which of the following interventions may help prevent hospitalization of this patient?

A. Continuous nebulized albuterol for 1 hour
B. Intravenous (IV) magnesium
C. Supplemental oxygen
D. Long-acting β-agonist (LABA)
E. Leukotriene receptor antagonist (LTRA)

271. A 9-year-old previously healthy male presents with rash and fever. The rash is present on his trunk and bilateral upper and lower extremities. The rash does not appear to bother him and did not improve with diphenhydramine. He had some hip discomfort yesterday, and his right knee is sore and swollen today. A few weeks ago, he complained of a sore throat, but his family did not seek medical care at the time. He has no recent travel history and is up to date on vaccinations.

On examination, he is tachycardic with a temperature of 39.1°C, but otherwise vital signs are normal for age. There are several circular lesions with a slightly raised red outline and a light pink center. His left knee has mild swelling and some discomfort with flexion, but he can bear weight on it without difficulty. Of the following, what is the best next laboratory test to aid in diagnosis?

A. Creatine kinase
B. Blood culture

C. Lyme serologies
D. Anti–streptolysin O (ASO) titer
E. Anti–double-stranded DNA titer

272. A 6-month-old male is transferred out of the intensive care unit after multiple head injuries related to nonaccidental trauma. His nurse reports his urine output has increased significantly to approximately 6 mL/kg/h, and he seems to be more fatigued. The laboratory reports a critical sodium level. What is the likely etiology of his sodium abnormality?

A. Deficiency of antidiuretic hormone (ADH) leading to polyuria and hypernatremia
B. Increased production of ADH leading to polyuria and hyponatremia
C. Renal resistance to ADH leading to polyuria and hypernatremia
D. Increased renal susceptibility vasopressin V2 leading to polyuria and hyponatremia
E. Deficiency of vasopressin V2 leading to polyuria and hyponatremia

273. A 3-year-old boy is admitted for pain management after splinting of a right supracondylar fracture. He continues to have agitation after receiving a dose of morphine. On examination he is fussy and crying, and his right arm is swollen, bruised, and cool to touch. He has a diminished distal pulse. While awaiting arrival of the on-call orthopedic surgeon, which of the following interventions should be done first?

A. Removal of the dressing and splint
B. Elevation of the limb
C. Heparin
D. Measurement of compartment pressure
E. Right upper extremity venous Doppler ultrasound

274. A 4-year-old previously healthy child is brought to the emergency department (ED) with acute onset of noisy, rapid breathing. The mother reports the child has had a low-grade fever, runny nose, mild cough, and decreased activity in the 3 days prior. In the ED, vital signs are notable for temperature 39.1°C, respiratory rate 56 breaths per minute, blood pressure 87/56 mm Hg, heart rate 160 beats per minute, and oxygen saturation 85% on room air. Physical examination reveals inspiratory stridor, diffuse rhonchi, and moderate abdominal retractions. No drooling is noted. He is given nebulized epinephrine without significant improvement. Supplemental oxygen is provided via nasal cannula with improvement in oxygen saturation to 90% but with persistently increased work of breathing. What is the next step in the management of this patient?

A. Obtain laboratory testing, including complete blood count, C-reactive protein, and arterial blood gas
B. Obtain imaging with chest and lateral neck radiographs
C. Give a one-time dose of oral dexamethasone 0.6 mg/kg
D. Start ceftriaxone
E. Prepare to obtain an advanced airway

275. A previously healthy 9-month-old girl presents with a rash. She has been fussier than usual for the past 2 days, especially when her parents pick her up or change her diaper. Today, she developed a diffuse red rash over most of her body and a fever of 38.1°C, so her parents brought her to the emergency department. She does not take any medications.

On evaluation, she is uncomfortable when examined but quickly calms afterward. She has an erythematous rash on her face, trunk, and extremities with diffuse desquamation as seen in Figure 1.15. There are no mucosal lesions. She is nontoxic and well hydrated. She is hospitalized for further care. In addition to appropriate pain control, which of the following is the best next step in management?

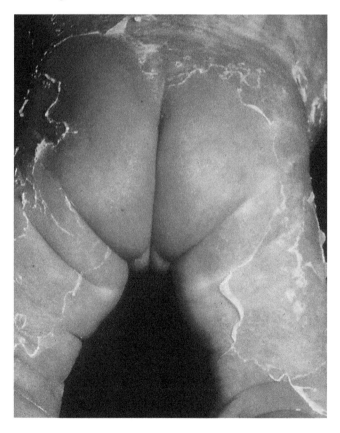

Figure 1.15

A. Topical mupirocin
B. Topical triamcinolone
C. Intravenous nafcillin
D. Intravenous methylprednisolone
E. Intravenous immunoglobulin (IVIG)

276. A previously healthy 1-year-old male is admitted to the hospital for hypoxia caused by right lower lobe pneumonia. On admission, a complete blood count (CBC) shows a white blood cell count of 18.5 × 10⁹/L, hemoglobin 12.3 g/dL, and platelets 32 × 10⁹/L. The patient is febrile and requires 1 liter per minute of oxygen via nasal cannula to maintain a saturation of 94%. His physical examination is significant for mild respiratory distress with subcostal retractions. The remainder of his examination is normal. The family denies any recent history of bleeding or bruising. Of the following, what is the most appropriate next step in management?

A. Repeat CBC with a peripheral smear
B. Bone marrow biopsy
C. Computed tomographic (CT) scan of the head
D. Coagulation tests
E. Transfuse platelets

277. A 6-week-old male presents to the emergency department (ED) for strong cough followed by post-tussive gasping for air and vomiting. He had 5 days of rhinorrhea prior to the development of cough. This evening during one such episode, his mother noticed his lips turn blue. On physical examination, he is afebrile and alert, with frequent forceful coughing. His laboratory testing is notable for a white blood cell (WBC) count of 32,000/μL with 12% neutrophils and 60% lymphocytes. Which of the following is the best next step?

A. Send nasopharyngeal polymerase chain reaction (PCR) testing
B. Observe for 4–6 hours in the emergency department
C. Administer inhaled racemic epinephrine
D. Give azithromycin
E. Perform chest radiograph

278. You are discussing a patient admitted with a nongap metabolic acidosis with the resident team. One resident asks how to differentiate between gastrointestinal (GI) versus renal losses of bicarbonate in a nongap metabolic acidosis. Which response best answers this question?

A. GI causes have a negative urinary anion gap (UAG), and renal causes have a positive UAG
B. GI causes have a negative UAG, and renal causes have a neutral UAG
C. GI causes have a positive UAG, and renal causes have a neutral UAG
D. GI causes have a positive UAG, and renal causes have a negative UAG
E. GI causes have a neutral UAG, and renal causes have a negative UAG

1. ANSWER: E

The patient's presentation is concerning for inflammatory bowel disease (IBD), which includes ulcerative colitis and Crohn's disease. Although a majority of patients will present with gastrointestinal symptoms, including abdominal pain, bloody diarrhea, anorexia, and nausea/vomiting, extraintestinal manifestations are present in up to 30% of patients. Common extraintestinal symptoms include fever, weight loss, malaise, uveitis, arthritis, and a variety of skin manifestations. Laboratory investigation may reveal anemia, elevated inflammatory markers, hypoalbuminemia, and elevated fecal calprotectin. Endoscopy/colonoscopy remains the gold standard diagnostic test for IBD. Findings typically include erythematous, friable, edematous, and ulcerated mucosa. While stool guaiac and abdominal ultrasound may be helpful screening tests for IBD, they are less specific than endoscopy/colonoscopy. Upper GI series with small bowel follow-through may be helpful in evaluation if there is concern for associated stricture or obstruction but would not confirm a diagnosis of IBD. Stool culture is not helpful in diagnosing IBD.

[ABP 1.E.12. Inflammatory bowel disease]

2. ANSWER: D

This patient has Wiskott-Aldrich syndrome (WAS). WAS has a wide range of phenotypes but classically presents with thrombocytopenia, eczema, and infections due to immunodeficiency. It is inherited in an X-linked pattern, and thus almost exclusively affects males. WAS can be easily misdiagnosed as immune thrombocytopenia (ITP) as both present with thrombocytopenia. This is especially true in younger patients, who may initially present with thrombocytopenia alone. A key distinction is that WAS typically causes thrombocytopenia with small platelets, while ITP presents with large or normal-size platelets. Of the answers provided, only a hematopoietic stem cell transplant would be curative for WAS. Anti-D immune globulin can be used to treat ITP for patients who are Rh+. Methylprednisolone and IVIG are treatments for ITP. IVIG is also sometimes used to provide immune protection to patients with WAS but is not curative. Clarithromycin, omeprazole, and metronidazole together are a treatment for *Helicobacter pylori*, a proposed cause of ITP in adults, but they have no role in the management of WAS.

[ABP 1.M.2. Immunodeficiencies]

3. ANSWER: B

Hypertrophic cardiomyopathy (HCM) is a genetic illness that accounts for about 42% of all pediatric cardiomyopathies. Abnormal thickening of the left ventricle (LV) can lead to left outflow tract obstruction, LV dysfunction, myocardial ischemia, and arrhythmias. Patients may be asymptomatic or may present with chest pain, dyspnea, presyncope/syncope, palpitations, symptoms of heart failure, or sudden cardiac death. Although the cardiac examination may be normal, the classic finding is a systolic ejection murmur heard best at the apex and lower left sternal border that increases in intensity with maneuvers that decrease preload and worsen the dynamic outflow tract obstruction. An ECG may show signs of LV hypertrophy and septal hypertrophy, as seen in this patient. The diagnosis is based on findings of LV wall thickening on echocardiogram and/or cardiac magnetic resonance imaging, without alternative explanations. Genetic testing that confirms known causal mutations can also be diagnostic. β-blockers are the most common first-line medical therapy in symptomatic children with LV outflow tract obstruction, to decrease heart rate and improve ventricular filling. Vasodilators such as amlodipine should be avoided as they can decrease systemic vascular resistance and exacerbate LV obstruction. In children who have had an arrhythmic event, an electrophysiology study and/or placement of an AICD would be an appropriate consideration; however, this was not seen in the patient described. Serial troponins do not have any utility in the diagnosis of HCM. Reassurance is not appropriate in this patient, as he has symptomatic HCM that requires close follow-up.

[ABP 1.D.1. Cardiomyopathies]

4. ANSWER: B

The decision to treat acetaminophen ingestions with *N*-acetylcysteine is based on where the patient's serum acetaminophen level falls on the Rumack-Matthew nomogram. Due to differences in absorption rates and metabolism, the nomogram is not accurate until peak values are obtained 4 hours after ingestion. Acetaminophen toxicity is typically not seen with levels below the treatment line. Therefore, acetaminophen levels should be obtained at least 4 hours postingestion prior to initiating treatment or finalizing disposition. The clinical presentation for acute acetaminophen toxicity can initially be nonspecific. In the first stage of toxicity (first 24 hours after ingestion), patients can be asymptomatic or have nonspecific gastrointestinal symptoms. Therefore, the decision to obtain new laboratory tests should not be solely based on clinical symptoms. Laboratory evidence of liver damage typically presents during the second stage (24–72 hours) and peaks during the third stage. If patients survive stage 3, they progress to complete recovery.

[ABP 1.N.1. Ingestions (intentional and unintentional)]

5. ANSWER: B

This patient's clinical picture is most concerning for a foreign body aspiration (FBA). This patient is presenting with acute onset of wheezing without any prodromal symptoms. In addition, she does not respond to albuterol nebulizer treatments or steroids, making the diagnosis of asthma or reactive airway unlikely. In patients who present with FBA, the most common chest radiograph finding is asymmetric air trapping due to the foreign object lodged in a part of the bronchial tree.

Foreign body aspiration may be missed if the aspiration event is not witnessed. In addition, patients who are developmentally delayed are at higher risk of FBA. Providers need to have a high level of suspicion for this, especially when patients do not respond to common treatments for respiratory issues.

Posterior rib fractures can be seen in child abuse cases; there is nothing concerning for abuse in this case. Bilateral symmetrical peribronchial thickening and cuffing is a finding that can be seen in bronchiolitis. Although wheezing can be associated with bronchiolitis, patients typically have other symptoms, such as fever, congestion, cough, and other lung findings, such as rhonchi or crackles. Lobar consolidations are associated with bacterial pneumonia, which can present with fever and increased work of breathing but are not typically associated with wheezing. An enlarged cardiac silhouette may be associated with multiple conditions, such as cardiomegaly, pericardial effusion, or anterior mediastinal mass. This patient does not present with any features that would cause an enlarged cardiac silhouette.

[ABP 1.C.6. Foreign body aspiration]

REFERENCE

1. Louie MC, Bradin S. Foreign body ingestion and aspiration. *Pediatr Rev.* 2009;*30*(8):295–301.

6. ANSWER: B

Lyme disease is a cause of peripheral facial nerve palsy and needs to be distinguished from central causes of facial nerve palsy such as stroke and other peripheral causes. This patient did not have forehead sparing of her facial weakness, which suggests a peripheral rather than central palsy. The associated systemic symptoms of fatigue and myalgia point to Lyme disease. In areas endemic for *Borrelia burgdorferi*, Lyme disease should be considered as an infectious cause of facial weakness, especially if there is associated erythema migrans (EM) rash, arthralgia, and systemic symptoms. Areas with high incidence of Lyme disease include the northeastern United States, Wisconsin, and Minnesota. Facial nerve palsy is a common manifestation of early disseminated Lyme disease, which occurs 1–4 weeks after infection. Other cranial nerve palsies may occur but are less common.

Presence of EM rash in an endemic region is sufficient for the diagnosis of early Lyme. Antibody testing should not be routinely obtained; however, if performed, a two-tier serologic approach should be used, with an enzyme-linked immunosorbent assay (ELISA) followed by a Western immunoblot or a second enzyme immunoassay to confirm.

Findings associated with stroke include being well immediately prior to presentation, an inability to walk, and focal findings of face or arm weakness. Bell's palsy can present with facial weakness but typically is not associated with fatigue and myalgia. Ramsay Hunt syndrome is often preceded by pain and is associated with vesicular lesions of the ear canal or pharynx on examination. Guillain-Barré syndrome presents with ascending weakness or paralysis and is associated with bilateral facial palsy. Distinguishing features of various diagnoses associated with facial palsy are seen in the Table 1.1.

[ABP 1.A.11. Other (cranial nerve palsies)]

Table 1.1 DIFFERENTIAL DIAGNOSIS OF ACUTE PERIPHERAL FACIAL NERVE PALSY

DISEASE	DISTINGUISHING FEATURES
Lyme disease	Tic exposure in high-incident area Unilateral weakness or paralysis of the facial, involves the forehead Rash (EM), arthralgia, systemic symptoms, carditis
Otitis media	Ear pain with erythematous tympanic membrane, purulent middle ear effusion
Bell's palsy	Possibly herpes simplex virus activation; infection with human immunodeficiency virus, cytomegalovirus, Epstein-Barr virus, adenovirus, rubella virus, mumps, influenza B, echovirus, and coxsackie virus
Ramsay Hunt (varicella-zoster virus reactivation) • Rare where primary herpes zoster vaccination occurs	Preceded by pain Vesicular lesions on examination of ear canal or pharynx
Guillain-Barré syndrome	Bilateral facial nerve palsy, ascending weakness/paralysis, diminished or absent reflexes, sensory abnormalities
Tumors	Typically more indolent and slowly progressive Primary parotid or facial nerve tumor

REFERENCE

1. Shapiro ED. Borrelia burgdorferi (Lyme disease). *Pediatr Rev.* 2014;35(12):500–509.

7. ANSWER: A

Mumps is a viral illness caused by a paramyxovirus. Clinical symptoms may include parotitis, myalgia, anorexia, malaise, orchitis, and headaches. The most common presenting symptom of mumps is parotitis, which has been reported in up to 94% of cases in the prevaccine era in certain groups. Orchitis may be reported in 20%–30% of cases and can be a complicating feature. In 1967, the United States initiated an extensive vaccination program to vaccinate against mumps, leading to a 99% decrease in mumps cases nationally. The other answer choices are not associated with mumps infections.

[ABP 1.B.5. Parotitis]

REFERENCE

1. Centers for Disease Control and Prevention. Mumps. Updated March 8, 2021. Accessed June 1, 2021. https://ww.cdc.gov/mumps/hcp.html#clinical.

8. ANSWER: C

A BRUE is defined as an event occurring in an infant younger than 1 year of age when the observer reports a sudden, brief, and now resolved episode of 1 or more of the following: (1) cyanosis or pallor; (2) absence, decreased, or irregular breathing; (3) marked change in tone (hyper- or hypotonia); and (4) altered level of responsiveness. Patients can be risk stratified into higher-risk and "low-risk" categories, which can guide your workup and management. To be designated low risk, the following criteria should be met:

- Age more than 60 days
- Gestational age 32 weeks or older and postconceptional age 45 weeks or older
- First BRUE (no previous BRUE and not occurring in clusters)
- Duration of event less than 1 minute
- No cardiopulmonary resuscitation (CPR) required by trained medical provider

The patient presenting in this case is less than 60 days old and therefore does not meet low-risk criteria. Choices A, D, and E describe features that are included in the BRUE definition but are not used to determine risk stratification.

Choice B is incorrect due to the definition of higher risk being associated with an event lasting 1 minute or more.

Current evidence-based guidelines provide management recommendations only for low-risk patients. Higher-risk patients are managed off guidelines and need to be assessed more thoroughly to determine further workup and/or consultation needs. Those determined to be low risk can likely be managed without extensive diagnostic evaluation or hospitalization.

[ABP 1.O.1. Brief resolved unexplained events (BRUE)]

REFERENCE

1. Tieder JS, Bonkowsky JL, Etzel RA, et al. Brief resolved unexplained events (formerly apparent life-threatening events) and evaluation of lower-risk infants. *Pediatrics.* 2016;137(5):e20160590.

9. ANSWER: D

Beckwith-Wiedemann syndrome (BWS) is a disorder of genomic imprinting. Babies with BWS have macrosomia and are large for gestational age. Other characteristic findings include macroglossia, hemihypertrophy, visceromegaly, omphalocele, and transient neonatal hypoglycemia. Babies with BWS are at increased risk for Wilms tumor, hepatoblastoma, neuroblastoma, and rhabdomyosarcoma. Routine ultrasounds for serial monitoring of tumors are recommended.

Hypoglycemia seen in these babies is transient and due to excessive insulin production from pancreatic β-cell hyperplasia. It is not associated with insulinomas. BWS is not associated with retinoblastoma, brain tumors, or thyroid cancers.

[ABP 1.I.7. Hypoglycemia]

10. ANSWER: D

The finding of anogenital warts is suspicious for sexual abuse. The absence of other warts on examination makes nonsexual transmission less likely. In addition, sexual abuse can also be associated with behavioral changes such as constipation and encopresis. A thorough and confidential social history should be obtained in order to screen for abuse, and reporting of sexual abuse is recommended. Warts caused by HPV infection are clinically diagnosed without indication for biopsy or HPV testing. Anogenital warts are not associated with inflammatory bowel disease, although perianal disease such as skin tags, fistulae, and abscesses can be seen in Crohn's disease. Thyroid disorders, while potentially associated with constipation, are not associated with anogenital warts.

[ABP 1.J.2. Sexual abuse]

REFERENCE

1. Kellogg N, American Academy of Pediatrics Committee on Child Abuse and Neglect. The evaluation of sexual abuse in children. *Pediatrics.* 2005;*116*(2):506–512.

11. ANSWER: B

The patient above has a new diagnosis of nephrotic syndrome. Nephrotic syndrome is due to an injury to the glomerular filtration barrier and can be categorized as primary, secondary, congenital, or infantile. Patients may present with generalized edema, periorbital edema, hyperlipidemia, elevated blood pressure, hypoalbuminemia, or proteinuria. For diagnosis, only the last two laboratory findings are necessary. Complications include peritonitis due to increased susceptibility to encapsulated bacterial infection and weakened humoral immunity, cellulitis due to skin breakdown, anasarca, thrombosis due to hypercoagulable state, transient renal insufficiency, hypovolemic shock, and poor growth due to steroid use. Risk factors that increase a patient's risk of hypercoagulable state include immobility, infection, hemoconcentration, presence of central venous catheter, and thrombocytosis.

[ABP 1.F.5. Nephrotic syndrome]

12. ANSWER: D

Transient synovitis is a self-limited virus-related condition typically seen in children ages 3 to 8. Patients are often afebrile, limping, and with limited range of motion of the affected hip. A history of URI in the preceding 2–4 weeks is often present. The abrupt onset and lack of systemic symptoms make autoinflammatory conditions less likely; thus, steroids are not indicated.

Distinguishing between transient synovitis and early septic arthritis, which requires urgent surgical intervention and antibiotics, is often difficult. The Kocher criteria (Box 1.1) can be used to distinguish between septic arthritis and transient synovitis. Absence of all four criteria (e.g., this patient) yields a 0.2% probability of septic arthritis, with increased probability with increasing number of criteria. Septic arthritis often presents with a synovial fluid white blood cell count of more than 50,000 cells/mm.

Box 1.1 KOCHER CRITERIA[a]

Temperature >101.3°F (38.5°C)

White blood cell count >12,000/mL

Erythrocyte sedimentation rate >40 mm/h

Inability to ambulate

[a] Adapted from Reference 1.

In transient synovitis, nonsteroidal anti-inflammatory drugs are the mainstay of treatment, with expected resolution within 7 to 10 days. A surgical washout, intravenous antibiotics, and systemic steroids are all treatment options for septic arthritis, but not for transient synovitis. Further imaging is not indicated in this case.

[ABP 1.H.3. Inflammatory arthritis, 1.G.2. Bone and joint infections]

REFERENCES

1. Kocher MS, Zurakowski D, Kasser JR. Differentiating between septic arthritis and transient synovitis of the hip in children: an evidence-based clinical prediction algorithm. *J Bone Joint Surg Am.* 1999;*81*(12):1662–1670.
2. Herman MJ, Martinek M. The limping child. *Pediatr Rev.* 2015;*36*(5):184–197.

13. ANSWER: C

Open fractures can be classified using the Gustilo and Anderson classification system (see Table 1.2). The single most important factor in reducing infection rates of open fractures in pediatric patients is the early administration (within 3 hours) of appropriate antibiotics. A first-generation cephalosporin such as cefazolin is the antibiotic of choice for all open fractures; however additional gram-negative coverage with an aminoglycoside is recommended for type II and III fractures. Since the patient in this case meets criteria for a type II fracture, she should get a first-generation cephalosporin and an aminoglycoside. First-generation cephalosporins have been shown to be superior to penicillin and streptomycin in preventing open fracture infections. The benefits of routine coverage of methicillin-resistant staphylococcal aureus, which vancomycin would provide, have not been established in the literature. Such coverage should be based on individual risk factors. Regardless, vancomycin alone would not provide the gram-negative coverage indicated for a type II fracture.

[ABP 1.G.1. Fractures]

REFERENCES

1. Gustilo RB, Anderson JT. Prevention of infection in the treatment of one thousand and twenty-five open fractures of long bones: retrospective and prospective analyses. *J Bone Joint Surg Am.* 1976;*58*(4):453–458.
2. Gustilo RB, Mendoza RM, Williams DN. Problems in the management of type III (severe) open fractures: a new classification of type III open fractures. *J Trauma.* 1984;*24*(8):742–746.

14. ANSWER: B

This case describes a common presentation for cat scratch disease due to *Bartonella henselae.* Cat scratch disease is

Table 1.2 GUSTILO AND ANDERSON CLASSIFICATION OF OPEN FRACTURES AND RECOMMENDED
ANTIBIOTIC REGIMEN

FRACTURE TYPE	DEFINITION	RECOMMENDED ANTIBIOTICS
I	Wound <1 cm; minimal contamination, soft tissue damage, no comminution	First-generation cephalosporin (e.g., IV cefazolin)
II	Wound >1 cm; moderate soft tissue damage, minimal periosteal stripping	First-generation cephalosporin (e.g., IV cefazolin) + aminoglycoside (e.g., gentamicin)
IIIA	Wound >10 cm, extensive soft tissue damage, substantial contamination, adequate soft tissue coverage of bone	
IIIB	Wound >10 cm, extensive soft tissue damage, substantial contamination, inadequate soft tissue coverage of bone	
IIIC	Wound >10 cm, extensive soft tissue damage, vascular injury requiring repair	

one of the most common infectious causes of fever of un-known origin in children. Regional lymphadenopathy prox-imal to the inoculation site is the most common finding. Although many patients will have gradual resolution of symptoms without therapy, treatment is recommended to prevent serious complications, such as dissemination to the liver, spleen, eye, or central nervous system. For patients with lymphadenitis as the only manifestation, a 5-day course of azithromycin is the preferred treatment. Rifampin is added to azithromycin to treat disseminated *Bartonella* disease and may be given as monotherapy for patients unable to tolerate azithromycin. Ceftriaxone, clindamycin, and amoxicillin are not indicated in the treatment of cat scratch disease.

[ABP 1.O.5. Fever of unknown origin]

15. ANSWER: B

The findings in this patient are consistent with Alagille syn-drome. Alagille syndrome results primarily from mutations in the *JAG1* or *NOTCH2* genes and is characterized by de-ficiency of interlobular bile ducts, which results in chronic cholestasis. Patients classically present in the first 6 months of life with conjugated hyperbilirubinemia and/or poor growth. Other associated findings include congenital heart disease (CHD), butterfly vertebrae, dysmorphic fa-cies, renal dysplasia, poor growth, and developmental delay. Hypotonia, abdominal wall defects, immunodeficiency, and polydactyly are not typically associated with Alagille syndrome. Alagille syndrome is confirmed in patients with clinically suspected disease by performing a liver biopsy or specific genetic testing for *JAG1* or *NOTCH2* mutations.

[ABP 1.E.9. Hyperbilirubinemia]

16. ANSWER: C

Subcutaneous low-molecular-weight heparin (LMWH) and IV heparin are both effective at treating venous thromboemboli. A LMWH, such as enoxaparin, has several

advantages over IV heparin, making it the preferable agent for treating pediatric thrombophilia in the hospital setting. Since it is given via subcutaneous injection, families can be taught to administer the medication at home, making it easier to continue therapy on discharge. While once or twice daily monitoring of anti–factor Xa is required after initiation of LMWH to ensure adequate dosing, IV heparin typically requires monitoring of the activated partial thromboplastin time (aPTT) levels at least every 6 hours after initiation. Some potential disadvantages of LMWH that hospitalists should consider are that it has a longer onset of action than IV heparin and is only partially reversible by protamine.

[ABP 1.L.2. Deep venous thrombosis/pulmonary em-bolism/hypercoagulable states]

17. ANSWER: C

Biphasic anaphylaxis occurs when a patient receives proper treatment for anaphylaxis followed by an asymptomatic period of 1 hour or more before a recurrence of symptoms without further exposure to a suspected antigen. The time period between the resolution of the first reaction and the start of the second reaction ranges from 1 hour to up to 78 hours. It is suggested that patients with anaphylaxis be admitted for observation when they require more than one dose of epinephrine; have a severe initial presentation, in-cluding hypotension; or if they received epinephrine after a significant delay (>60 minutes) because these are thought to be possible risk factors for biphasic anaphylaxis. The other an-swer choices listed are not associated with an increased risk of biphasic anaphylaxis. The use of glucocorticoids has been as-sociated with a slightly increased risk of biphasic anaphylaxis.

[ABP 1.M.1. Anaphylaxis]

18. ANSWER: E

This patient is presenting with a URI followed by signs and symptoms of heart failure likely due to dilated cardiomyopathy (DCM). DCM is the most common form of cardiomyopathy. At this time, it would be important to obtain an echocardiogram to evaluate the degree of heart failure and cardiac dysfunction and assess for ventricular dilation. A chest radiograph may show cardiomegaly and pulmonary edema suggestive of DCM but would not confirm the diagnosis. Viral etiologies for DCM include parvovirus B19, influenza, Epstein-Barr virus, human immunodeficiency virus, coxsackie virus, herpes simplex virus, and adenovirus, among others. DCM may also be idiopathic or secondary to a genetic predisposition or toxicity from medications, including chemotherapeutics. Several viral and bacterial causes of DCM are not included in an RVP or blood culture, and it is more important to determine the degree of heart failure first. With the murmur and gallop on cardiac examination, it is less likely that her hepatomegaly is an intrinsic liver issue, making an abdominal ultrasound less helpful.

[ABP 1.D.3. Heart failure]

19. ANSWER: B

This patient meets the diagnostic criteria of exertional heat stroke (EHS), which is defined as a core temperature greater than 40°C with findings of neurologic dysfunction. Core body temperatures should be obtained rectally, as axillary or oral temperatures are unreliable in the diagnosis of EHS. Central nervous system dysfunction can range from mild confusion and disorientation to seizures and coma. Additional clinical features include tachycardia, tachypnea, gastrointestinal symptoms, and flushed skin. Sweating is often absent in the setting of nonexertional (or classic) heat stroke, but notably can be present with EHS. EHS complications also include cardiac dysfunction, hepatic injury, renal insufficiency, rhabdomyolysis, and disseminated intravascular coagulation.

Rapid initiation of cooling is the most effective strategy to limit the effects of EHS. Cooling measures include ice water immersion, evaporative cooling techniques, and application of cold towels or ice packs. While fluid resuscitation is commonly required in the management of EHS, cooling measures remain the definitive treatment for this condition. Importantly, antipyretics such as acetaminophen or ibuprofen have no utility in the care of patients with EHS and may worsen any associated hepatic or renal injury. Dantrolene is used for treatment of malignant hyperthermia, but it is not routinely used for EHS. Sepsis may be included in the differential diagnosis for patients presenting with a high temperature; however, it is less common for core temperatures to exceed 41°C with bacterial infections alone.

[ABP 1.N.4. Hypo- and hyperthermia]

20. ANSWER: E

Viral bronchiolitis is one of the most common reasons for pediatric admission, particularly in the winter months. This patient's presentation with fever, viral upper respiratory symptoms, increased work of breathing, and various lung sounds on auscultation are most consistent with this diagnosis. The American Academy of Pediatrics (AAP) published updated recommendations in 2014 with clear changes in terms of the management of bronchiolitis. Nebulized hypertonic saline may be considered in hospitalized children to help with symptoms. Although choices A–D were commonly used in the past for bronchiolitis, they are no longer recommended by the AAP.

[ABP 1.C.1. Bronchiolitis]

REFERENCE

1. Ralston SL, Lieberthal AS, Meissner HC, et al. Clinical practice guideline: the diagnosis, management, and prevention of bronchiolitis. *Pediatrics*. 2014;*134*(5):e1474–e1502.

21. ANSWER: C

This patient has an increased risk for epilepsy. Febrile seizures occur in patients between the ages of 6 months and 5 years in the setting of a febrile illness without evidence of central nervous system infection. This patient has had two seizures within a 24-hour period and therefore meets the diagnostic criteria for complex febrile seizure (Table 1.3). Characteristics of patients with febrile seizures that increase the risk of epilepsy include neurodevelopmental impairment, complex febrile seizures, and family history of epilepsy. Patients with this condition are at risk for having another episode with future febrile illnesses. Younger age at presentation is associated with a higher risk of experiencing another febrile seizure.

Table 1.3 CHARACTERISTICS OF SIMPLE VERSUS COMPLEX FEBRILE SEIZURES

SIMPLE FEBRILE SEIZURE	COMPLEX FEBRILE SEIZURE
Generalized tonic-clonic	Focal features
<15 minutes	>15 minutes
One in 24 hours	Recurs within 24 hours
Typically return to baseline mental status in about 1 hour	

For simple febrile seizures, the American Academy of Pediatrics' Subcommittee on Febrile Seizures has recommended the following:

1. A lumbar puncture should be performed in any child who presents with concerns for meningitis or intracranial infection.
2. A lumbar puncture should be considered in
   a. Any underimmunized infant between 6 and 12 months of age
   b. A child who is pretreated with antibiotics.
3. Serum electrolytes, calcium, phosphorus, magnesium, blood glucose, complete blood cell count, EEG, and neuroimaging should not be performed routinely for evaluation of simple febrile seizures.

Because this patient had a complex febrile seizure and underlying developmental delay, it may be appropriate for him to have additional workup. While there is no role for inpatient EEG and it will not predict recurrences, an outpatient EEG is appropriate for this patient with multiple risk factors for epilepsy. A CT of the head may be helpful in identifying intracranial bleeding, gross anatomic abnormalities, a space-occupying lesion, or risk for herniation. However, it is unlikely to find an underlying condition in this patient because he did not have focal features on examination. There has been no evidence to support benefit of intermittent acetaminophen in preventing recurrent febrile seizures.

[ABP 1.A.2. Seizures]

REFERENCES

1. Subcommittee on Febrile Seizures; American Academy of Pediatrics. Neurodiagnostic evaluation of the child with a simple febrile seizure. *Pediatrics*. 2011;*127*(2):389–394.
2. Offringa M, Newton R, Cozijnsen MA, Nevitt SJ. Prophylactic drug management for febrile seizures in children. *Cochrane Database Syst Rev*. 2017;*2*:CD003031.

22. ANSWER: E

According to the Centers for Disease Control and Prevention, gonorrhea is the second most reported communicable disease. Some of these infections may be asymptomatic and thus can be spread without a patient's knowledge. It is common in the adolescent population and should be on the differential, particularly when other studies have been negative. This patient's throat findings are consistent with pharyngitis. Uncomplicated gonococcal pharyngitis is treated with a single dose of ceftriaxone. This patient has knee pain in addition to pharyngitis, which can be a symptom of a disseminated gonococcal infection. Disseminated infections can present with skin lesions and various joint complaints, such as polyarthralgias, tenosynovitis, or septic arthritis. In patients with disseminated disease, the treatment course consists of ceftriaxone and azithromycin. Her initial studies were negative, thus making streptococcal infection and EBV infections less likely. Imaging is not useful in diagnosing gonococcal infection. Continuing symptomatic treatment would not lead to the diagnosis.

[ABP 1.B.3. Oropharyngeal infections]

REFERENCE

1. Workowski KA, Bolan GA; Centers for Disease Control and Prevention. Sexually transmitted diseases treatment guidelines, 2015. *MMWR Recomm Rep*. 2015;*64*(RR-03):1–137.

23. ANSWER: A

As seen Table 1.4, current American Academy of Pediatrics (AAP) guidelines for the management of brief resolved unexplained events (BRUEs) do not recommend extensive workup for patients with a "low-risk" BRUE; rather they may be monitored on a continuous pulse oximeter with

Table 1.4 RECOMMENDATIONS FOR PATIENTS WITH LOW-RISK BRUE[a]

Should	Should not
• Educate caregivers about BRUEs and engage in shared decision-making to guide evaluation, disposition, and follow-up • Offer resources for cardiopulmonary resuscitation (CPR) training to caregiver	• Obtain a white blood cell count, blood culture, or cerebrospinal fluid analysis or culture, basic metabolic panel, ammonia, blood gases, urine organic acids, plasma amino acids or acylcarnitines, CXR, echocardiogram, electroencephalogram, studies for gastroesophageal reflux, or laboratory evaluation for anemia • Initiate home cardiorespiratory monitoring • Prescribe acid suppression therapy or antiepileptic medications

May	Need not
• Obtain pertussis testing and 12-lead electrocardiogram • Briefly monitor patients with continuous pulse oximetry and serial observations	• Obtain viral respiratory test, urinalysis, blood glucose, serum bicarbonate, serum lactic acid, or neuroimaging • Admit the patient to the hospital *solely* for cardiorespiratory monitoring

[a] Adapted from Reference 1.

serial examinations. These guidelines do not recommend a CXR (evidence quality grade B, moderate recommendation), an echocardiogram (evidence quality grade C, moderate recommendation), or a CBC (evidence quality grade B, strong recommendation) for low-risk infants. While discharge home with close follow-up with the primary care provider within 24 hours is a reasonable option, current guidelines do not recommend home cardiopulmonary monitoring (evidence quality grade B, moderate recommendation).

[ABP 1.O.1. Brief resolved unexplained events (BRUE)]

REFERENCE

1. Tieder JS, Bonkowsky JL, Etzel RA, et al. Brief resolved unexplained events (formerly apparent life-threatening events) and evaluation of lower-risk infants. *Pediatrics.* 2016;*137*(5):e20160590.

24. ANSWER: C

The most helpful laboratory test for ruling out type 1 diabetes is the absence of pancreatic islet autoantibodies. These include anti–tyrosine phosphatase (IA2) antibodies, anti–glutamic acid decarboxylase (GAD), and a β-cell–specific autoantibody to zinc transporter 8 (ZnT8).

A high C-peptide level supports a diagnosis of type 2 diabetes, but values may overlap between type 1 and type 2 diabetes. Anti-insulin antibodies can be useful to diagnose type 1 diabetes in patients who have received insulin for less than 2 weeks. While a high BMI is a risk factor for developing type 2 diabetes, it cannot be used to differentiate between type 1 and type 2. Finally, while there are an increasing number of genetic variants that are known to be associated with type 2 diabetes, they are not useful for diagnostic purposes.

[ABP 1.I.6. Diabetes mellitus]

25. ANSWER: D

This scenario is concerning for medical child abuse due to a discrepancy between the mother's insistence on an invasive procedure and the lack of any objective findings to suggest an underlying pathology. Medical child abuse occurs when caregivers induce, falsify, or exaggerate symptoms in their children to obtain unnecessary and potentially harmful medical treatment for them. The diagnosis is often challenging to make. Treatment involves a multidisciplinary team meeting to obtain consensus that medical child abuse is occurring and to develop a new care plan to present to the family. When this information is not accepted by the family, medical child abuse is more likely and should be reported to CPS to help develop a treatment and safety plan. The history does not suggest an organic cause for the patient's malnutrition given the negative workup and normal weight gain and oral intake with prior hospitalizations; therefore, a repeat CT, pH probe study, chromosomal analysis, or G-tube placement would not be recommended.

[ABP 1.J.3. Medical child abuse]

REFERENCE

1. Jenny C, Metz JB. Medical child abuse and medical neglect. *Pediatr Rev.* 2020;*41*(2):49–60.

26. ANSWER: A

In a patient with nephrotic syndrome who does not respond to steroid therapy, a renal biopsy is recommended. About 10%–20% of patients with idiopathic nephrotic syndrome initially do not respond to steroids. There are three common causes of nephrotic syndrome: minimal change disease, focal segmental glomerulosclerosis, and membranous nephropathy. Because of the increased risk of developing end-stage renal disease, the histopathology on a kidney biopsy may help guide other treatment modalities. In addition, a patient who is younger than 1 year of age or older than 10 years of age, is hypertensive, has abnormal complement levels, has gross hematuria, or has extrarenal symptoms such as purpura, a kidney biopsy is recommended.

[ABP 1.F.5. Nephrotic syndrome]

27. ANSWER: D

Immunoglobulin A (IgA) vasculitis (formerly known as Henoch-Schönlein purpura) is the most common vasculitis of childhood, with the greatest incidence between 4 and 6 years of age. The diagnosis is made clinically in the presence of rash and gastrointestinal (GI), renal, and/or musculoskeletal involvement. Laboratory findings, unlike in disseminated intravascular coagulation or immune thrombocytopenia, reveal normal coagulation studies and platelet counts.

Arthritis or arthralgias occur in 75% of affected individuals, with arthritis usually occurring in an oligoarticular pattern in the large joints. GI symptoms are due to inflammation of the GI vasculature and result in colicky abdominal pain in up to 57% of children. GI bleeding or ileo-ileal intussusception may also occur. Kidney disease occurs in 30%–50% of children. Urinalysis with microscopy should be obtained at time of diagnosis and periodically after clinical improvement. One percent of children with renal involvement progress to chronic kidney disease.

Nonsteroidal anti-inflammatory drugs are the mainstay of treatment. Most children improve in 4–6 weeks without further intervention, though one-third have a relapse in the first year. Steroids are indicated in the setting of renal disease or severe abdominal pain, but should be tapered to prevent relapse. In children with well-controlled pain, adequate oral intake, and absence of renal disease, steroids are not generally recommended. While steroids may alleviate symptoms, this must be weighed against the effect of long-term steroid use in noncomplicated and self-limiting cases. Watchful waiting would not be appropriate, as this patient's pain should be alleviated. Antibiotics and intravenous immunoglobulin are not indicated to treat IgA vasculitis.

[ABP 1.H.1. Henoch-Schönlein purpura]

REFERENCES

1. Reid-Adam J. Henoch-Schonlein purpura. *Pediatr Rev.* 2014;35(10): 447–449.
2. Oni L, Sampath S. Childhood IgA vasculitis (Henoch Schonlein purpura)—advances and knowledge gaps. *Front Pediatr.* 2019;7:257.
3. Bowman P, Quinn M. Question 1: should steroids be used to treat abdominal pain caused by Henoch-Schonlein purpura? *Arch Dis Child.* 2012;97(11):999–1000.

28. ANSWER: A

The patient's presentation, including single-joint arthritis, fever, inability to bear weight, elevated inflammatory markers, and synovial fluid with leukocytosis and PMN predominance is concerning for septic arthritis of his left knee. Rapid diagnosis and treatment are critical as it has devastating sequelae if left untreated. Staphylococcus aureus (gram-positive cocci in clusters) has been the most common cause of culture-positive septic arthritis. Streptococci (including α-hemolytic pneumococcus and β-hemolytic streptococcus) are the next most common gram-positive infections. *Kingella kingae* (gram-negative coccobacilli), which has been increasingly found in recent studies, has a more indolent course and can be associated with mouth ulcers. Although *Haemophilus influenzae* type B (Hib) (gram-negative coccobacilli) had been a prominent cause of septic arthritis in children under 2 years of age, it is rarely seen now due to vaccines. In neonates and sexually active adolescents, *Neisseria gonorrhea* (gram-negative diplococci) should be considered. About 35% of joint aspirates are sterile in patients with other clinical and laboratory findings of a septic joint, including positive blood cultures.

[ABP 1.G.2. Bone and joint infections]

29. ANSWER: C

This patient's presentation of poor growth, pancytopenia, multiple episodes of otitis media, easy bruising, and pneumonia is likely due to Shwachman-Diamond syndrome (SDS). SDS is a rare bone marrow failure multisystem disorder that is autosomal recessive and is the second most common cause of exocrine pancreatic insufficiency in childhood. This condition is characterized by nutrient malabsorption and abnormal hematopoiesis. Patients commonly present in infancy with failure to thrive, steatorrhea, deficiencies of fat-soluble vitamins, recurrent infections, and less often tooth enamel defects, cleft palate, and neurocognitive dysfunction. They are at increased lifetime risk of myelodysplastic syndrome (MDS) and acute myeloid leukemia (AML). Management is based on the degree of neutropenia and includes granulocyte colony-stimulating factor, pancreatic enzyme replacement therapy, and hematopoietic cell transplantation. None of the other answer choices are consistent with SDS.

[ABP 1.M.2. Immunodeficiencies]

30. ANSWER: B

Tetralogy of Fallot is the most common cyanotic congenital heart disease. It includes a ventricular septal defect (VSD) and right ventricular outflow tract (RVOT) obstruction. The degree of cyanosis is dependent on the amount of RVOT obstruction. Infants who are not prenatally diagnosed, such as the patient in this case, may present with hypercyanotic episodes or "Tet spells" during periods of agitation, crying, or other stress that increases pulmonary vascular resistance (PVR) and heart rate, which worsen RVOT obstruction. Initial management strategies for Tet spells include soothing the patient, increasing systemic vascular resistance (SVR) with measures such as knees-to-chest positioning, and initiating oxygen. Other therapies that can be trialed if initial strategies fail include narcotics for sedation and pain management, a fluid bolus to improve right ventricular filling and pulmonary flow, phenylephrine to increase SVR, or β-blockers to decrease heart rate and improve right ventricular filling. Prostaglandins have no role in the management of Tet spells, although they may be required on initial presentation to maintain the patency of the ductus arteriosus if the RVOT obstruction is severe.

[ABP 1.D.2. Congenital heart disease]

31. ANSWER: C

This patient is most likely suffering from anticholinergic toxicity. Many over-the-counter medications that are easily accessible such as antihistamines, cold medications, and sleep aids may contain ingredients that can lead to anticholinergic toxicity when ingested in large quantities. Competitive inhibition of the neurotransmitter acetylcholine at muscarinic receptors results in predictable symptoms. A common mnemonic for this toxidrome is "mad as a hatter (agitation/delirium), blind as a bat (mydriasis), dry as a bone (anhidrosis), hot as a hare (hyperthermia), full as a flask (urinary retention), and red as a beet (cutaneous vasodilation to compensate for anhidrosis)." Tachycardia is also common. Anticholinergic toxicity can be reversed with physostigmine, which is an acetylcholinesterase inhibitor that can cross the blood-brain barrier. This increases the amount of acetylcholine within the synaptic cleft to overcome the postsynaptic receptor inhibition. Given the potency of this medication, it is generally only used for severe cases and requires close monitoring for adverse effects, including cholinergic effects. Dantrolene is used to treat malignant hyperthermia, *N*-acetylcysteine for acetaminophen overdose, cefepime for infection, and atropine for organophosphate poisoning, none of which would treat this patient's underlying illness.

[ABP 1.N.1. Ingestions (intentional and unintentional)]

32. ANSWER: E

Foreign body aspiration (FBA) is an issue that occurs most often in younger children. These children are more likely to place small objects in their mouths and run with these objects, making an aspiration event more likely. These aspirations can lead to serious complications. Various factors are important in obtaining the history, which includes timing of ingestion, type of object, size of object, and current symptoms. Physical examination can reveal respiratory distress, coughing, wheezing, stridor, and cyanosis. Aspirated objects are commonly radiolucent; therefore, providers must maintain a high index of suspicion for FBA even when no object is visualized on a chest radiograph.

This patient is symptomatic with cough and stridor in the setting of a likely button battery aspiration in the mainstem bronchus as these are found in small toys. The next most appropriate step is immediate removal. Foreign body ingestions are important to distinguish from foreign body aspirations as some ingested objects can be monitored for passage without intervention. Button batteries are an important exception to this as they commonly require removal if in the esophagus given their caustic nature.

[ABP 1.C.6. Foreign body aspiration]

REFERENCE

1. Salih AM, Alfaki M, Alam-Elhuda DM. Airway foreign bodies: a critical review for a common pediatric emergency. *World J Emerg Med*. 2016;7(1):5–12.

33. ANSWER: B

For children 1 month of age and older suspected to have bacterial meningitis, empiric antimicrobial therapy should consist of vancomycin in addition to a third-generation cephalosporin, such as ceftriaxone or cefotaxime. Bacterial meningitis in this age group is most frequently caused by *Streptococcus pneumoniae*, *Neisseria meningitidis*, and *group B Streptococcus*. Due to increasing *S. pneumoniae* resistance, monotherapy with penicillin or a third-generation cephalosporin is no longer recommended. Most experts now recommend adding vancomycin to a third-generation cephalosporin. In neonatal bacterial meningitis, empiric antimicrobial therapy should consist of ampicillin and gentamicin. Bacterial meningitis in neonates is commonly caused by pathogens such as *group B Streptococcus*, *Escherichia coli*, and *Listeria monocytogenes*. Targeted antimicrobial therapy should only be employed once a causative pathogen has been identified during the diagnostic workup. Duration of antimicrobial therapy is ultimately dependent on the causative pathogen. In complicated cases, consultation with an infectious disease specialist should be strongly considered. Rifampin would be indicated as chemoprophylaxis for close contacts in the case of meningococcal disease.

[ABP 1.A.3. Meningitis]

REFERENCE

1. Tunkel AR, Hartman BJ, Kaplan SL, et al. Practice guidelines for the management of bacterial meningitis. *Clin Infect Dis*. 2004;39(9):1267–1284.

34. ANSWER: A

This patient's clinical picture is most consistent with an Epstein-Barr virus (EBV) infection. EBV infections can present with fevers, fatigue, pharyngitis, lymphadenopathy, hepatosplenomegaly, head and body aches, and rash. The symptoms can appear 4 to 6 weeks after exposure. EBV is most commonly spread through body fluids such as saliva and is referred to as the "kissing disease." Diagnosis can be made on clinical symptoms, although laboratory testing is commonly done, including EBV titers and the monospot test.

Treatment of EBV infections is mainly supportive. The majority of infections are self-resolved, but patients may be admitted for issues related to decreased oral intake, dehydration, and various complications related to the infection, such as peritonsillar abscess, sinusitis, mastoiditis, and sialadenitis. EBV infections can also be complicated by myocarditis, pancreatitis, pneumonia, and interstitial lung disease. Of the choices that are listed, only myocarditis is associated with EBV infections.

[ABP 1.B.3. Oropharyngeal infections]

35. ANSWER: C

When hospitalized, pediatric patients should be evaluated for growth to ensure patients with failure to thrive can be identified early. Failure to thrive should be considered when an infant or child crosses two or more major growth percentile lines on growth charts. In this scenario, this child has only moved down one major percentile line for weight (from 10th percentile at birth to 5th percentile) and has maintained the same percentile line (25th percentile) for length. The best course of action in this case is to reassure the parents that the infant is growing as expected. Given that the infant's weight and length do not have a disproportionate decrease, no other intervention or diagnostic workup is indicated at this time.

[ABP 1.O.2. Failure to thrive]

REFERENCE

1. National Center for Health Statistics. Clinical growth charts. Centers for Disease Control and Prevention. June 16, 2017. Accessed June 1, 2021. https://www.cdc.gov/growthcharts/clinical _charts.htm.

36. ANSWER: C

Medical neglect is the most common form of child maltreatment. It is the failure to identify signs of serious illness or to follow a physician's instructions, resulting in harm to a child. Although many states have religious exemption laws, the American Academy of Pediatrics still recommends reporting suspected medical neglect, even if motivated by religion, when the refused treatment is likely to prevent death or serious disability. Medical neglect is often challenging to diagnose, and many physicians are reluctant to report it for fear of harming the parent-physician alliance. The use of complementary medicine is increasing in popularity; when there is no evidence of harm, continued use may help in developing a therapeutic alliance with patients. The parents have demonstrated an understanding of the recommended treatment and have given no indication that they are not competent to make medical decisions. Finally, given the degree of hyperglycemia and prior history of missed clinic visits, it would be harmful to defer diabetes management and discussion to the outpatient setting.

[ABP 1.J.1. Physical abuse and child neglect]

REFERENCE

1. Jenny C, Metz JB. Medical child abuse and medical neglect. *Pediatr Rev.* 2020;*41*(2):49–60.

37. ANSWER: A

This patient presents with abnormal uterine bleeding. Causes of abnormal uterine bleeding include complications of pregnancy, sexually transmitted infections, foreign bodies, clotting and platelet disorders, polycystic ovarian syndrome (PCOS), medications, thyroid disease, and anatomical abnormalities such as polyps. Patients with a history of prolonged or heavy menstruation are more likely to have an underlying clotting or platelet disorder. All of the answer choices evaluate clotting and platelet disorders, and several choices might be part of an appropriate evaluation of abnormal uterine bleeding. Because von Willebrand disease is the most common cause of abnormal uterine bleeding, a workup for this disease is most likely to lead to the correct diagnosis. Prothrombin time and activated partial thromboplastin time evaluate for various clotting factor deficiencies. A bleeding time evaluates platelet function but is rarely used because it is highly user dependent, and results are difficult to interpret. A low platelet count might suggest a quantitative platelet deficiency but would not confirm a specific diagnosis. A dilute Russell viper venom time is part of the evaluation for antiphospholipid syndrome, a condition associated with an increased risk of thrombosis but not bleeding.

[ABP 1.F.7. Dysfunctional uterine bleeding]

38. ANSWER: B

This adolescent girl has systemic lupus erythematosus (SLE). Twenty percent of cases of SLE are diagnosed in the first two decades of life, with a strong female predominance. The 2019 consensus guideline specifies that a current or past ANA titer of 1:80 or greater is required to diagnose SLE, along with the presence of sufficient clinical, laboratory, and/or histologic features based on a scoring system. This patient has fever, arthritis, malar rash, leukopenia, thrombocytopenia, pericarditis, and nephritis, providing sufficient clinical criteria to support a diagnosis of SLE. Obtaining an ANA is the best next step to diagnose SLE in this case.

Antineutrophil cytoplasmic antibodies and rheumatoid factor are not useful in diagnosing SLE. EBV infection can present with an acute febrile illness followed by a prolonged postviral syndrome with fatigue but would not include many of the clinical findings noted. The ASO titer can be useful to provide evidence of past group A streptococcal infection if considering rheumatic fever, although this girl's presentation is more consistent with SLE.

[ABP 1.H.4. Systemic lupus erythematosus]

REFERENCES

1. Weiss JE. Pediatric systemic lupus erythematosus: more than a positive antinuclear antibody. *Pediatr Rev.* 2012;*33*(2):62–74.
2. Aringer M, Costenbader K, Daikh D, et al. 2019 European League Against Rheumatism/American College of Rheumatology classification criteria for systemic lupus erythematosus. *Arthritis Rheumatol.* 2019;*71*(9):1400–1412.

39. ANSWER: B

The patient's diagnosis is consistent with acute hematogenous osteomyelitis (AHO) without abscess formation. In older infants and children, cefazolin or nafcillin are the empiric antibiotics of choice to cover methicillin-sensitive *Staphylococcus aureus* (MSSA), *Kingella kingae*, and group A streptococcus. *Kingella kingae* is more common in children up to 5 years, especially those under 3 years. Nafcillin or oxacillin with the addition of a broad-spectrum cephalosporin such as cefepime would be appropriate in neonates for coverage of group B strep, MSSA, and gram-negative bacteria. The decision to empirically cover for MRSA depends on severity of illness, risk factors for MRSA, and local prevalence. Some reports have recommended MRSA coverage if the community prevalence is greater than 10%–15%. The *addition* of vancomycin to a β-lactam should also be considered if the patient is critically ill. In this case, the MRSA prevalence is 3% in a clinically stable child with no known risk factors. Antibiotics can be transitioned from intravenous to oral administration when there is clinical and laboratory improvement and bacteremia has resolved, but cephalexin and amoxicillin-clavulanate would not be appropriate initial antibiotic choices.

[ABP 1.G.2. Bone and joint infections]

40. ANSWER: E

This infant's presentation is consistent with transient neonatal pustular melanosis (TNPM). TNPM is a benign, self-limited condition that is typically present at birth and more common in African American infants. The lesions progress from pustules to ruptured pustules with a collarette of fine scale and finally to hyperpigmented macules. These hyperpigmented macules may last for a few months but eventually will resolve without intervention. TNPM can be diagnosed clinically, and no treatment is required; however, if done, a Wright stain of a pustule will show neutrophils, rare eosinophils, and cellular debris. A culture of a pustule will be sterile.

The differential diagnosis for TNPM includes neonatal herpes simplex virus (HSV) infection, which is a serious and life-threatening condition. The lesions of neonatal HSV typically present after birth as clusters of vesicles with an erythematous base. A Wright stain, if done, will show multinucleated giant cells. The diagnosis of HSV can be made with polymerase chain reaction testing. Given the potential for progression to severe disease and death, intravenous acyclovir should be started empirically while awaiting testing results in cases of suspected HSV.

[ABP 1.K.1. Skin and soft tissue infections, ABP 3.B.4. Neonatal infections, including exposure]

REFERENCE

1. In: Prose NS, Kristal L, eds. *Weinberg's Color Atlas of Pediatric Dermatology.* 5th ed. New York: McGraw-Hill; 2017.

41. ANSWER: E

The patient's clinical presentation is consistent with gastroesophageal reflux (GER). GER is the physiologic process of gastric contents moving retrograde into the esophagus and is extremely common in infants less than 1 year of age. In a large majority of infants, GER is benign and will resolve by 18 months of age, with symptoms peaking in the first 4 months of life. In a small number of patients, GER can be complicated by irritation to the esophagus, poor growth, or respiratory distress due to microaspiration. For patients with uncomplicated GER, such as this patient, no additional diagnostic evaluation is necessary. Management for uncomplicated GER includes reflux precautions, such as keeping infants upright for 20 minutes postfeeds and giving smaller volume feeds. Thickening feeds with rice cereal is used in some cases. Formula changes are not recommended unless cow's milk protein allergy is suspected. For patients with complicated GER, acid suppression with H_2 antagonists or proton pump inhibitors can be trialed on a limited basis. For patients started on acid suppression, symptoms should be reevaluated after 6–8 weeks to determine if continuation is warranted.

[ABP 1.E.5. Gastroesophageal reflux]

42. ANSWER: D

The most common abnormality of red blood cell metabolism is glucose-6-phosphate dehydrogenase (G6PD) deficiency. The G6PD enzyme protects red blood cells from oxidative damage. While fava beans and medications such as nitrofurantoin are classically associated with G6PD deficiency, infection or acidosis alone can trigger hemolysis in affected individuals. The disorder is X linked and more common in males of Mediterranean, Asian, and African descent. The classic presentation is acute hemolysis with anemia, jaundice, and dark urine. G6PD deficiency also should be suspected with prolonged neonatal hyperbilirubinemia. Heinz bodies on the smear reflect precipitated hemoglobin from oxidative damage. Results of the G6PD assay may be falsely normal during active hemolysis and should be repeated in 3 months if suspicion is high. Therapy for this patient is supportive, and a transfusion is not indicated.

The osmotic fragility test is used to identify hereditary spherocytosis, Hb electrophoresis is useful for identifying hemoglobinopathies such as sickle cell disease, and direct Coombs detects antibody-related hemolytic anemia. Ristocetin cofactor testing is used in the diagnosis of von Willebrand disease, which is a clotting disorder.

[ABP 1.L.1. Anemias]

43. ANSWER: A

Reactions to contrast agents are common. Anaphylactoid reactions range from mild to severe and can include hives, swelling (including swelling of the airway), and hypotension with reflex tachycardia. While not considered true allergic reactions because they are not mediated by immunoglobulin E, anaphylactoid and allergic reactions are treated the same. There are also physiologic reactions to contrast media, which include hypertension, hypotension with bradycardia (due to a vagal effect), cardiac arrhythmias, chest pain, seizures, nausea, and vomiting. Anaphylactoid reactions to contrast media are idiosyncratic and not related to the dose of contrast. While a reaction may occur on the first exposure to contrast, the most significant risk factor for future reactions is a history of a past reaction. For patients with that history, pretreatment with corticosteroids is indicated when possible as this has been shown to significantly reduce the rate of reactions. Conversely, corticosteroids do not reduce the rate of physiologic reactions. Of the answer choices listed, hypertension is consistent with a physiologic rather than an anaphylactoid reaction.

[ABP 1.M.1. Anaphylaxis]

44. ANSWER: E

Transposition of the great arteries (TGA) is the most common cyanotic congenital heart disease manifesting in the first week of birth, often presenting with cyanosis from birth. In TGA, the aorta arises from the right ventricle (RV), and the pulmonary artery (PA) arises from the left ventricle (LV). Mixing, such as via a patent ductus arteriosus (PDA), is required to allow systemic oxygenation, making this lesion ductal dependent. In this newborn, the PDA is likely closing, leading to poor mixing, with hypoxemia that is unresponsive to oxygen. This patient's chest radiograph shows the classic "egg-shaped" cardiac silhouette caused by a narrow mediastinum. Confirmation of the diagnosis with an echocardiogram should not delay initiation of PGE_1, which will keep the PDA open and raise the arterial oxygen saturation until the patient can undergo an atrial septostomy or cardiac surgery. If cyanosis persists despite an open PDA, inotropic support may help improve saturations; however, PGE_1 would be indicated first. Cyanosis from birth in a calm neonate is not consistent with a hypercyanotic "Tet" spell, which would be treated with knees-to-chest positioning. Additionally, in tetralogy of Fallot, the chest radiograph classically demonstrates a boot-shaped heart. If there is evidence of heart failure on the pending echocardiogram, diuretics may be indicated, although this does not usually present in the first few hours of life. Antibiotics would not address the underlying issue.

[ABP 1.D.2. Congenital heart disease]

45. ANSWER: A

Organophosphates are commonly found in pesticides or fertilizer. These compounds act as cholinesterase inhibitors, resulting in increased acetylcholine activation at neuronal synapses. A common mnemonic used for this toxidrome is DUMBBBELS (defecation, urination, miosis, bronchorrhea, bronchospasm, bradycardia, emesis, lacrimation, salivation). Additional effects include weakness or paralysis. Organophosphate toxicity should be treated with an anticholinergic, such as atropine, which is a competitive inhibitor of acetylcholine. Sepsis can be mediated by an endotoxin release that subsequently activates cytokine pathways in the host. This inflammation is typically associated with a fever and tachycardia rather than bradycardia. Guillain-Barré syndrome can be a result of peripheral nerve demyelination, but it is more likely to have a slower onset and would not be associated with increased lacrimation and salivation. Deficiency in lactase found on the intestinal brush border can cause diarrhea, but it is unlikely to cause the other symptoms found in this patient.

[ABP 1.N.1. Ingestions (intentional and unintentional)]

46. ANSWER: D

This patient has recurrent pneumonia in the same location. This patient had a prior chest CT that showed normal lung anatomy, making an anatomical cause of her symptoms unlikely. When patients have recurrent pneumonias in the setting of normal anatomy, foreign body aspiration should be taken into consideration. The most commonly aspirated foreign bodies in children are foods such as peanuts, popcorn, and hot dogs. The patients may describe a history of a choking episode, although this is not always recalled by the caregivers. Signs and symptoms may include asymmetric breath sounds, wheezing, stridor, or frequent cough.

This patient is clinically stable and has been improving, but her presentation warrants further investigation given that six admissions for pneumonia over 1 year is concerning for an underlying cause. Prolonged antibiotics or prophylactic antibiotics would not be recommended at this point as the patient is clinically improving. In addition, an emergent bronchoscopy is not indicated at this point as the patient is stable without any signs of respiratory distress.

[ABP 1.C.6. Foreign body aspiration]

47. ANSWER: C

This patient most likely has Sturge-Weber syndrome (SWS), a rare neurocutaneous disorder characterized by a facial vascular malformation with associated leptomeningeal angiomas involving the brain and eye on the affected side. It is important that the facial vascular malformation, also known as a port wine stain, is differentiated from a benign nevus or ecchymosis caused by a traumatic delivery. Patients with port wine stains involving the upper branch (ophthalmic branch) of the fifth cranial nerve (trigeminal nerve) have a 50% risk for developing glaucoma.[1] In addition, this group of patients has a 10%–35% risk for brain involvement. As glaucoma can cause optic nerve damage and threaten vision, these children warrant close monitoring. Treatment options for patients with SWS who develop glaucoma include ophthalmic medications to decrease intraocular pressure and surgical intervention. Plexiform neurofibromas are typically seen in patients with neurofibromatosis type 1. Cardiac rhabdomyomas may occur in children with tuberous sclerosis. Hypercalcemia may be present in Williams syndrome, an autosomal dominant disorder with clinical features including "elfin-like" facial features, long philtrum, prominent chin, mandibular hypoplasia, stellate pattern in the iris, supravalvular aortic stenosis, and mild-to-moderate intellectual disability.

[ABP 1.A.11. Other (central nervous system vascular disorder)]

REFERENCES

1. Faux BM, Suhr AW, Hsieh DT. Visual diagnosis: newborn with a facial vascular birthmark. *Pediatr Rev.* 2015;36(9):e30–e34.
2. Korf BR, Bebin EM. Neurocutaneous disorders in children. *Pediatr Rev.* 2017;38(3):119–128.

48. ANSWER: E

Group A streptococcus (GAS) is a common cause of pharyngitis and accounts for about 1.78 million cases annually. GAS is spread mainly by droplets, direct contact, contaminated fomites, or foodborne contaminations. Clinical symptoms include sore throat, fevers, lymphadenopathy, vomiting, headache, and abdominal pain. Complications of GAS infection include scarlet fever, erysipelas, cellulitis, toxic shock syndrome, and necrotizing fasciitis. In addition, these infections can cause acute rheumatic fever, poststreptococcal glomerulonephritis, and pediatric autoimmune neuropsychiatric disorders. The majority of acute infections are treated as an outpatient but can present in the inpatient setting.

According to the Centers for Disease Control and Prevention, testing for streptococcal infections in patients under 3 years of age is not routinely indicated. Acute rheumatic fever is rare in children under 3 years, and classic streptococcal pharyngitis is unusual in this population. However, testing should be considered if the patient had symptoms classic for streptococcal pharyngitis and a close contact with the illness. Rapid streptococcal antigen tests are highly specific, but in this case the positive test result likely indicates asymptomatic colonization, which does not require antibiotics.

[ABP 1.B.3. Oropharyngeal infections]

REFERENCE

1. Pharyngitis (strep throat): information for clinicians. Centers for Disease Control and Prevention. Updated November 1, 2018. Accessed June 1, 2021. https://www.cdc.gov/groupastrep/diseases-hcp/strep-throat.html.

49. ANSWER: C

The patient has developed exertional rhabdomyolysis with a resulting acute kidney injury. In the setting of dehydration and her kidney injury, she has become hyperkalemic with peaked T waves seen in multiple leads on her ECG. While the most important intervention for her underlying illness is fluid resuscitation, the more pressing issue currently is her hyperkalemia, with a need for cardiac membrane stabilization with intravenous calcium gluconate to avoid arrhythmias. This is preferred over calcium chloride if the patient has peripheral vascular access due to a lower risk of tissue necrosis if the fluid extravasates. Once the cardiac membrane has been stabilized, other interventions may be indicated to help decrease the serum potassium level. Intravenous furosemide would help eliminate the potassium via diuresis, but given the patient's acute kidney injury and ECG changes, this would not be the appropriate next step. Oral Kayexalate is a potassium-binding medication that can also help eliminate potassium from the body through stool, but this takes longer to act. Subcutaneous insulin would shift potassium intracellularly. This should be given with dextrose-containing fluids to avoid hypoglycemia. In addition, inhaled albuterol and sodium bicarbonate are medications that would act similarly to insulin to shift potassium intracellularly. Ultimately, if her kidney injury does not improve and her potassium remains elevated, she may require dialysis. Other electrolyte abnormalities may also result in ECG changes as seen in Table 1.5.

[ABP 1.O.6. Electrolyte abnormalities]

Table 1.5 ELECTROLYTE IMBALANCES THAT MAY RESULT IN ECG CHANGES

ELECTROLYTE IMBALANCE	COMMON ELECTROCARDIOGRAM FINDINGS
Hyperkalemia	Flat P waves, prolonged PR intervals, QRS widening, peaked T waves
Hypokalemia	ST depression, flattened/inverted T waves, U waves
Hypercalcemia	Shortened ST segments, widened T waves
Hypocalcemia	Prolonged ST segments, prolonged QT intervals
Hypermagnesemia	Prolonged PR intervals, QRS widening
Hypomagnesemia	Tall T waves, ST depression

50. ANSWER: D

Early morning serum sodium, serum osmolality, and urine osmolality can help confirm a diagnosis of diabetes insipidus (DI). This patient's presentation along with his normal blood glucose and dilute urine should raise suspicion for this diagnosis. Diabetes insipidus is caused by inadequate antidiuretic hormone (ADH) activity, due to either decreased secretion from the pituitary (central DI) or impaired action in the kidneys (peripheral DI). While he will need to refrain from drinking prior to collection of these tests, limiting his water intake alone without further testing would not be helpful. In patients with DI, limiting intake for prolonged periods can lead to severe and potentially life-threatening hypernatremia. Desmopressin is the treatment of choice for central DI, but that diagnosis has not yet been confirmed. Finally, while his clinical presentation would be concerning for diabetes, his normal glucose levels make the diagnosis unlikely, so further testing would not be helpful.

[ABP 1.I.1. Diabetes insipidus]

51. ANSWER: B

This patient's findings are consistent with urethral prolapse, which is treated supportively with Sitz baths and estrogen cream. Within pediatrics, it is most commonly seen between the ages of 4 and 8 years. Because it presents with vaginal bleeding, it is often mistaken for sexual abuse. However, the most common finding in sexual abuse is a normal genitourinary examination. Other mimickers of sexual abuse include lichen sclerosis, which causes bleeding and itching and is treated with steroid cream. A foreign body, most commonly toilet paper in a young female patient, can present with foul-smelling vaginal discharge, thus raising suspicion for sexually transmitted infections; this is treated with vaginal irrigation if the child is able to tolerate it. There is no indication for a pelvic ultrasound in urethral prolapse.

[ABP 1.J.2. Sexual abuse]

REFERENCE

1. Hornor G. Common conditions that mimic findings of sexual abuse. *J Pediatr Health Care*. 2009;23(5):283–288.

52. ANSWER: C

This patient most likely has a urinary tract infection (UTI). The presence of an indwelling urinary catheter greatly increases the risk of urine infection. Such patients are at risk for infection with a wide range of organisms that rarely cause urine infection in the general population. The patient's age and the results of the Gram stain suggest that *Enterococcus* is the most likely infective organism. *Enterococcus* UTI is rare outside of patients with catheters, obstruction, or anatomical abnormalities. Of the available choices, ampicillin is the best empiric option. *Enterococcus* species are inherently resistant to most cephalosporins, including ceftriaxone. Nitrofurantoin is an effective choice for simple cystitis due to *Enterococcus* but is not the best choice for this febrile UTI, which may represent pyelonephritis. Gentamicin is included in some regimens for *Enterococcus* infections, but it is not used as monotherapy. *Enterococcus* resistance to trimethoprim-sulfamethoxazole is very common.

[ABP 1.F.10. Pyelonephritis/urinary tract infections]

53. ANSWER: C

This patient has a clinical picture concerning for acute bone or soft tissue infection with fever, inability to bear weight, swelling in his lower extremity, and elevated inflammatory markers. Plain radiographs should be obtained first. Radiographic changes occur in three stages, with the first two being changes in soft tissue. Radiographic evidence of bone destruction is usually not detected until 2–3 weeks after symptom onset. MRI is the imaging study of choice for evaluation for osteomyelitis after plain radiograph; it has a sensitivity of more than 90% as well as the ability to delineate subperiosteal and soft tissue fluid collections. Radionuclide scan or bone scan has been used historically to evaluate for osteomyelitis; however, it has overall lower sensitivity and specificity than MRI. Ultrasound is helpful in evaluating for a joint effusion that may indicate septic arthritis; however, the patient has full range of motion at the hip making this less likely. CT scans may be useful in delineating subperiosteal abscesses or in children with compromised MRI quality, such as those with implanted medical devices.

[ABP 1.G.2. Bone and joint infections]

54. ANSWER: D

This patient's rash is consistent with erythema migrans, an annular, erythematous lesion with central clearing. This is the most common manifestation of Lyme disease in children. Factors that help distinguish erythema migrans from a localized allergic reaction to a tick bite include lesion expansion, size greater than 5 cm, slower onset, and lack of pruritis. Erythema migrans is classified as part of early localized Lyme disease, but without treatment the disease can progress to early disseminated and late disease (Table 1.6).

Diagnostic testing is not required for uncomplicated erythema migrans. Empiric treatment should be started with amoxicillin or doxycycline. For early localized disease, antibiotic treatment duration is 10 to 14 days, whereas for early

Table 1.6 CLINICAL MANIFESTATIONS OF LYME DISEASE

STAGE	SYMPTOMS
Early localized	Erythema migrans, malaise, headache, fever, myalgias, arthralgias
Early disseminated	Multiple erythema migrans lesions, fatigue, myalgia, fever, cranial nerve palsies, headache, meningitis, myocarditis
Late	Arthritis (monoarticular, large joint), central nervous system involvement (less common in children)

disseminated and late disease treatment duration is 14 to 28 days depending on the specific extracutaneous disease.

In cases suspicious for Lyme disease but lacking the characteristic rash, diagnostic testing is a two-test approach with an enzyme-linked immunosorbent assay (ELISA) and confirmatory Western blot, although antibodies to *Borrelia burgdorferi* are often not yet detectable in the early localized stage. In this vignette, antibody testing is not indicated and would only delay treatment. Skin biopsy, inflammatory markers and emollients would not be helpful.

[ABP 1.K.2. Dermatologic manifestations of systemic disease]

REFERENCES

1. Bhanja DB, Sil A. Erythema migrans: the cutaneous manifestation of Lyme disease. *QJM.* 2020;*113*(8):580.
2. Lantos PM, Rumbaugh J, Bockenstedt LK, et al. Clinical practice guidelines by the Infectious Diseases Society of America (IDSA), American Academy of Neurology (AAN), and American College of Rheumatology (ACR): 2020 guidelines for the prevention, diagnosis and treatment of Lyme disease. *Clin Infect Dis.* 2021;*72*(1):e1–e48.

55. ANSWER: B

The patient's clinical presentation is suggestive of intussusception. Intussusception has rarely been associated with the rotavirus vaccine, typically occurring within 1 week of the first or second dose. The mechanism is unclear. Intussusception occurs when a portion of the bowel invaginates into itself, most commonly involving the small bowel. It is one of the most common abdominal emergencies in children and occurs most frequently between the ages of 6 months and 6 years. Patients typically present with episodes of severe abdominal pain or inconsolability that last for 10–30 minutes. Additionally, patients may present with emesis and stools with blood and mucus or "currant jelly stools." Between episodes, patients can be completely asymptomatic. Intussusception is most frequently identified using ultrasound. Treatment for patients with intussusception includes reduction through the use of either barium or pneumatic enema. For patients with bowel perforation or for whom reduction is unsuccessful, operative treatment may be required. None of the other answer choices are risk factors for intussusception.

[ABP 1.E.6. Gastrointestinal bleeding, ABP 1.E.8. Obstruction]

56. ANSWER: D

The patient has developed acute chest syndrome (ACS), which is a leading cause of morbidity and mortality in children with sickle cell disease (SCD). ACS is defined by fever; respiratory symptoms (hypoxemia relative to baseline, tachypnea, cough, or wheezing); and a new infiltrate on chest x-ray. All febrile patients with SCD should undergo a 24-hour evaluation for bacteremia as their functional asplenia puts them at higher risk for invasive bacterial infections. Ceftriaxone is the preferred empiric agent because it provides coverage against encapsulated bacteria such as *Streptococcus pneumoniae, Haemophilus influenzae,* and *Neisseria meningitidis.* Clindamycin is used in patients with cephalosporin allergies, and vancomycin may be added for patients with severe disease or risk of resistant organisms. The infectious etiology of ACS is most often *Chlamydia, Mycoplasma,* or viruses. Therefore, the addition of a macrolide such as azithromycin is needed for coverage of atypical bacterial pathogens. Ampicillin is a first-line antibiotic for uncomplicated community-acquired bacterial pneumonia. Penicillin is an important prophylactic agent for patients with SCD who are under the age of 5 or in older children who are incompletely vaccinated or have undergone splenectomy, but penicillin is not the preferred agent in suspected bacteremia or ACS.

[ABP 1.L.4. Sickle cell disease]

57. ANSWER: E

This patient has leukocyte adhesion deficiency (LAD) type 1. There are several different types of LAD. Type 1 is due to a mutation in leukocyte integrin β_2 (CD18), which leads to a delay in neutrophil response to infections and may present with delayed separation of the umbilical cord. Clinical manifestations in childhood include recurrent bacterial sinopulmonary infections, skin infections, periodontitis, gingivitis, and poor wound healing. Type 2 LAD is less severe. While clinical manifestations include recurrent bacterial sinopulmonary and skin infections, type 2 LAD is also associated with small stature, abnormal facies, and cognitive impairment. None of the other conditions is associated with LAD.

[ABP 1.M.2. Immunodeficiencies]

58. ANSWER: E

This infant presents with symptoms of heart failure secondary to an increasing degree of left-to-right shunting through the VSD. In a large VSD, there is a loss of separation between the ventricles, leading to equalized pressures; thus, the degree of left-to-right shunting is dependent on the relative pulmonary and systemic vascular resistances (PVR and SVR, respectively). As the infant's PVR declines over the first several weeks of life, left-to-right shunting increases, which leads to increased pulmonary blood flow (Q_p) compared to systemic flow (Q_s). Q_p:Q_s less than 1 implies that the pulmonary flow is less than the systemic flow and suggests right-to-left shunting, and Q_p:Q_s = 1 implies equal pulmonary and systemic flow and suggests no shunting is occurring.

[ABP 1.D.3. Heart failure]

59. ANSWER: C

There are approximately 30 species of venomous snakes that can be found across the United States, except in Maine, Alaska, and Hawaii. First aid care of victims of snakebites should focus on transporting the patient to a medical facility as soon as possible. Prehospital interventions such as tourniquets, pressure immobilization, or incision and suction of the bite site have not been proven to be beneficial and often can lead to further complications. Hospital management of snakebites should focus on stabilization of a patient's airway, breathing, and circulation. Antivenom should be considered in patients with moderate-to-severe envenomation as determined by clinical signs and laboratory abnormalities (Table 1.7). Despite relatively mild clinical findings, this patient's thrombocytopenia, tachycardia, and tachypnea would classify him as having a moderate degree of envenomation.

[ABP 1.N.2. Insect and animal bites]

REFERENCE

1. Goto CS, Feng SY. Crotalidae polyvalent immune Fab for the treatment of pediatric crotaline envenomation. *Pediatr Emerg Care.* 2009;25(4):273–282.

60. ANSWER: A

This patient's story is concerning for an aspiration event given the choking event while eating popcorn. Foreign body aspirations are more common in the toddler age group. There are multiple factors that are important to consider when evaluating these cases, including patient age, type and size of foreign body, and location and degree of airway obstruction.

Patients classically present with a triad of paroxysmal cough, wheezing, and decreased air movement. Increased work of breathing and crackles more commonly represent lung findings in pneumonia. Rhonchi are low-pitched sounds, more common during expiration, that occur with some component of airway obstruction. Mediastinal crunch, also called Hamman crunch, is a sign of pneumomediastinum. Pleural friction rubs are seen when there is inflammation of the pleura, which would not be seen in aspiration. Stridor is an upper airway sound seen in conditions such as croup. Transmitted upper airway sounds are referred sounds that can be heard through auscultation but are from the upper airway such as the nose and mouth. Rales are lung sounds that can be heard from the small airway spaces when they are atelectatic or filled with fluid; they would not be consistent with a foreign body aspiration.

[ABP 1.C.6. Foreign body aspiration]

Table 1.7 DETERMINING THE DEGREE OF ENVENOMATION[a]

DEGREE OF ENVENOMATION	EXAMINATION FINDINGS	SYSTEMIC SYMPTOMS	LABORATORY ABNORMALITIES
None	Puncture wounds, no significant erythema or swelling	None	None
Mild	Puncture wounds, local erythema, edema, ecchymosis, pain	None	None
Moderate	Puncture wounds, progression of erythema, edema, ecchymosis, but not involving the entire extremity	Nausea, vomiting, metallic taste, oral paresthesia, tachycardia, tachypnea, mild hypotension	Abnormal coagulation parameters (e.g., elevated prothrombin time, low platelets)
Severe	Puncture wounds, significant progression of erythema, edema, ecchymosis involving the entire extremity; blisters and necrosis common	Nausea, vomiting, metallic taste, oral paresthesia, tachycardia, tachypnea, mild hypotension; serious bleeding may be noted	Abnormal coagulation parameters (e.g., elevated prothrombin time, low platelets)

[a] Adapted from Reference 1.

NOTE: All findings listed are not required to qualify for the specific degree of envenomation.

REFERENCE

1. Sarkar M, Madabhavi I, Niranjan N, Dogra M. Auscultation of the respiratory system. *Ann Thorac Med*. 2015;*10*(3):158–168.

61. ANSWER: C

This patient has developed a brain abscess as a complication from sinusitis. The most appropriate empiric antibiotic choice is ceftriaxone and metronidazole because this covers common causes of brain abscesses, including *Streptococcus, Staphylococcus* species, anaerobic organisms, and gram-negative bacteria. Up to a third of brain abscesses can be polymicrobial. Vancomycin may be added if methicillin-resistant staphylococcus aureus (MRSA) is suspected. Aminoglycosides and first-generation cephalosporins are generally not used as first-line therapy to treat brain abscesses because of poor penetration across the blood-brain barrier. Vancomycin and metronidazole are incorrect because this combination of medications inadequately covers gram-negative organisms. Tobramycin with nafcillin would not provide adequate coverage against anaerobic organisms.

Patients with brain abscesses can present nonspecifically, with only a small proportion having the classic triad of fever, headache, and focal neurologic deficits. Surgical aspiration through a burr hole is typically preferred over surgical excision to limit sequelae of neurologic deficits; however, excision may be necessary in the setting of multiloculated abscesses or encapsulated abscesses or to remove foreign material associated with a traumatic brain abscess.

[ABP 1.A.4. Abscesses]

REFERENCE

1. Brouwer MC, Coutinho JM, van de Beek D. Clinical characteristics and outcome of brain abscess: systematic review and meta-analysis. *Neurology*. 2014;*82*(9):806–813.

62. ANSWER: D

Peritonsillar abscesses (PTAs) and retropharyngeal abscesses (RPAs) are commonly seen in the inpatient setting. PTAs are the most common deep space neck infections in the pediatric population. The incidence peaks at 13 years of age. These infections typically present with fevers, voice change, drooling, trismus, uvula deviation, tonsillar swelling, and lymphadenopathy. The treatment of choice is incision and drainage and generally antibiotic therapy as well.

Retropharyngeal abscesses occur in the retropharyngeal space, which is a potential space anterior to the prevertebral fascia and contains lymph nodes. Abscesses in this space can lead to complications and spread of infection into the surrounding structures, such as the mediastinum. These abscesses may also spread laterally and form a parapharyngeal abscess. The peak incidence of RTA is at 3–5 years of age given that they have an increased number of lymph nodes in this space. As patients age, these lymph nodes atrophy, and thus these infections become less likely. Both PTAs and RPAs are typically polymicrobial infections and can include aerobes and anaerobes. Both PTAs and RPAs are treated with medical or surgical management, depending on their clinical course. PTAs typically require drainage as a part of treatment, but medical management alone may be appropriate for small abscesses less than 1 cm without voice changes, trismus, or drooling. In patients who present with RPA, medical management is typically attempted first, with 24–48 hours of antibiotics. If there is no improvement in symptoms, patients will need surgical management.

[ABP 1.B.3. Oropharyngeal infections]

REFERENCE

1. Bochner RE, Gangar M, Belamarich PF. A clinical approach to tonsillitis, tonsillar hypertrophy, and peritonsillar and retropharyngeal abscesses. *Pediatr Rev*. 2017;*38*(2):81–92.

63. ANSWER: E

This child has maintained the same length percentile of 25% on the growth chart. However, her weight crossed 2 major percentile lines, which meets the definition of failure to thrive (FTT), and her *z* score for weight-for-height of 3 or less indicates severe malnutrition. Given this decline in growth and severe malnutrition, inpatient evaluation and treatment are recommended. Other indications for admission for FTT include a child who has failed outpatient management, concern for abuse or neglect, or concern about the ability of the caregiver. Laboratory evaluation, supplementation, and gastroenterology consultation may all be appropriate steps to pursue for this patient in the inpatient setting.

[ABP 1.O.2. Failure to thrive]

REFERENCES

1. Clinical growth charts. Centers for Disease Control and Prevention. Published June 16, 2017. Accessed June 1, 2021. https://www.cdc.gov/growthcharts/clinical_charts.htm.
2. Becker P, Carney LN, Corkins MR, et al. Consensus statement of the Academy of Nutrition and Dietetics/American Society for Parenteral and Enteral Nutrition: indicators recommended for the identification and documentation of pediatric malnutrition (undernutrition). *Nutr Clin Pract*. 2015;*30*(1):147–161.

64. ANSWER: A

This infant has a presentation most concerning for DiGeorge syndrome. Clinical features of this disorder include thymic aplasia or hypoplasia, parathyroid aplasia or hypoplasia leading to hypoparathyroidism, cardiac defects, developmental delay, and characteristic facial features. Hypoparathyroidism may lead to hypocalcemia during either the neonatal period or later in life when increased demands for parathyroid hormone (PTH) cannot be met by the patient's diminished parathyroid reserve. Although DiGeorge syndrome may cause immunoglobulin deficiency, this is not directly related to calcium levels. CHARGE (coloboma of the eye, heart anomalies, choanal atresia, retardation, genital and ear anomalies) association shares features with DiGeorge syndrome, but these diagnoses can be differentiated by the characteristic eye involvement of CHARGE association, which this child does not have.

[ABP 1.I.4. Hypo and hypercalcemia]

65. ANSWER: C

This patient presented with a focal seizure and was found to have new-onset intracranial bleeding on imaging. As part of the evaluation for abuse, additional laboratory tests were sent, including coagulation studies, which revealed a markedly elevated PTT. This presentation is most concerning for severe hemophilia, with hemophilia A being the most common type. Given the concern for a brain bleed, a trial of factor 8 infusion is indicated, with a follow up PTT to confirm appropriate response. While a sepsis workup would be initiated in this patient with fever and seizure, the presence of significant intracranial bleeding as well as suspected coagulopathy would preclude performance of a lumbar puncture at the time of presentation. In light of the otherwise negative workup for abuse and with a suspected coagulopathy as the cause for this patient's intracranial bleed, a report to CPS is not the best next step. An abdominal ultrasound is unlikely to yield additional information with normal AST and lipase. A brain MRI is also unlikely to change management of this patient's hemophilia.

[ABP 1.J.1. Physical abuse and child neglect]

66. ANSWER: A

This patient most likely has *Streptococcus pneumoniae*–associated hemolytic uremic syndrome (HUS), which is well known for its classic triad of acute kidney injury, microangiopathic hemolytic anemia, and thrombocytopenia. It is due to a thrombotic microangiopathy where abnormalities in the vessel wall of arterioles and capillaries lead to the creation of microvascular thrombosis. The etiology is categorized into two categories: hereditary and acquired. Hereditary causes include complement gene mutations and inborn errors of cobalamin C metabolism. Acquired causes include infections due to Shiga toxin–producing *Escherichia coli* (STEC), *Streptococcus*

pneumoniae, and human immunodeficiency virus (HIV), as well as drug toxicity.

Shiga toxin–producing *Escherichia coli* is the most common cause of HUS in the pediatric population and accounts for 90% of cases. Patients typically present with abdominal pain, vomiting, and diarrhea. *Streptococcus pneumoniae*–associated HUS occurs mainly in infants and younger children, whose symptoms develop 3 to 13 days after an initial infection, most commonly pneumonia. These patients have a more severe hospital course, longer periods of oligo- and anuria, and an increased need for acute dialysis. Complications of HUS include end-stage renal failure, pancreatitis, purpura fulminans, cholecystitis, thrombosis, cardiac dysfunction, and hearing loss. Management is mainly supportive, with fluid support to maintain adequate intravascular volume, electrolyte monitoring and repletion, nutritional supplementation, and transfusions as needed as well as early evaluation by nephrology for dialysis.

[ABP 1.F.1. Hemolytic-uremic syndromes]

67. ANSWER: B

Juvenile dermatomyositis (JDM) is the most common inflammatory myopathy of childhood and is characterized by pathognomonic rashes, proximal muscle weakness, and elevated muscle enzymes. Since the publication of the 2017 consensus guideline, the diagnosis of JDM is made based on symptoms, physical examination findings, and laboratory testing.

This patient exhibits symmetrical proximal muscle weakness and heliotrope rash. Characteristic rashes of JDM, including Gottron papules and heliotrope rash, are the first symptom to be recognized in half of children. Gottron papules are erythematous-to-violaceous lesions that may include scale and often occur over the extensor surfaces of joints, especially the knuckles, elbows, knees, malleoli, and toes. Heliotrope rash is a purple to erythematous patch over the eyelids or in a periorbital distribution. Laboratory findings that support a JDM diagnosis include anti-Jo-1 (anti-histidyl-tRNA synthetase) antibodies and increased muscle enzyme levels (CK and LDH). The other answer choices are not part of the diagnostic criteria for JDM.

Treatment of JDM varies and may include corticosteroids, methotrexate, intravenous immunoglobulin (IVIG), mycophenolate mofetil, and/or cyclosporine.

[ABP 1.K.2. Dermatologic manifestations of systemic disease]

REFERENCES

1. Huber AM, Kim S, Reed AM, et al. Childhood Arthritis and Rheumatology Research Alliance consensus clinical treatment plans

for juvenile dermatomyositis with persistent skin rash. *J Rheumatol.* 2017;*44*(1):110–116.
2. Pachman LM. Juvenile dermatomyositis: a clinical overview. *Pediatr Rev.* 1990;*12*(4):117–125.

68. ANSWER: A

This boy is experiencing an annular cutaneous eruption that is most consistent with a serum sickness-like reaction (SSLR). SSLRs are typically polycyclic with central clearing, involving most of the body, but sparing the palms and soles. High fevers as well as facial and acral edema are common. Antibiotics are the most common trigger. Symptomatic management includes antihistamines and nonsteroidal anti-inflammatory drugs, though systemic steroids can be considered in severe cases. Parabens may cause contact dermatitis but would not be expected to cause an annular eruption. HSV and mycoplasma are common causes of erythema multiforme (EM), though the clinical features of this case are more suggestive of SSLR. Urticaria multiforme, SSLR, and EM have overlapping features and can be differentiated with historical features and examination findings.

[ABP 1.M.3. Drug reactions, ABP 1.K.3. Erythema multiforme and Stevens-Johnson syndrome]

REFERENCES

1. Cohen BA, Davis HW, Gehris RP. Dermatology. In: Zitelli BJ, McIntire S, Nowalk AJ, eds. *Atlas of Pediatric Physical Diagnosis.* 6th ed. Philadelphia, PA: Saunders/Elsevier; 2012.
2. Shah KN, Honig PJ, Yan AC. "Urticaria multiforme": a case series and review of acute annular urticarial hypersensitivity syndromes in children. *Pediatrics.* 2007;*119*(5):e1177–e1183.

69. ANSWER: D

The patient's presentation is concerning for pancreatitis. Acute pancreatitis can be idiopathic or secondary to a broad range of underlying causes, including systemic disease, trauma, toxins, medications, and biliary obstruction. Given this patient's history of multiple episodes and family history, she should be evaluated for causes of recurrent pancreatitis, including heritable pancreatitis. The most common autosomal dominant form of hereditary pancreatitis involves the *PRSS1* gene. The reported history of similar episodes in the patient's mother suggests an autosomal dominant pattern of inheritance, making *PRSS1* the most likely associated gene. The *SPINK1* gene is implicated in autosomal recessive hereditary pancreatitis, while the *CFTR* gene is affected in patients with cystic fibrosis, who can also suffer from recurrent pancreatitis. The *JAG1* and *NOTCH2* genes are associated with Alagille syndrome.

[ABP 1.E.10. Pancreatitis]

70. ANSWER: C

The patient has a pulmonary embolism. Risk factors include venous stasis, endothelial injury, and hypercoagulability, known as the Virchow triad. Obesity and certain medications, including oral contraceptives are also risk factors. Historically, ventilation/perfusion scintigraphy was the preferred diagnostic test, but imaging interpretation is challenging and often confounded by underlying pulmonary and cardiac disease processes. Helical CT pulmonary angiography is now the preferred imaging modality in both adults and children due to its speed and high sensitivity and specificity. Magnetic resonance pulmonary angiography avoids radiation exposure, but the long study time is a disadvantage. Echocardiogram is useful for assessing ventricular function and may allow visualization of large-vessel thrombi but would offer limited visualization of other pulmonary vessels. D-dimer is used widely as a screening test in adults, but its negative predictive value in children is poor.

[ABP 1.L.2. Deep venous thrombosis/pulmonary embolism/hypercoagulable states]

71. ANSWER: B

This baby likely has food protein–induced proctitis/proctocolitis of infancy. This is a non–immunoglobulin (Ig) E immune response commonly due to cow's milk and soybean. Inflammation occurs in the distal colon and rectum, while the proximal intestinal mucosa is unaffected, allowing for absorption of nutrients to continue. Patients present between 2 and 8 weeks of age with diarrhea or bloody stools. Unlike IgE-mediated food allergies, non–IgE-mediated food allergies will present with chronic symptoms often isolated to the skin or gastrointestinal tract. Lactose intolerance is rare in children under the age of 6 and typically presents with abdominal pain, nausea, and bloating rather than the bloody stools seen in this vignette. Young children with eosinophilic gastroenteritis typically present with eating dysfunction, including an inability to progress from liquids to solids. Older children will present with dysphagia and food impaction. Bloody stools are not consistent with eosinophilic enterocolitis. A child with malrotation with volvulus or necrotizing enterocolitis would not have a reassuring physical examination.

[ABP 1.M.2. Immunodeficiencies]

72. ANSWER: B

Dilated cardiomyopathy (DCM) is the most common cardiomyopathy in children, with an estimated incidence of 0.56 cases per 100,000 per year. The most frequently recognized familial form is associated with DMD. DCM has a high risk of mortality, with progression to congestive heart failure, as seen in this patient. An echocardiogram may demonstrate markedly dilated ventricles, reduced ejection fraction, and enlarged left atrium. Hypertrophic cardiomyopathy is usually familial (about 50% inherited as autosomal dominant) and is characterized by a hypertrophied left ventricle, sometimes with a dynamic obstruction of the left outflow tract. Patients with severe hypertrophy and obstruction may experience anginal chest pain, syncope, and arrhythmias, which may lead to sudden death. Restrictive cardiomyopathy is extremely rare and may be idiopathic or associated with systemic infiltrative diseases or inborn errors of metabolism. Arrhythmogenic cardiomyopathy is also rare and may present at any age with palpitations, syncopal episodes, or cardiac death. Noncompaction cardiomyopathy may present with signs and symptoms of heart failure during infancy, but most are asymptomatic.

[ABP 1.D.1. Cardiomyopathies]

73. ANSWER: B

The timing and need for removal of any ingested foreign body depends on (1) the type of foreign body ingested, (2) the location of the foreign body, and (3) the presence or absence of symptoms. The timing of removal can be divided into emergent (within 2 hours, regardless of nil per os [NPO; nothing by mouth] status); urgent (within 24 hours, adhering to common NPO guidelines); and elective (>24 hours, adhering to common NPO guidelines).

Coins are the most common type of foreign body ingested by children. Most are found in the stomach by the time of presentation. Both anterior/posterior and lateral images should be obtained to distinguish coins from button batteries, as these can often resemble each other on radiographs and have significantly different management strategies. Coins located in the esophagus in an asymptomatic child may be removed via endoscopy after a period of observation of up to 24 hours. Repeat radiographs should be obtained prior to the procedure as an estimated 25% of esophageal coins pass spontaneously within the time of observation. Emergent endoscopic removal would be indicated for symptomatic patients. Observation with serial x-rays or discharge would not be appropriate for a patient with objects retained in the esophagus, as these objects may require removal.

[ABP 1.N.1. Ingestions (intentional and unintentional)]

74. ANSWER: B

This patient is presenting with a severe asthma exacerbation. She has received appropriate initial therapy with steroids and bronchodilators. Her initial blood gas shows a mixed respiratory alkalosis (due to mild hypocarbia resulting from tachypnea) and metabolic acidosis. While the subsequent decrease in her respiratory rate may initially seem like an improvement, the follow-up blood gas shows a worsening respiratory status with evidence of acute respiratory acidosis due to CO_2 retention. This is concerning for impending respiratory failure, and preparation for an advanced airway should begin.

While continuous albuterol, intravenous (IV) magnesium, and heliox therapy are all used in the treatment of severe asthma exacerbations, this patient's rapid decline over the span of an hour is concerning for impending respiratory failure, and thus these other therapies should be initiated after an airway is secured. Anti-inflammatory effects from IV steroids take several hours to reach peak effect; a second dose of IV steroids is not indicated.

[ABP 1.C.2. Asthma]

REFERENCE

1. Vasileiadis I, Alevrakis E, Ampelioti S, Vagionas D, Rovina N, Koutsoukou A. Acid-base disturbances in patients with asthma: a literature review and comments on their pathophysiology. *J Clin Med.* 2019;8(4):563.

75. ANSWER: C

This patient has suffered a cerebellar stroke, which can present with nonspecific symptoms such as vertigo, dizziness, nausea, and headache. Posterior circulation strokes present differently from the more commonly known syndromes associated with anterior circulation strokes. Due to the mild signs and symptoms, patients and their families may seek care later, and healthcare professionals may not think about this diagnosis. The best next diagnostic step is to obtain imaging. Ischemic stroke has a slightly higher incidence than hemorrhagic stroke in the pediatric population, and thus MRI is the preferred imaging modality because it is more sensitive and specific for ischemic insult. There is no concern based on the clinical vignette to suggest a cardiac source for an embolic event; therefore, an echocardiogram would not likely be helpful in the diagnosis. This patient has been afebrile and has not had any preceding illness symptoms prior to the acute onset of neurologic symptoms, so he is less likely to have a central nervous system infection. It is possible he has a different neurologic condition in which a lumbar puncture would aid in the diagnosis, such as a demyelinating disorder, but this would not be the most appropriate next step in evaluation. The patient has symptoms of vestibular dysfunction; quantitative vestibular tests such as electro-oculography would confirm the presence of vestibular dysfunction but would not aid in the diagnosis of the underlying cause. Rapid diagnosis of acute ischemic stroke is critical because it improves outcomes.

Risk factors for pediatric ischemic stroke include arteriopathies, cardiac disease, prothrombotic disorders, sickle cell disease, infection, and dehydration.

[ABP 1.A.10. Cerebrovascular accident]

REFERENCE

1. Rivkin MJ, Bernard TJ, Dowling MM, Amlie-Lefond C. Guidelines for urgent management of stroke in children. *Pediatr Neurol.* 2016;56:8–17.

76. ANSWER: A

This patient's presentation is most consistent with acute suppurative parotitis. Parotitis can be viral, bacterial, chronic, or recurrent in nature. The most common age for presentation is early elementary age. The majority of cases present with unilateral facial swelling, but bilateral facial swelling is also possible. Patients may have pain with mastication. Physical examination findings in these patients include erythema over the parotid gland, swelling, pain, and tenderness. The Stenson duct connects the parotid gland to the mouth. Pus in the duct indicates an infection and possible abscess of the parotid gland. Acute suppurative parotitis is treated with antibiotics and sometimes drainage of the site. Imaging is indicated if there is a concern about an abscess that would require surgical intervention.

Given that the facial nerve passes directly through the gland, inflammation or infection of the parotid can lead to facial nerve palsy. The location of the facial nerve must also be taken into consideration when surgical drainage is performed. The other answer choices would not be complications commonly seen with parotitis.

[ABP 1.B.5. Parotitis]

REFERENCE

1. Iro H, Zenk J. Salivary gland diseases in children. *GMS Curr Top Otorhinolaryngol Head Neck Surg.* 2014;13:Doc06.

77. ANSWER: E

This patient has *E. coli* pyelonephritis with bacteremia, which has improved on ceftriaxone. A treatment course is determined based on the organism and sensitivities. There is evidence to support shorter durations of antibiotic therapy and earlier transition to oral therapy in uncomplicated pyelonephritis, even with bacteremia. Historically, bacteremia indicated the need for a prolonged intravenous antibiotic course requiring placement of a PICC; however, studies citing the risks of secondary infection and thrombus formation with PICCs support earlier transition to oral therapy. A renal bladder ultrasound to look for anatomic anomalies predisposing to development of pyelonephritis would be appropriate. A VCUG would only be recommended if the ultrasound is abnormal. A repeat urine culture to document clearance is not indicated. An echocardiogram is not indicated because *E. coli* is not a typical organism associated

with endocarditis, and the patient is now well appearing without persistent bacteremia.

[ABP 1.O.3. Bloodstream infections (bacteremia)]

78. ANSWER: C

Given this patient's age, the presence of a goiter on examination and his normal development, the most likely etiology of his hypothyroidism is Hashimoto thyroiditis. This is the most common cause of acquired hypothyroidism in children in the United States. While thyroid antibodies help confirm the diagnosis, the best next step for this patient is to initiate treatment. Prior to starting thyroid hormone replacement therapy, it is important to rule out concurrent adrenal insufficiency (AI) to avoid precipitating an adrenal crisis. However, adrenal testing in this patient was normal. Thyroid biopsy, thyroid scan, and brain imaging to look for pituitary causes are not helpful in Hashimoto thyroiditis and would only delay necessary treatment.

[ABP 1.I.3. Hypo and hyperthyroidism]

79. ANSWER: E

This patient's osteopenia raises concern for an organic diagnosis rather than nonaccidental trauma. Proximal renal tubular acidosis (RTA), including Fanconi syndrome, can result in growth failure and bony abnormalities due to renal losses of phosphate with subsequent osteodystrophy. It can be diagnosed using serum and urine electrolytes showing hyperchloremic metabolic acidosis, hypophosphatemia, hypokalemia, proteinuria, and glucosuria. A femur fracture without a reasonable mechanism of injury would typically raise concern for abuse. Similarly, posterior rib, scapular, sternal, spinous process, and metaphyseal avulsion fractures in children are also concerning for abuse. However, in this case, the fracture is likely to be pathological secondary to an underlying medical diagnosis leading to osteopenia. In the setting of abuse, a skeletal survey would be beneficial in evaluating for other fractures; head CT would also be indicated to evaluate for occult brain injury in this age group. Both of these would likely confirm the presence of osteopenia and may show additional fractures but would not help elucidate the underlying etiology in this patient. A social history would be beneficial to evaluate for other risk factors but would not yield the diagnosis of RTA. A peripheral blood smear would be beneficial in diagnosing a malignancy, which can present with pathologic fractures, but would not account for diffuse osteopenia.

[ABP 1.J.1. Physical abuse and child neglect]

80. ANSWER: A

This patient most likely has pelvic inflammatory disease (PID) given her pain, fever, discharge, and adnexal tenderness. Definitive diagnosis requires laparoscopy, but PID is usually a clinical diagnosis. This patient's high fever and severe pain indicate severe PID. PID is a polymicrobial infection that may include *Chlamydia trachomatis*, *Neisseria gonorrhoeae*, and anaerobic organisms, so treatment involves broad-spectrum antibiotics. This patient requires hospitalization and parenteral antibiotics given the severity of her symptoms and inability to tolerate anything by mouth. There are two preferred parenteral regimens that have the most evidence supporting their use: doxycycline with either cefotetan or cefoxitin or clindamycin and gentamicin. Quinolones have been considered for PID in the past, but quinolone-resistant *Neisseria gonorrhoeae* is increasingly common. Piperacillin-tazobactam has not been evaluated for the treatment of PID. Ampicillin-sulbactam with doxycycline is an acceptable alternative treatment, but ampicillin without a β-lactamase inhibitor is insufficient. Azithromycin with or without metronidazole is an alternative regimen for mild-to-moderate PID, but it has not been studied in severe PID.

[ABP 1.F.6. Pelvic inflammatory disease]

81. ANSWER: C

This patient's presentation of oligoarthritis, enthesitis, conjunctivitis, and sacroiliitis is most consistent with reactive arthritis, formally known as Reiter syndrome. Reactive arthritis is a spondylarthritis arising after infection elsewhere in the body, typically a gastrointestinal or urogenital infection. However, as in this case, patients may not always report a preceding infection. The classic triad of arthritis, conjunctivitis, and urethritis is uncommon in children.

Enteric pathogens such as *Yersinia*, *Campylobacter*, *Salmonella*, and *Shigella* commonly incite reactive arthritis; however, in healthy patients without diarrhea, treatment of these pathogens is not necessary. *Chlamydia trachomatis* is a common precipitating infection in patients with reactive arthritis and is important to test for and treat, especially in sexually active patients. *S. aureus* is a common cause of septic arthritis; however, this patient's constellation of symptoms is more consistent with a reactive arthritis.

[ABP 1.H.2. Inflammatory arthritis]

82. ANSWER: C

Atopic dermatitis (AD) is a common condition that is diagnosed clinically based on distribution and characteristics of skin lesions. AD is characterized by the presence of pruritis and eczematous skin lesions. In infants and children, facial, neck, and extensor involvement is common, and the groin and axillary regions are often spared. Flexural lesions can be present in any age group. AD is often chronic or relapsing. Baseline care involves good hygiene and use of emollients and/or topical corticosteroids.

In this case, the patient's chronic AD symptoms are likely due to noncompliance, and hospitalization for WWT is appropriate. WWT involves application of medium-potency corticosteroids or emollients followed by two layers of cotton pajamas, gauze, or other such dressings. The first layer is moist with water, while the second is dry. Inpatient application of WWT may help to establish control of symptoms and demonstrate effectiveness of treatment. Hospitalization may also provide an opportunity for education and establishment of a written plan to support the family, which may help with compliance. Antibiotics are not indicated due to lack of evidence of superinfection. Systemic steroids or referral to dermatology for escalation of therapy, such as immunomodulators or biologics, may be needed if WWT and continued adherence to treatment is not effective, but these are not first-line treatments.

[ABP 1.K.4. Complicated eczema]

REFERENCES

1. Eichenfield LF, Tom WL, Chamlin SL, et al. Guidelines of care for the management of atopic dermatitis: section 1. Diagnosis and assessment of atopic dermatitis. *J Am Acad Dermatol.* 2014;70(2):338–351.
2. Sidbury R, Tom WL, Bergman JN, et al. Guidelines of care for the management of atopic dermatitis: section 4. Prevention of disease flares and use of adjunctive therapies and approaches. *J Am Acad Dermatol.* 2014;71(6):1218–1233.

83. ANSWER: B

The patient's clinical presentation is concerning for malrotation with midgut volvulus. Most commonly occurring in patients less than 1 year of age, malrotation occurs as a result of incomplete rotation of the embryonic gut. Volvulus can occur with malrotation if the mesentery twists in a way that compromises blood flow to bowel through the superior mesenteric artery. Patients typically present with vomiting, which can be bilious, hemodynamic instability, abdominal distension, peritonitis, and hematochezia. The diagnosis of malrotation should be a primary consideration in patients with emesis and hemodynamic instability. If the patient is clinically stable, diagnosis can be confirmed through imaging with an upper gastrointestinal series. However, in cases of hemodynamic instability, patients should be taken emergently to the operating room for surgical exploration and correction following resuscitation. Definitive correction occurs with the Ladd procedure, which is meant to prevent future episodes of malrotation. Although corticosteroids, gastric decompression, broad-spectrum antibiotics, and packed red blood cells may be considerations for this patient, surgical intervention is the most appropriate next step in management.

[ABP 1.E.8. Obstruction]

84. ANSWER: B

The patient most likely has iron deficiency anemia given her age and dietary history. Iron deficiency anemia is characterized by low hemoglobin and hematocrit, microcytosis, and elevated red blood cell distribution width. Additional laboratory findings include low plasma iron, low ferritin, normal-to-high total iron-binding capacity, and low transferrin saturation. A trial of oral elemental iron 3 mg/kg/d is indicated for mild iron deficiency anemia. The patient's anemia likely was gradual in onset, and she is asymptomatic and clinically stable. Therefore, blood transfusion and intravenous iron are not indicated. Cow's milk consumption greater than 24 ounces per day has been associated with anemia due to low bioavailability of iron in cow's milk as well as potential microscopic intestinal blood loss. There are no red flags on the patient's history or laboratory data (e.g., pancytopenia) to necessitate hematology referral. Primary care follow-up is appropriate to monitor for rising hemoglobin within several weeks, and iron supplementation should occur for at least 3 months to replenish iron stores. Vitamin B_{12} deficiency presents with macrocytic rather than microcytic anemia.

[ABP 1.L.1. Anemias]

85. ANSWER: B

This patient most likely has a serum sickness-like reaction (SSLR) secondary to trimethoprim-sulfamethoxazole. SSLR can be triggered by medications, viral infections (including hepatitis B), and some bacterial infections. Medications commonly implicated include cephalosporins (especially cefaclor) and trimethoprim-sulfamethoxazole. Though the exact mechanism is poorly understood, SSLR tends to be much milder than true serum sickness. The timing of onset of symptoms is important for diagnosing SSLR, typically occurring 1–2 weeks after starting a medication. Typical symptoms of SSLR include low-grade fever and an urticarial rash that may start in the flexural areas. The rash can have many appearances, but a slowly evolving urticarial rash is most typical. In general, discontinuing the offending agent is sufficient to treat SSLR, but in severe cases with extension rash and high fevers (as in this vignette) a short course of corticosteroids should be given. Discontinuing trimethoprim-sulfamethoxazole alone, or switching to clindamycin, would be appropriate for someone with milder symptoms. Stevens-Johnson syndrome and toxic epidermal necrolysis are also drug reactions that cause a severe rash and may necessitate transfer to a burn center for treatment, but these typically have mucosal involvement. Skin testing is not useful in the evaluation of SSLR. Patients with drug-induced SSLR are at risk for recurrent reactions if they are treated with that medication in the future.

[ABP 1.M.3. Drug reactions (e.g., serum sickness)]

86. ANSWER: C

The infant's ECG demonstrates supraventricular tachycardia (SVT), which is the most common tachyarrhythmia seen in infants and children. Reentry SVT is characterized by a heart rate greater than 180 beats/min in older children or greater than 220 beats/min in infants, without variability. It is classically abrupt in onset and termination with an absent P wave and narrow QRS complex. Initial management depends on the stability of the patient. In a well-appearing patient with otherwise stable vital signs, it is appropriate to try vagal maneuvers such as placing an ice-water bag on the face to produce a diving reflex. If the vagal maneuver is ineffective, as in the case of this infant, the medication of choice for SVT is adenosine, which acts on the atrioventricular node. Due to its short half-life, it must be given by rapid intravenous bolus followed by a saline flush. If the patient is unstable or showing signs of heart failure, management would be immediate synchronized cardioversion. A β-blocker or normal saline bolus would not be first-line treatment for SVT. Verapamil should be avoided in infants younger than 12 months of age due to the risk of extreme bradycardia and hypotension. SVT can be idiopathic or due to Wolff-Parkinson-White (WPW) preexcitation, congenital heart defects, or cardiac surgery.

[ABP 1.D.4. Dysrhythmias]

87. ANSWER: D

Esophageal impaction of an ingested button battery is the leading indication for emergent endoscopic intervention. The hydroxide radicals generated by the battery may lead to severe complications, such as esophageal perforation, tracheoesophageal fistula, esophageal strictures, vocal cord paralysis, mediastinitis, or aortoenteric fistula. Continued injury may occur even after battery removal. The other objects listed need to be removed if they remain in the esophagus but can be removed urgently after following appropriate nil per os (nothing by mouth) guidelines rather than emergently within 2 hours of arrival.

[ABP 1.N.1. Ingestions (intentional and unintentional)]

88. ANSWER: E

This patient presents with a moderate asthma exacerbation and is started on appropriate treatment with a short-acting β-agonist (SABA) and inhaled anticholinergic. SABAs may transiently cause hypoxemia by worsening the ventilation-perfusion (V/Q) mismatch. This occurs when the drug is systemically absorbed, causing pulmonary vasodilation, thereby increasing perfusion to areas of the lung that may be underventilated due to bronchial constriction. This effect is temporary, often lasting less than 30 minutes, and should be treated with supplemental oxygen to maintain an oxygen saturation of 92% or greater.

An arterial blood gas is not necessary given the likely transient nature of the hypoxemia and may delay the start of treatment with oxygen. An advanced airway is not indicated as the patient is not showing signs of impending respiratory failure (including significant fatigue, hypercarbia, refractory hypoxemia, or altered mental status). While magnesium sulfate is used in the treatment of moderate-to-severe asthma exacerbations, it does not take priority over oxygen in this patient with mild hypoxia. When used appropriately, treatments with nebulizers versus metered dose inhalers are similar in efficacy.

[ABP 1.C.2. Asthma]

REFERENCE

1. Patel SJ, Teach SJ. Asthma. *Pediatr Rev.* 2019;*40*(11):549–567.

89. ANSWER: B

This patient is presenting with infantile spasms (ISs), also known as West syndrome, and tuberous sclerosis complex (TSC). The clues in this vignette are the descriptions of episodes that are classic for infantile spasms, a common age of presentation for West syndrome (4–7 months), and hypomelanotic macules (also called ash-leaf spots) that point toward TSC. Tuberous sclerosis complex is a heterogeneous genetic disorder with multisystem manifestations summarized in the Table 1.8. Epilepsy prevalence in TSC is as high as 90%. Patients with TSC can have cortical/subcortical tubers, subependymal nodules, cortical dysplasias, subependymal giant cell astrocytomas, or other types of neuronal migration defects on neuroimaging. Subependymal nodules are tumors along the ependymal linings of the lateral ventricles. Lissencephaly, absent corpus collosum, and pituitary hypoplasia are not classically associated with TSC. This patient's presentation is not consistent with acute stroke.

Table 1.8 MANIFESTATIONS OF TSC

Gene Mutations	TSC1, TSC2
Neurologic	Cortical/subcortical tubers, subependymal nodules, cortical dysplasias, subependymal giant cell astrocytomas, or other types of neuronal migration defects Infantile spasms, focal seizures, and other epilepsy syndromes Aggressive behaviors, autism spectrum disorders, intellectual disabilities, psychiatric and neuropsychological disorders
Renal	Renal angiomyolipomata, polycystic disease, renal cell carcinoma, or other tumors Secondary hypertension
Pulmonary	Pulmonary lymphangioleiomyomatosis
Dermatologic	Facial angiofibromas, fibrous cephalic plaques, hypomelanotic macules (ash-leaf spots) or confetti lesions, ungual fibromas, shagreen patch, defects in tooth enamel, and intraoral fibromas
Cardiac	Rhabdomyomas Arrhythmias
Ophthalmologic	Hamartomas and hypopigmented lesions of the retina
Other	Vascular aneurysms, gastrointestinal polyps, bone cysts, and endocrinopathies

[ABP 1.A.2. Seizures]

REFERENCE

1. Davis PE, Filip-Dhima R, Sideridis G, et al. Presentation and diagnosis of tuberous sclerosis complex in infants. *Pediatrics.* 2017;*140*(6):e20164040.

90. ANSWER: B

This clinical situation is most consistent with parotitis caused by a sialolith or stone. This patient has the clinical signs and symptoms of parotitis with unilateral facial swelling, erythema, and swelling over the parotid gland. Bimanual intraoral palpation is a technique that allows for detection of stones in the ducts. The Stenson duct, sometimes called the parotid duct, connects the parotid gland to the mouth and carries saliva into the oral cavity. Obstruction of this duct can lead to parotitis.

As in the patient described, once a stone has been identified, conservative or medical management is typically tried first, including the use of sialagogues such as lemons to stimulate the production of saliva and flush out the stone. If medical management is not successful, surgical or shock-wave lithotripsy can be attempted. Further imaging of the patient would not be helpful as the diagnosis can be made based on physical examination alone. Massage of the duct on the opposite side would not be helpful in promoting movement of the stone. Dental issues are a common cause of facial swelling, but in this case the physical examination findings are clearly consistent with a sialolith.

[ABP 1.B.5. Parotitis]

91. ANSWER: D

This patient with a central line presenting with fever is at risk for having a central line–associated bloodstream infection (CLABSI). The diagnosis requires isolation of an organism from a blood culture of the central line. It is standard to obtain both a central line culture and a peripheral blood culture to confirm that there is clinically significant bacteremia originating from the central line and admit for empiric broad-spectrum antibiotics while awaiting results. If the central line has multiple lumens, cultures from each lumen should be obtained. Cultures should continue to be collected every 24 hours while febrile or if there is growth of an organism.

The most common sign of a CLABSI in a patient with a central line is fever. The line site may show physical examination findings to support an infection, but this is not always the case. Risk factors for CLABSI include the presence of the central line allowing organisms to migrate into the catheter and then the bloodstream, as well as chronic TPN use and short-gut syndrome, leading to risk of bacterial translocation.

It is unsafe to treat the fever and discharge without any cultures or antibiotics, as these patients can rapidly decompensate. It is also inappropriate to treat with antibiotics before obtaining cultures and to remove a central line before obtaining more information, especially in a child who depends on parenteral nutrition.

[ABP 1.O.3. Bloodstream infections (bacteremia)]

92. ANSWER: D

The most common cause of hyperthyroidism in pediatric patients is Graves' disease. Diagnosis can be confirmed by the presence of TSI antibodies. Patients with Hashimoto thyroiditis may present with hyperthyroidism before they develop hypothyroidism. It is important to differentiate these two conditions, as they are treated differently. The hyperthyroidism in early Hashimoto thyroiditis is caused by a release of preformed hormone, so antithyroid medications will not be helpful.

A biopsy is not necessary to diagnose Graves' disease. Although thyroidectomy can be an effective treatment for Graves' hyperthyroidism, it is not first-line treatment and should be reserved for cases in which antithyroid drug therapy fails or causes intolerable side effects. Treatment should be initiated as soon as the diagnosis is confirmed. The antithyroid drug of choice is methimazole. Propylthiouracil is also effective but has more frequent and severe side effects, including a small risk of severe hepatotoxicity. While propranolol can be helpful as an adjunctive therapy to both decrease adrenergic symptoms and slow the conversion of T_4 to T_3, it is not first-line therapy and would be contraindicated in a child with asthma.

[ABP 1.I.3. Hypo and hyperthyroidism]

93. ANSWER: D

This patient's physical examination findings are consistent with an abusive burn injury through intentional immersion. A burn with a sharp line of demarcation on the lower back or a "donut" pattern on the buttocks with central sparing are both concerning for intentional immersion in boiling water. In addition to fluid resuscitation, wound care, and other supportive measures, a skeletal survey is indicated as part of the evaluation for abuse, especially in a nonverbal infant. Staphylococcal scalded skin syndrome can have the appearance of burns, though this distribution is not typical; therefore, antibiotics or bacterial cultures are not indicated. Of note, severe burns can result in fever even in the absence of infection. Both Stevens-Johnson syndrome and autoimmune conditions such as bullous pemphigoid can also have the appearance of burn injuries, though this patient's distribution is not typical of either of these conditions, so drug history or skin biopsy are unlikely to change management.

[ABP 1.J.1. Physical abuse and child neglect]

94. ANSWER: E

This patient most likely has epididymitis, as suggested by his acute onset of scrotal pain with dysuria. Normal testicular lie, negative Doppler ultrasound, and intact cremaster reflex make testicular torsion unlikely. Therefore, a urology consultation is not necessary. The causes and management of epididymitis vary depending on whether the patient is sexually active and at risk for urinary tract infections. In non–sexually active males, including prepubertal males, the most common causes of epididymitis are viral, with enteroviruses and adenoviruses being most common. Treatment for these infections is supportive and includes analgesia, rest, and scrotal support. Patients may have an associated urinary tract infection (UTI), so a urinalysis and urine culture should be sent. For patients with pyuria, abnormal genitourinary anatomy, or other risk factors for a UTI, empiric antibiotics such as cephalexin may be initiated. This patient had no risk factors for UTI and no pyuria, so cephalexin is not indicated. For sexually active males, the most common causes of epididymitis are chlamydia and gonorrhea as well as *Escherichia coli*. There is increased risk for infection with gram-negative rods in males who practice insertive anal sex. Ceftriaxone and azithromycin are the treatment for gonorrhea and chlamydia, while ofloxacin can be used to treat epididymitis caused by a gram-negative rod, none of which are suspected in this case.

[ABP 1.F.9. Testicular mass and torsion]

95. ANSWER: A

The patient's presentation is most consistent with sarcoidosis. Sarcoidosis is a granulomatous inflammatory disease that can affect nearly any organ system, depending on the location of granulomas. In children, the lung, eyes, liver, and lymph nodes are most commonly affected. There are no standardized diagnostic criteria for sarcoidosis. The diagnosis is made when a patient has a consistent clinical presentation, typical radiographic features, nonnecrotizing granulomatous inflammation in tissue samples, and other causes of granulomatous disease have been excluded. While an ACE level may be elevated, this is a nonspecific finding.

As the diagnosis is often delayed due to the disease's many nonspecific signs and symptoms, it is important to obtain baseline serum calcium levels to diagnose associated hypercalcemia. This can lead to hypercalciuria and treatment-resistant renal injury if left untreated. Sarcoidosis is more common in African American children. In early-onset sarcoidosis, the most common presenting symptoms are extrathoracic and include rash, uveitis, and arthritis. In older children and teenagers, pulmonary involvement and lymphadenopathy are more predominant.

[ABP 1.C.5. Chronic respiratory conditions]

REFERENCES

1. Nathan N, Marcelo P, Houdouin V, et al. Lung sarcoidosis in children: update on disease expression and management. *Thorax.* 2015;70(6):537–542.
2. Crouser ED, Maier LA, Wilson KC, et al. Diagnosis and detection of sarcoidosis. An official American Thoracic Society clinical practice guideline. *Am J Respir Crit Care Med.* 2020;201(8):e26–e51.

96. ANSWER: D

This patient's presentation is suggestive of inflammatory bowel disease. Erythema nodosum (EN) is a panniculitis that presents as tender erythematous subcutaneous nodules that are typically found on the anterior surfaces of the lower extremities. It can be associated with various infectious, autoimmune, and oncologic causes or can be idiopathic. EN may be associated with inflammatory bowel disease, and in some cases EN may be the presenting sign. Erythema infectiosum, also known as fifth disease, is a "slapped cheek" rash associated with parvovirus B19. Erythema migrans is associated with Lyme disease. It is an erythematous targetoid lesion that typically appears at the site of a tick bite, usually 7–10 days after the bite. Erythema migrans lesions may be diffuse in disseminated disease. Erythema multiforme is a hypersensitivity reaction to drugs or infectious agents. It typically presents as diffuse erythematous macular lesions with central clearing. Erythema toxicum is a benign transient rash in newborns. It presents as multiple small migratory yellow macules on an erythematous base. It generally resolves within the first 2 weeks after birth.

[ABP 1.K.2. Dermatologic manifestations of systemic disease, ABP 1.E.12. Inflammatory bowel disease]

REFERENCE

1. Schwartz RA, Nervi SJ. Erythema nodosum: a sign of systemic disease. *Am Fam Physician.* 2007;75(5):695–700.

97. ANSWER: C

The patient's clinical presentation is consistent with Hirschsprung disease, which is caused by a congenital absence of ganglion cells in the distal rectum. Patients with Hirschsprung disease often fail to pass meconium within the first 24 hours of life. Those with severe disease often present in infancy with signs of intestinal obstruction. However, patients with less severe disease can present later in childhood with chronic constipation and, occasionally, poor growth. The diagnosis of Hirschsprung disease can be confirmed through rectal biopsy, which shows the absence of ganglion cells in the distal rectum. The management for Hirschsprung disease involves surgical resection of the affected portion of bowel. Other common causes of chronic constipation in children outside the neonatal period include functional constipation and lack of adequate fiber or fluid intake. These diagnoses would not be expected to reveal any abnormalities on intestinal biopsy. Villous atrophy is commonly associated with celiac disease, another potential cause of constipation in children. Hirschsprung disease should be suspected in this case over the other diagnoses listed given the delayed passing of meconium as well as the protracted nature of the patient's constipation, which began at an early age and has persisted for years despite an adequate bowel regimen.

[ABP 1.E.3. Constipation]

98. ANSWER: E

Fever and neutropenia in an oncology patient constitute a medical emergency. Fever is defined as a single temperature of 38.3°C or higher or a temperature of 38.0°C or greater lasting more than 1 hour or obtained twice within 24 hours. Neutropenia in this case refers to severe neutropenia, defined as an absolute neutrophil count less than 500 cells/mm³. Appropriate empiric antibiotics include cefepime, piperacillin-tazobactam, or meropenem. Vancomycin should be considered in patients with an infectious source concerning for methicillin-resistant *Staphylococcus aureus* (MRSA), a history of MRSA, or hemodynamic instability. For cephalosporin-allergic patients, appropriate empiric therapy includes meropenem, aztreonam plus clindamycin, or aztreonam plus vancomycin. Antifungal therapy is indicated for high-risk patients with fever and neutropenia persisting four or more days. Micafungin is an appropriate empiric antifungal agent. Liposomal amphotericin B also may be used but has a less-favorable side-effect profile. In the absence of localizing signs, lumbar puncture, stool culture, and repeat urine culture are not indicated.

[ABP 1.L.6. Fever and neutropenia]

99. ANSWER: C

The patient above likely has X-linked agammaglobulinemia caused by a mutation in the gene responsible for producing the BTK enzyme. This leads to a significant reduction or absence of B cells, which in turn leads to a decrease in immunoglobulin classes and a defective antibody response. Absence of the B-cell–rich adenoids and tonsils is the only characteristic physical examination finding, as is seen in this patient. Symptoms present after 6–9 months of age when maternal immunoglobulins decrease. Past medical history may reveal recurrent bacterial respiratory tract infections, sinusitis, or otitis media as well as family history of males affected with chronic infections. Additionally, patients may have sequelae of chronic infections, such as failure to thrive, growth delay, chronic cough, chronic rhinitis, postnasal drainage, and digital clubbing.

Workup includes complete blood count with differential as well as serum immunoglobulin levels. Once low immunoglobulin levels are noted, T lymphocytes, B lymphocytes, and natural killer cell subsets should be assessed by flow cytometry. The flow cytometry provides a screening tool for diagnosis that will be confirmed with BTK genotyping.

A dihydrorhodamine assay is useful for diagnosis of chronic granulomatous disease, which presents with recurrent pneumonias and skin infections. Patients typically have hepatomegaly, splenomegaly, or lymphadenitis. IgA deficiency can present with recurrent sinopulmonary infections, although the majority of patients are asymptomatic. Absence of tonsillar tissue is not characteristic. A lymphocyte enumeration panel can aid in the diagnosis of immunodeficient states characterized by decreased cellular immunity, but is a nonspecific test that would not confirm the diagnosis in this case.

[ABP 1.M.2. Immunodeficiencies]

100. ANSWER: C

Salt-wasting congenital adrenal hyperplasia (CAH) can present with vomiting and severe dehydration in early infancy. 21-Hydroxylase deficiency is the most common type of CAH to present in infancy. Adrenal insufficiency from CAH classically presents with hyponatremia, hyperkalemia, hypoglycemia, and acidosis. Renin levels are increased in salt-wasting CAH, while aldosterone levels are decreased or normal.

Females are typically born with clitoral enlargement and labial fusion due to the effects of androgen excess. Males may have a hyperpigmented scrotum and enlarged phallus at birth or may have a normal examination. If the condition is not identified on newborn screening, males will often present as in this vignette with vomiting and severe dehydration.

[ABP 1.I.5. Adrenal disorders]

101. ANSWER: A

The finding of a frenulum laceration in a nonambulatory patient is concerning for abuse. Specifically, this can be seen with force-feeding behaviors, with either a bottle or a pacifier. This injury pattern is consistent with a sentinel injury, which is considered a "warning injury" for abuse. In addition, sentinel injuries often escalate to more life-threatening abusive behaviors. In this case, the patient's irritability on examination further raises concern for an occult head injury, which should be evaluated with CT of the head. A social work consult and skeletal survey should also be obtained in this age group. If bruising was present on examination or if intracranial hemorrhage was confirmed on imaging, a complete blood count and coagulation studies could be helpful to exclude thrombocytopenia or coagulopathy as the etiology. Unlike liver enzymes and lipase, which may suggest abdominal trauma, serum electrolytes are not routinely recommended for evaluation of abuse. Finally, a full skeletal survey is more effective in evaluating for occult fractures than a chest and abdomen radiograph, also known as a "babygram."

[ABP 1.J.1. Physical abuse and child neglect]

102. ANSWER: C

This patient has nephrotic syndrome, as evidenced by his proteinuria and hypoalbuminemia. While a 24-hour urine collection is the gold standard for assessing proteinuria, it is cumbersome and time consuming. The urine protein-to-creatinine ratio measured on a random urine sample is a useful substitute. While a normal urine protein-to-creatinine ratio is less than 0.2, nephrotic range proteinuria is considered to result in a ratio greater than 3, as seen in this patient. Hypoalbuminemia is another key diagnostic feature of nephrotic syndrome. Other common findings that are not necessary for the diagnosis include edema and hyperlipidemia. The most common cause of nephrotic syndrome in children is minimal change disease, which is responsible for about three-fourths of all cases. Because minimal change disease responds very well to a course of corticosteroids, renal biopsy can be deferred in most patients. Such patients should be 1–12 years of age and prepubescent, have normal complement factors, and have no gross hematuria, hypertension, marked elevation in serum creatinine, and no extrarenal findings that would suggest an alternative cause. Patients who do not meet these criteria should undergo renal biopsy rather than empiric treatment. This patient's hypertension is an indication for renal biopsy. Elevated triglycerides and edema are expected findings in nephrotic syndrome of any cause. Microscopic hematuria is not an indication for biopsy. The patient's age is within the range in which empiric treatment can be considered.

[ABP 1.F.5. Nephrotic syndrome]

103. ANSWER: A

The patient above most likely has selective immunoglobulin (Ig) A deficiency (sIgAD). It is the most common immunologic defect and is diagnosed in patients older than 4 years with low serum IgA and normal IgG and IgM. Other causes of hypogammaglobulinemia, such as common variable immunodeficiency (CVID), transient agammaglobulinemia of infancy, and X-linked agammaglobulinemia, must be excluded. Most patients are asymptomatic. Those with symptoms present with a history of recurrent sinopulmonary and gastrointestinal infections or rarely anaphylaxis after blood transfusions due to presence of antibodies directed against IgA. Patients are at higher risk of having asthma, celiac disease, inflammatory bowel disease, and autoimmune disorders, including systemic lupus erythematosus, rheumatoid arthritis, and immune thrombocytopenia. A CBC with differential and bacterial blood culture could be useful for diagnosing serious bacterial infections; both would be unlikely to diagnose this patient's underlying condition. A dihydrorhodamine assay is useful for diagnosis of chronic granulomatous disease, which presents with recurrent pneumonias and skin infections. Patients typically have hepatomegaly, splenomegaly, or lymphadenitis.

[ABP 1.M.2. Immunodeficiencies]

104. ANSWER: D

The rhythm shows atrial and ventricular beats that are completely independent of each other, representing third-degree AV block. The P waves are regular with a normal heart rate for the patient's age. The QRS complex is also regular but at a slower rate. In sinus rhythm, the P wave would come before every QRS complex, and every QRS complex would follow a P wave. Second-degree heart block may show increasing PR intervals with or without dropped QRS complexes. PVCs are represented by wide, abnormal-appearing, early QRS complexes. Of *congenital* heart block cases, 60% to 90% are caused by neonatal lupus erythematosus, which is likely the cause in this case given the mother's history. Maternal anti-Ro and anti-La antibodies can cross the placenta and persist up to 9 months in the infant; thus, there is potential for late development of complete heart block at several months of age. The most common *acquired* cause of third-degree AV block is cardiac surgery. Other causes include severe myocarditis, acute rheumatic fever, cardiomyopathies, tumors, Lyme carditis, and certain drugs. Untreated infants may develop congestive heart failure (CHF). Management options are variable, depending on cause and symptoms. Permanent pacemaker therapy is indicated if the patient is symptomatic, develops CHF, has an average ventricular rate less than 50–55 beats per minute, has ventricular dysfunction, or has heart block caused by surgery that is not expected to resolve.

[ABP 1.D.4. Dysrhythmias]

105. ANSWER: D

Hydrocarbon ingestion is associated with a significant risk of aspiration. Products with low viscosity, low surface tension, and high volatility are more likely to be aspirated. Patients presenting with mild-to-moderate respiratory symptoms are likely to have aspirated some amount of the product and are therefore at risk for chemical pneumonitis. Antibiotics are not indicated for chemical pneumonitis but can be considered if fevers continue for 48 hours, as this could indicate bacterial superinfection. This patient does not warrant intubation at this time given his lack of respiratory distress and stable neurologic examination. Corticosteroids are not indicated in cases of chemical pneumonitis.

[ABP 1.N.1. Ingestions (intentional and unintentional)]

106. ANSWER: E

While patients with acute asthma require intravenous (IV) fluids for dehydration and insensible losses, their fluid balance should be frequently evaluated and IV fluid rate adjusted accordingly, as they are at risk of pulmonary edema from overhydration. This patient's new oxygen requirement after several days of IV fluids, along with crackles on examination, is concerning for pulmonary edema and can be treated with a one-time dose of diuretic, such as furosemide. Positive fluid balances in patients with acute asthma exacerbations have been linked to longer lengths of stay, oxygen utilization, and treatment duration. In addition to decreasing the rate of IV fluids, the patient should be advised to get out of bed frequently and/or use an incentive spirometer to reduce atelectasis, which may worsen edema and hypoxia.

Broad-spectrum antibiotics are not indicated in this patient without other clinical signs of bacterial infection, such as fever or focal lung examination. If the clinical examination is not clear, a chest radiograph may be helpful to differentiate between infection and edema. While short-acting β-agonists (SABAs) can cause transient hypoxia due to increased ventilation-perfusion mismatch, this is generally seen at the start of therapy. There is no clear evidence that levalbuterol has less of an effect on heart rate than albuterol, and it does not improve hypoxia. Heliox (a helium-oxygen blend) improves laminar flow of air into the airways, thereby improving dyspnea and delivery of inhaled therapies. However, it should be used with caution in patients with hypoxia who require oxygen to maintain appropriate levels of saturation. It is also not indicated in this patient, who is showing evidence of pulmonary edema. Increasing the frequency of corticosteroids would not be expected to improve this new oxygen requirement.

[ABP 1.C.2. Asthma]

REFERENCE

1. Kantor DB, Hirshberg EL, McDonald MC, et al. Fluid balance is associated with clinical outcomes and extravascular lung water in children with acute asthma exacerbation. *Am J Respir Crit Care Med.* 2018;*197*(9):1128–1135.

107. ANSWER: A

The child in this clinical vignette is most likely experiencing symptoms secondary to *Clostridium botulinum* infection. A gram-positive, anaerobic, spore-producing bacteria, *C. botulinum* is commonly found in soil and dust. In the United States, the most common source is ingestion of spores in dust from nearby construction or agricultural sites, leading to bacterial colonization in the gastrointestinal tract with resulting toxin production. Foodborne botulism from either honey or inappropriate canning of food can also lead to botulism in children less than 12 months of age. The potent *C. botulinum* toxin blocks transmission of acetylcholine at the presynaptic membrane of the neuromuscular junction. Botulism classically presents with descending acute paralysis. Patients will typically have facial, ocular, and swallowing deficits, such as ptosis, diplopia, difficulty feeding, dysphagia, decreased gag reflex, and a weak suck. In addition, these patients will demonstrate generalized weakness and hypotonia. Progression of the paralysis can ultimately lead to respiratory compromise. Constipation is a common gastrointestinal symptom.

Infant botulism can be mimicked by many other conditions. An abnormal mutation in the *SMN1* gene is seen in patients with spinal muscular atrophy (SMA). Patients with SMA typically have a more progressive history of weakness. Neonatal myasthenia gravis is caused by maternally acquired antibodies against postsynaptic membranes acetylcholine receptors. Symptoms can be very similar to botulism, but there is typically a maternal history of myasthenia gravis, and clinical signs are usually present within hours to days of birth. Many mitochondrial myopathies are caused by genetic mutations in mitochondrial DNA, which subsequently alter mitochondrial metabolism. The acute nature of this patient's presentation makes mitochondrial myopathy less likely. IgG anti–GQ1b antibody and molecular mimicry is thought to be responsible for Miller Fisher syndrome, a rare variant of Guillain-Barré syndrome. Classically, this condition presents following an acute infection that triggers an abnormal autoimmune response and presents with ophthalmoplegia, ataxia, and areflexia.

[ABP 1.A.9. Neuromuscular disorders]

REFERENCE

1. Rosow LK, Strober JB. Infant botulism: review and clinical update. *Pediatr Neurol.* 2015;*52*(5):487–492.

108. ANSWER: B

This patient's presentation is most concerning for suppurative cervical lymphadenitis with abscess formation. Infectious causes of cervical lymphadenopathy include acute reactive, subacute/chronic, mycobacterial, fungal, and parasitic. Common viruses that can trigger acute reactive lymphadenopathy include rhinovirus, adenovirus, influenza, parainfluenza, and respiratory syncytial virus. Suppurative cervical lymphadenitis is most often caused by *Staphylococcus aureus*, group A *Streptococcus*, rarely anaerobes, and (in neonates) group B *Streptococcus*. While neck ultrasound is noninvasive with no radiation exposure, high suspicion of abscess formation (along with concern for deep-space neck involvement) should prompt more detailed contrast-enhanced imaging. CT remains popular for lymph node imaging due to its wide availability, speed, and excellent spatial resolution. While viral lymphadenitis will resolve without treatment within 7 days, antibiotic coverage is indicated for bacterial causes. As this patient has failed outpatient treatment with amoxicillin/clavulanate, IV antibiotic treatment with clindamycin or vancomycin to cover methicillin-resistant staphylococcus aureus (MRSA) is indicated. If there is insufficient improvement after 48–72 hours, broadening antibiotics to include coverage of anaerobes and gram-negative organisms would be appropriate. To date, no predictive factors for the need of surgery have been identified, including size and location of suppurated nodes. Therefore, image-guided aspiration or surgical drainage should be reserved for patients who fail appropriate second- and third-line antibiotics.

[ABP 1.B.2. Neck masses and infections]

REFERENCE

1. Weinstock MS, Patel NA, Smith LP. Pediatric cervical lymphadenopathy. *Pediatr Rev.* 2018;*39*(9):433–443.

109. ANSWER: A

Many factors play a role in the decision for central line removal for patients with a central line–associated bloodstream infection (CLABSI). In a patient who depends on the line for nutrition, there are risks associated with removal, with limited vascular access sites in addition to the baseline risks associated with the procedure and repeat anesthesia. Indications for removal of a tunneled central line are if the line is irreparably disrupted (e.g., broken or occluded), the patient is significantly ill appearing, the infection is disseminated, bacteremia cannot be cleared after 48–72 hours of treatment, or there is evidence of fungemia.

Not all infections with gram-negative species require line removal, though line salvage attempts with certain organisms such as *Pseudomonas* or drug-resistant gram-negative bacilli are often unsuccessful. This is also the case for *Staphylococcus aureus* infections. The most common bacteria isolated in CLABSIs is coagulase-negative *Staphylococcus*, which can usually be treated with antibiotics alone. Time to positivity of a culture and timing of central line placement are not indications for removal.

[ABP 1.O.3. Bloodstream infections (bacteremia)]

110. ANSWER: E

Although the placenta is impermeable to maternal TSH, maternal thyroid-stimulating immunoglobulins and medications for maternal Graves' disease can both cross the placenta and influence the newborn's thyroid function. While prematurity and low birth weight are both associated with immaturity of the thyroid axis, there are set reference ranges for these populations that should allow the results to be properly interpreted. Because of the TSH surge that occurs within the first 12 hours of life, a newborn screen that is collected too early can lead to a false-positive result, but a screen obtained after 24 hours of life would not.

[ABP 1.I.3. Hypo and hyperthyroidism]

111. ANSWER: A

Surface PCR from open lesions is the preferred test to diagnose an active HSV infection. HSV serology is less preferred as a test for HSV infection as studies have shown that up to 30% of infants of mothers with HSV-1 may seroconvert by 30 months of age without a clear history of HSV lesions. In children and adolescents, vulvar ulcers may have many other causes, including Epstein-Barr virus and cytomegalovirus infection, neither of which are sexually acquired. Therefore, testing is important prior to concluding that sexual abuse has occurred or before initiation of empiric therapy. In addition, in young children who still require assistance from caretakers with hygiene and toileting, HSV-1– or HSV-2–related genital ulcers may be acquired through nonsexual contact. Genital HSV infections are therefore still considered indeterminate for sexual abuse. A forensic genital examination should be conducted after a sexual abuse allegation is made, ideally within 24 hours of sexual contact, but is not likely to yield results in this case.

[ABP 1.J.2. Sexual abuse]

REFERENCE

1. Adams JA. Guidelines for medical care of children evaluated for suspected sexual abuse: an update for 2008. *Curr Opin Obstet Gynecol*. 2008;20(5):435–441.

112. ANSWER: B

This patient has an AKI, as evidenced by his serum creatinine of 1.4 mg/dL. While his baseline creatinine is unknown, the upper limit of normal for his age is 1.0 mg/dL. He has no history of kidney disease and no evidence of CKD on ultrasound, so CKD is unlikely. AKI is classified as prerenal, intrinsic, and postrenal. Postrenal AKI is characterized by an obstruction in the collecting system, which this patient has no evidence of by ultrasound. Prerenal AKI is characterized by decreased perfusion to the kidneys. Intrinsic AKI is characterized by damage to the renal parenchyma that reduces kidney function. This patient's watery diarrhea suggests a prerenal AKI due to hypovolemia, while his frequent use of ibuprofen puts him at risk for intrinsic AKI due to drug nephrotoxicity. The fractional excretion of sodium (FENa) is the standard formula used for differentiating between prerenal and intrinsic AKI for pediatric patients. The formula is

Percentage FENa = (Urine Sodium × Serum Creatinine)/(Urine Creatinine × Serum Sodium) × 100

A FENa of less than 1% suggests a prerenal etiology, while a FENa greater than 2% suggests an intrinsic AKI. This patient's FENa is 3%, suggesting that his AKI is intrinsic. His relatively low urine specific gravity, relatively high urine sodium, and the epithelial cell casts in his urine all support a diagnosis of acute tubular necrosis (ATN). FENa may be less accurate in neonates and patients who have received intravenous fluids or diuretics.

[ABP 1.F.2. Acute kidney injury]

113. ANSWER: B

The patient likely has oligoarticular juvenile idiopathic arthritis (JIA). Criteria for the diagnosis of JIA include age less than 16 years and at least 6 weeks of symptoms. JIA is classified into subcategories, with this patient having oligoarticular JIA due to fewer than four joints affected. Oligoarticular is the most common form of JIA and most often presents with monoarticular arthritis of the knee. It is more common in girls than boys. Children with oligoarticular JIA often do not have systemic symptoms or significant pain and usually have a good overall prognosis. Inflammatory markers may be normal.

While these patients will often be followed by a rheumatologist, the diagnosis and initial treatment with NSAIDs is often done by hospitalists after ruling out infectious and oncologic causes. The initial treatments of oligoarticular JIA are NSAIDs and/or intra-articular corticosteroid injections. If symptoms do not improve, the next steps in JIA management may include systemic corticosteroids, disease-modifying antirheumatic drugs, and/or biologic agents. Children with oligoarticular JIA are at risk for anterior uveitis and should be referred to an ophthalmologist.

[ABP 1.H.3. Inflammatory arthritis]

114. ANSWER: B

This girl's skin lesion is most consistent with a cutaneous abscess without surrounding cellulitis. According to guidelines from the Infectious Diseases Society of America (IDSA), purulent skin and soft tissue infections (SSTIs) such as abscesses should be treated with incision and drainage. Mild SSTIs such as this one can be treated with incision and drainage alone. Signs of systemic illness (e.g., fever, tachypnea, tachycardia, or abnormal white blood cell count); evidence of deeper or more serious infection (e.g., bullae, skin sloughing, hypotension, or organ dysfunction); or SSTI in an immunocompromised patient are indications for systemic antibiotics. Intravenous antimicrobials are indicated in cases of treatment failure or severe systemic symptoms. Antimicrobial therapy should be tailored to the local antibiogram. If the incision and drainage can be completed in the emergency department and follow-up ensured, this patient does not require hospitalization.

[ABP 1.K.1. Skin and soft tissue infections]

REFERENCE

1. Stevens DL, Bisno AL, Chambers HF, et al. Practice guidelines for the diagnosis and management of skin and soft tissue infections: 2014 update by the Infectious Diseases Society of America. *Clin Infect Dis.* 2014;59(2):e10–e52.

115. ANSWER: B

Appendicitis usually presents with diffuse abdominal pain that localizes to the right lower quadrant and is often accompanied by vomiting. However, children under the age of 5 may not localize their pain as well as older children. They are also more likely to have diarrhea due to an inflamed appendix causing irritation of the colon. This is less common in older children. Lactase deficiency is unlikely to present acutely and would not be accompanied by a fever. Transient lactase deficiency may follow a gastroenteritis, although fever and vomiting have usually resolved. Some viruses cause a large increase in the amount of secreted water in the intestines, often leading to large-volume diarrhea. *Escherichia coli* infections can dramatically remodel the lining of the intestines, leading to a loss of surface area available for absorption. While these viral and bacterial infections could account for some of this patient's symptoms, they rarely cause guarding on physical examination.

[ABP 1.E.1. Appendicitis]

116. ANSWER: A

Von Willebrand disease is the most common inherited bleeding disorder. Inheritance may be autosomal dominant or autosomal recessive, and children may present at any age depending on the level of reduction in von Willebrand factor activity. It is characterized by mucocutaneous bleeding. Common manifestations include petechiae, ecchymoses, epistaxis, prolonged bleeding following trauma or surgery, and menorrhagia in females. In contrast, patients with hemophilia typically present with bleeding in joints and muscles. Inheritance of hemophilia is X linked, such that males are affected and females are asymptomatic carriers. Bernard-Soulier and Wiskott-Aldrich are inherited platelet function disorders and relatively uncommon. Both syndromes may present with thrombocytopenia. Patients with Bernard-Soulier may have large platelets noted on peripheral smear, whereas patients with Wiskott-Aldrich will have small platelets.

[ABP 1.L.3. Bleeding disorders]

117. ANSWER: C

Hyperimmunoglobulin E recurrent infection syndrome is a rare autosomal dominant condition in which patients have recurrent skin and pulmonary infections as well as chronic eczema. It is due to genetic mutations of the JAK-STAT signaling pathway that lead to impaired T-helper cells and decreased neutrophil chemotaxis, causing increased susceptibility to fungal and bacterial infections. Clinical manifestations include chronic dermatitis, upper airway infections, sinusitis, and suppurative otitis media. Hyperimmunoglobulin E recurrent infection syndrome is associated with poor osteoclastogenesis and osteopenia, which may lead to skeletal abnormalities, including delay in shedding of primary teeth, recurrent fractures, hyperextensible joints, and scoliosis.

Aphthous ulcers are associated with selective immunoglobulin (Ig) A deficiency. Facial tetany can be a symptom of DiGeorge syndrome due to hypocalcemia caused by underdevelopment of the parathyroid gland. DiGeorge syndrome can be associated with T-cell immunodeficiency due to aplasia or hypoplasia of the thalamus. Thrombocytopenia is associated with Wiskott-Aldrich syndrome (WAS), which typically presents with eczema, thrombocytopenia, and recurrent infections. Because it is X linked, WAS almost exclusively effects males. Peripheral neuropathy can be seen in common variable immunodeficiency (CVID). Patients with CVID present with recurrent sinopulmonary and gastrointestinal infections; diagnosis before age 6 should be classified as preliminary due to immunologic immaturity and, in some children, the persistence of agammaglobulinemia.

[ABP 1.M.2. Immunodeficiencies]

118. ANSWER: E

Myocarditis is an inflammatory disease of the myocardium that can be precipitated by bacterial and viral infections, toxins, autoimmune diseases, and hypersensitivity reactions. The clinical presentation can range from sudden death, arrythmias, symptoms mimicking myocardial infarction, and acute heart failure. Endocardial biopsy remains the gold standard for a true confirmatory diagnosis of myocarditis. A chest x-ray may aid diagnosis by showing signs of heart failure such as cardiomegaly or pulmonary edema. An ECG will often have variable abnormalities, such as sinus tachycardia, ventricular hypertrophy, ST-segment and T-wave abnormalities, or arrythmias. An echocardiogram can show left ventricular dysfunction, decreased ejection fraction, atrioventricular valve regurgitation, and wall motion abnormalities. Cardiac MRI can show myocarditis findings such as myocardial edema, inflammation, and fibrosis. Despite the relatively high sensitivity and specificity of cardiac MRI for the diagnosis of myocarditis, it is not the gold standard.

[ABP 1.D.5. Endocarditis, myocarditis, and pericarditis]

119. ANSWER: B

The combination of mild hypotension, bradycardia, altered mental status, respiratory depression, and miosis is concerning for acute opioid toxicity, which is treated with naloxone. Many synthetic opioids, such as methadone, may not be detected on urine drug screens. Since methadone's half-life far exceeds that of naloxone, this patient should be admitted in case of need for additional doses or a continuous infusion of naloxone. Naltrexone is a longer-acting opioid antagonist used for maintenance of abstinence, but naloxone is preferred for acute opioid intoxication reversal. Flumazenil would be indicated in benzodiazepine ingestion; however, in cases of benzodiazepine overdose, the respiratory depression is not as profound, and the pupils are generally not affected. Gastrointestinal decontamination techniques such as gastric lavage are not indicated in patients with altered mental status due to their unclear benefit as well as the risk of aspiration. Atropine and pralidoxime are used in combination for cases of organophosphate exposure. These patients generally have additional symptoms such as excess salivation and sweating.

[ABP 1.N.1. Ingestions (intentional and unintentional)]

120. ANSWER: A

This patient has a history and presentation that is concerning for cystic fibrosis (CF), and discharge planning should include a chloride sweat test to assess this further. Sweat testing should be done at a certified center given the need for skilled sample collection and handling.

Clues from this patient's history include constipation, chronic cough, and poor weight gain. His presentation with mild hypoxia and likely mucus plugging on chest radiograph is concerning for an acute pulmonary exacerbation. While all 50 states screen for cystic fibrosis with newborn screening tests, screening may miss between 2% and 5% of cases.

In patients with clinical suspicion for CF, the chloride sweat test remains the preferred method for diagnosis. Subsequent testing for *CFTR* gene mutations can aid diagnosis if the sweat test results are unclear or help guide the development of genotype-specific treatment plans. A CT scan is unnecessary in this patient who is beginning to recover from his acute illness. In patients with CF, advanced imaging is not likely to show any chronic changes at this early age. Immunoglobulin testing is used for patients with suspicion for common variable immune deficiency (CVID) and other primary immunodeficiencies that may present with recurrent bacterial infections of the respiratory tract. While this patient and his family may benefit from additional social services, including assistance with establishing a pediatrician, a referral to Child Protective Services would be premature.

[ABP 1.C.5. Chronic respiratory conditions]

REFERENCE

1. Farrell PM, White TB, Ren CL, et al. Diagnosis of cystic fibrosis: consensus guidelines from the Cystic Fibrosis Foundation. *J Pediatr.* 2017;*181S*:S4–S15.e1.

121. ANSWER: C

Clinical symptoms of anti-NMDA encephalitis may mimic psychiatric disorders or substance-induced psychosis. Anti-NMDA encephalitis, one of many autoimmune encephalitides, can present with a constellation of neuropsychiatric symptoms, including abnormal or bizarre behavior, delusions, hallucinations, agitation, psychosis, disrupted sleep patterns, short-term memory deficits, fluctuating levels of arousal, and dyskinesias. These neuropsychiatric symptoms may be preceded by a viral-like illness and occur progressively over several weeks to months. In addition, these patients may have notable autonomic instability causing abnormal temperature regulation, hypertension, tachycardia, and bradycardia. Anti-NMDA encephalitis has been associated with ovarian teratomas and herpes simplex virus (HSV) encephalitis. Diagnostic workup typically reveals cerebrospinal fluid (CSF) pleocytosis, magnetic resonance imaging findings suggestive of encephalitis, and/or new-onset seizures on electroencephalography. The presence of anti-NMDA receptor antibodies in the CSF confirms the diagnosis.

Synthetic cathinone intoxication would manifest with sympathomimetic toxidrome symptoms such as tachycardia, hyperthermia, hypertension, mydriasis, agitation, and seizures. Synthetic compounds, such as bath salts, may not be detected on routine urine drug screening. The patient's subacute presentation with no clear infectious symptoms such as fever, rash, or meningeal signs makes viral encephalitis less likely. She has not had any specific risk factors for HIV infection. A progressive stepwise neuropsychiatric decline is not consistent with a cerebrovascular accident.

[ABP 1.A.5. Encephalitis]

REFERENCE

1. Barbagallo M, Vitaliti G, Pavone P, Romano C, Lubrano R, Falsaperla R. Pediatric autoimmune encephalitis. *J Pediatr Neurosci.* 2017;*12*(2):130–134.

122. ANSWER: B

Etiologies of subacute (lasting 2 to 6 weeks) and chronic (lasting greater than 6 weeks) neck masses include *Bartonella henselae*, toxoplasmosis, viruses (e.g., Epstein-Barr virus, cytomegalovirus, human immunodeficiency virus), mycobacteria, and malignancy. Immediately or several weeks after exposure, *B. henselae* causes granulomatous inflammation, often through the scratch or bite of a cat, and can involve multiple organ systems, including the central nervous system. *Toxoplasma gondii* may present with nontender, nonsuppurative LAD and can be diagnosed with serum polymerase chain reaction (PCR). Nontuberculous mycobacteria (NTM) typically cause afebrile, chronic, nontender, unilateral cervical LAD in the submandibular region of immunocompetent children. Increased incidence of NTM lymphadenitis has been linked to age less than 3 years, female gender, and colder environmental temperatures. Purified protein derivative skin testing is often negative, and fine-needle aspiration with acid-fast bacillus staining is often necessary to confirm diagnosis. While treatment options are variable, with combinations of medical and surgical interventions, complete surgical excision results in greater than 95% cure rates compared to 66% with medical therapy alone. *Mycobacterium tuberculosis* can also cause chronic cervical LAD, termed scrofula, typically in the supraclavicular area. Incision and drainage of mycobacterial lesions should be avoided due to the potential for fistula formation. Historical and clinical features of LAD can be helpful in distinguishing infectious from oncologic etiologies (Table 1.9). While CT scans can be helpful for diagnosing and staging malignancy, CT is not indicated for this patient initially. Panoramic radiographs would be low yield in the absence of dental findings.

[ABP 1.B.2. Neck masses and infections]

Table 1.9 COMPARISON OF TYPICAL HISTORICAL AND CLINICAL FEATURES OF LYMPHADENOPATHY CAUSED BY INFECTIOUS AND ONCOLOGIC PROCESSES

	INFECTIOUS	ONCOLOGIC
History	Preceding upper respiratory infection	Night sweats, fatigue, easy bleeding/bruising, weight loss
Location	Bilateral or unilateral	Unilateral
Consistency	Soft, fluctuant	Firm, indurated, rubbery
Mobility	Freely mobile	Fixed, matted
Duration	<2 weeks	>2 weeks
Location	Submandibular, anterior/posterior cervical	Supraclavicular
Tenderness	Usually tender, can be nontender	Usually nontender

REFERENCE

1. Zimmermann P, Curtis N, Tebruegge M. Nontuberculous mycobacterial disease in childhood—update on diagnostic approaches and treatment. *J Infect.* 2017;*74*(suppl 1):S136–S142.

123. ANSWER: B

When considering prolonged fever, one should differentiate fever without a source (FWS), fever of unknown origin (FUO), pseudo-FUO, and factitious fever. Pseudo-FUO is the result of serial infections in which the fevers abate and recur with persistent vague symptoms. This case is most consistent with pseudo-FUO. Therefore, reassurance and monitoring are all that are indicated at this time. FWS is defined as fever for less than 1 week without an explanation after a thorough history and examination. Although the time cutoff varies, FUO is generally defined as daily fever for greater than 1–2 weeks, during which a cause has not been identified despite a thorough clinical evaluation. Factitious fever is defined by false manipulation of the thermometer or misinterpretation of the actual temperature.

An echocardiogram should be done if there is a concern for Kawasaki disease with prolonged fever. Toxic-appearing, clinically unstable patients may require empiric antibiotics without a clear source of infection. Consultation with a rheumatologist could be considered if there are specific findings such as rash, joint pain/swelling, relapsing fevers, or family history concerning for autoimmune disease. CRP and ESR can be used as screening laboratory tests for FUO, but are nonspecific.

[ABP 1.O.5. Fever of unknown origin (prolonged/recurrent)]

124. ANSWER: D

This child most likely has ketotic hypoglycemia of childhood, a condition which typically presents by age 5 and remits in preadolescence. High ketones with appropriately decreased insulin are expected. Other gluconeogenic precursors, such as free fatty acids and amino acids, are high. Cortisol and growth hormone, which are counterregulatory hormones, are also high.

This patient's presentation is classic, with episodes occurring in the morning after a prolonged fast. Concurrent stress, high activity levels, and viral illnesses can also be precipitating factors. This condition is a diagnosis of exclusion. Ideally, a critical sample including a confirmatory serum glucose, ketones, growth hormone, cortisol, insulin, lactate, free fatty acids, ammonia, and free/total carnitine should be collected before giving glucose replacement. Once the diagnosis is established, the family should be advised to provide frequent high-protein, high-carbohydrate meals and avoid periods of prolonged fasting. Normal or high insulin levels and low ketones would be consistent with hyperinsulinism, which is much less likely to present at this age.

[ABP 1.I.7. Hypoglycemia]

125. ANSWER: E

In this patient, the reported history of complaints is not congruent with the reassuring physical examination and laboratory data seen on evaluation. This raises concern for medical child abuse. In these situations, caregivers may falsify symptoms by creating the appearance of blood in the stools. Hospitalization for close observation of parent-child interactions is often recommended, with close communication among hospital care providers regarding any unusual or inappropriate parental behaviors. While food allergies and infections can present with bloody stools, further testing for these conditions with allergy testing or stool culture, respectively, is unlikely to yield the diagnosis due to a discrepancy between the caregiver's report of symptoms and objective data. In particular, a normal hemoglobin would not be expected with prolonged bloody stools in this age group. Additionally, the patient's normal weight gain is reassuring against inflammatory bowel disease, making colonoscopy and fecal calprotectin testing unnecessary.

[ABP 1.J.3. Medical child abuse]

126. ANSWER: E

This patient most likely has a benign, mature teratoma (also called a dermoid cyst). Teratomas are the most common ovarian masses in the second and third decades of life. Benign teratomas classically appear as complex cystic masses arising from the ovary; these masses may contain a range of tissues, including teeth (which appear as calcified foci on this patient's CT scan). They are most often unilateral but can be bilateral. Malignant (also called immature) teratomas are more likely to be completely solid lesions and are much less common. Though uncommon, rupture of a benign teratoma can occur, allowing the typically sebaceous cystic fluid to leak into the abdomen, causing a shock-like presentation with hypotension as well as chemical peritonitis with pain and fever. As with any adnexal mass, there is a risk of ovarian torsion. Malignant transformation of a benign teratoma is uncommon but can occur in 0.2%–2% of all benign teratomas. Anti-NMDA receptor encephalitis is a rare but serious complication of both mature and immature teratomas. While in exceedingly rare cases benign teratomas can secrete hormones, the presence of or removal of the mass is not likely to cause Addison disease.

[ABP 1.F.8. Ovarian cysts and torsion]

127. ANSWER: A

This patient's clinical presentation is concerning for macrophage activation syndrome (MAS), an emergent and life-threatening complication of sJIA and other inflammatory conditions. It may be idiopathic or triggered by a disease flare, infection, or medication. MAS presents with high unremitting fevers; central nervous system dysfunction (headache, lethargy, seizure, or coma); and joint symptoms. MAS may occur at any time in the sJIA course. Lymphadenopathy, hepatomegaly, splenomegaly, and petechiae may be present.

A paradoxically falling ESR can be an important clue and can help distinguish MAS from infection or sJIA flare. In MAS, liver dysfunction and fibrin consumption lead to hypofibrinogenemia, which decreases the ESR. In MAS, ferritin, CRP, triglycerides, LDH, and transaminases are often elevated, while cell counts, ESR, and albumin are typically decreased. Comparing results with baseline values is important, as white blood cell counts, platelets, and inflammatory markers are often elevated in patients with sJIA at baseline and may be within the laboratory reference range during MAS.

Expert consensus suggests the following diagnostic criteria for MAS diagnosis:

1. Fever, and
2. Ferritin level greater than 684 ng/mL, and
3. Any two of the following:
   a. Platelets less than 182×10^9/L
   b. AST greater than 48 units/L
   c. Triglycerides greater than 156 mg/dL
   d. Fibrinogen less than 361 mg/dL

Treatment of sJIA-associated MAS typically involves high-dose corticosteroids. Other treatments include cyclosporine, cyclophosphamide, intravenous immunoglobulin, anakinra, and interleukin 6 inhibitors.

[ABP 1.H.3. Inflammatory arthritis]

REFERENCE

1. Ravelli A, Minoia F, Davì S, et al. 2016 classification criteria for macrophage activation syndrome complicating systemic juvenile idiopathic arthritis: a European League Against Rheumatism/American College of Rheumatology/Paediatric Rheumatology International Trials Organisation collaborative initiative. *Arthritis Rheumatol.* 2016;68(3):566–576.

128. ANSWER: D

Enteroviral vesicular stomatitis, also known as hand, foot, and mouth disease (HFMD), is a common illness caused by nonpolio enteroviruses such as coxsackie viruses. Clinical manifestations include oral enanthem and rash on the hands, feet, and diaper region. The rash can be vesicular, macular, or papular. The clinical course for HFMD is self-limiting, although children may require hospitalization for supportive care, including intravenous fluids and pain control, until oral lesions and fluid intake improve. Laboratory testing, antiviral therapy, antibiotic therapy, and skin biopsy are not indicated. HFMD is a clinical diagnosis.

[ABP 1.K.2. Dermatologic manifestations of systemic illnesses]

129. ANSWER: C

Hemolytic uremic syndrome (HUS), while uncommon, can occur in up to 10% of patients infected with the O157:H7 strain of enterohemorrhagic *E. coli*. HUS is more common in children under the age of 5, and symptoms often present 5–10 days after a prodrome of abdominal pain, vomiting, and bloody diarrhea. HUS presents with the sudden onset of hemolytic anemia, thrombocytopenia, and acute kidney injury. Children may present with paleness or fatigue due to anemia, bruising due to thrombocytopenia (though rarely bleeding), and decreased urine output. Central nervous system symptoms may be present in up to 25% of patients and include lethargy and seizures. Other bacterial (and viral) infections can lead to bloody stools, although the relationship with HUS is much less common. Treatment is supportive care, with some patients requiring blood transfusions and dialysis.

[ABP 1.E.4. Gastroenteritis]

130. ANSWER: C

Immune thrombocytopenia purpura is defined by a platelet count less than $100,000/mm^3$ in the absence of other causes of thrombocytopenia. In ITP, antiplatelet antibodies cause severely shortened platelet survival time. ITP may be a primary process or secondary to a viral infection, live vaccine, or other condition. The physician in this vignette selected glucocorticoids as first-line therapy, which is appropriate when bleeding risks are not severe. In contrast, intravenous immune globulin (IVIG) is the preferred therapy when a rapid rise in platelets is desired. The clinician should be aware that both therapies have significant side effects. Given their overlapping age distribution and presenting signs, acute leukemia and aplastic anemia must be excluded in cases of suspected ITP. Steroids can induce a temporary remission in patients with acute lymphoblastic leukemia, delaying the diagnosis of malignancy. Thus, it is crucial to obtain a peripheral smear before initiating steroids. Anti-D immune globulin is another common therapy for ITP in patients with Rh-positive blood types, so Rh status must be determined before using this therapy. Prothrombin time and partial thromboplastin time may be included in the general evaluation of a suspected coagulation disorder but are not specifically needed before starting corticosteroids in this patient. A fibrinogen level may be obtained in systemically ill patients where disseminated intravascular coagulation is suspected. The indirect Coombs test detects antibodies against foreign red blood cells. It is used prior to red blood cell transfusion and in prenatal testing of pregnant women. Complications of IVIG include anaphylaxis, aseptic meningitis, hemolysis, and thromboembolic events.

[ABP 1.L.5. Isolated thrombocytopenia]

131. ANSWER: A

Fever in a 6-week-old patient should prompt consideration of bacterial infections, such as urinary tract infection (UTI), bacteremia, and meningitis. Any ill-appearing infant in this age group should receive a full sepsis workup, including urinalysis and urine culture, blood culture, and cerebrospinal fluid analysis. However, well-appearing infants older than 28 days are generally able to safely receive a more limited initial workup. Several recommendations have been made regarding the management of these infants, including most recently the American Academy of Pediatrics (AAP) Clinical Practice Guideline (CPG) on Febrile Infants. Virtually all sources call for a urinalysis, as UTI is the most common cause of bacterial infection in this age group.

While an LP is usually indicated for infants younger than 28 days, the risk of missing meningitis is lower after the first month of life, so most sources (including the recent AAP CPG) recommend initial testing to determine the risk of invasive bacterial infection (IBI) prior to an LP. Previous studies have suggested using white blood cell count for this risk assessment; the most recent AAP CPG recommends using procalcitonin, absolute neutrophil count, and/or C-reactive protein. Patients with elevated inflammatory markers may be candidates for LP. There is no role for ESR in the workup of febrile infants. There is currently no evidence that detection of a virus can effectively rule out a bacterial process, so a respiratory pathogen panel would not be the most important test. A chest radiograph would only be indicated if there were respiratory symptoms concerning for pneumonia or other pulmonary pathology.

[ABP 1.O.4. Fever in infants less than 60 days]

REFERENCE

1. Pantell RH, Roberts KB, Adams WG, et al. Evaluation and management of well-appearing febrile infants 8 to 60 days old. *Pediatrics.* 2021;*148*(2):e2021052228.

132. ANSWER: A

This patient presents with classic symptoms for pericarditis, including fever and chest pain that worsens with deep breathing and improves with sitting upright and leaning forward. Her prodrome of upper respiratory symptoms makes this presentation highly suspicious for viral pericarditis. In children with viral pericarditis, inflammation of the pericardium can lead to increased membrane permeability and resultant fluid accumulation between the visceral and parietal pericardial layers. The first-line treatment for viral pericarditis is a high-dose NSAID. Colchicine is not indicated as a first-line treatment, although it may be a possible adjunct in cases of recurrent pericarditis. A pericardiocentesis is typically only indicated for diagnostic purposes if the etiology of pericarditis is under question or for therapeutic purposes if there is evidence of tamponade. Corticosteroids are reserved for consideration if an NSAID does not work. Empiric antibiotics may be indicated if a bacterial source is suspected; in this case the patient's presentation is more consistent with a viral process.

[ABP 1.D.5. Endocarditis, myocarditis, and pericarditis]

133. ANSWER: D

Antifreeze contains compounds to decrease a solution's freezing point. Some of these compounds can include toxic alcohols such as ethylene glycol. Toxic alcohol ingestion leads to an anion gap metabolic acidosis. This may indirectly lead to a respiratory alkalosis with a low (<40 mm Hg) rather than elevated $PaCO_2$. While ethanol ingestion can also lead to an anion gap metabolic acidosis, ethylene glycol is more likely to be found in antifreeze and would not cause an elevated ethanol level. Evidence of liver or kidney injury is not generally seen early in the course of toxic alcohol ingestion.

[ABP 1.N.1. Ingestions (intentional and unintentional)]

134. ANSWER: E

This patient's upper respiratory symptoms and physical examination findings on auscultation (often described as "washing machine sounds") are concerning for acute bronchiolitis. In 2014, the American Academy of Pediatrics

(AAP) released guidelines with recommendations about how to diagnose and treat bronchiolitis.

Previously, it was thought that steroids would help to decrease inflammation and improve the course of the disease. This has been studied extensively and found not to be the case; steroids of any kind are not recommended.

Bronchiolitis is a clinical diagnosis and does not require further imaging or laboratory work in order to diagnosis it. Chest radiographs are commonly obtained when patients present with respiratory symptoms but are not needed when the patient's diagnosis can be made from history and physical examination. Given that wheeze is a common symptom in bronchiolitis, inhaled short-acting β-agonists such as albuterol and levalbuterol have been commonly used in the past. While some initial studies demonstrated improvement in clinical symptom scores, larger randomized controlled trials found no benefit. Thus, they are not recommended for routine use in bronchiolitis.

A large Cochrane review of nine randomized controlled trials studying the effects of chest physiotherapy found no evidence of clinical benefit. Oxygen saturations are a common reason for admission in patients who are diagnosed with bronchiolitis. Placing patients on continuous pulse oximetry has been shown to increase length of stay without improving outcomes and is thus not routinely recommended in patients admitted with bronchiolitis.

[ABP 1.C.1. Bronchiolitis]

REFERENCE

1. Roqué i Figuls M, Giné-Garriga M, Granados Rugeles C, Perrotta C. Chest physiotherapy for acute bronchiolitis in paediatric patients between 0 and 24 months old. *Cochrane Database Syst Rev.* 2012;(2):CD004873.

135. ANSWER: D

This patient is suffering from a migraine headache. She is presenting with classic symptoms of headache associated with nausea, vomiting, and photophobia. Patients may also experience visual changes, such as auras, scintillations, or scotomas, prior to the migraine. Usually, there is a known family history of migraines. In the acute setting, an abortive therapy such as a triptan is typically used with an antiemetic and fluids. Of the options available, the best combination of medications is intravenous ketorolac and intravenous prochlorperazine. Her headache is severe and refractory to outpatient oral acetaminophen with caffeine and has been going on for more than 24 hours. Acetaminophen and ibuprofen are not likely to treat her refractory headache, and she likely will not tolerate oral medications given her persistent nausea and vomiting. There is no role for opioids in the treatment of migraines. Intravenous promethazine can cause severe tissue damage, and its use should be avoided, if possible. Topiramate is used as a daily preventive medication, as are propranolol and amitriptyline; none of these would be helpful in acute management.

[ABP 1.A.6. Headaches]

REFERENCE

1. Oskoui M, Pringsheim T, Holler-Managan Y, et al. Practice guideline update summary: acute treatment of migraine in children and adolescents: report of the Guideline Development, Dissemination, and Implementation Subcommittee of the American Academy of Neurology and the American Headache Society. *Neurology*. 2019;93(11):487–499.

136. ANSWER: D

This patient's clinical presentation is highly suspicious for epiglottitis, with abrupt onset of respiratory distress, drooling, and dysphagia (the "3 Ds"). Due to the rapid progression of this disease, management of epiglottitis revolves on securing the airway and should be done with the assistance of a critical airway team.

The incidence of epiglottitis has decreased significantly due to vaccination against the main pathogen, *Haemophilus influenzae* type B. Still, it can be found in unvaccinated and immunocompromised children and adults. The onset of symptoms is usually abrupt, with only a mild and very short prodrome, if any. Patients commonly have drooling, dysphagia, sore throat, anxiety, stridor, and a muffled or "hot potato" voice. Cough is typically absent. Children are generally toxic appearing and may present in "tripod or sniffing position" to maximally open the airway. The diagnosis is typically clinical, and while lateral neck radiographs may support the diagnosis with evidence of an enlarged epiglottis ("thumb sign") or thickened aryepiglottic folds, it is not required and may even delay urgent management. Direct visualization by an otolaryngologist can confirm the diagnosis and assess severity of obstruction. An experienced specialist or team should initiate endotracheal intubation, preferably in a controlled setting prior to worsening decompensation. Subsequently, antibiotics should be initiated with a third-generation cephalosporin and antistaphylococcal agent. Corticosteroids do not have a role in the treatment of epiglottitis.

[ABP 1.B.1. Upper airway infections and conditions]

137. ANSWER: D

This patient is presenting with prolonged fevers consistent with fever of unknown origin (FUO). The quotidian fever with associated self-resolving evanescent, salmon-pink rash is strongly suggestive of juvenile idiopathic arthritis (JIA). This is further supported by fatigue, lymphadenopathy, mild anemia, and elevated inflammatory markers. Arthralgias are common early in the course of JIA, but arthritis is not always prominent until later. Consultation with a rheumatologist is recommended for guidance to make the definitive diagnosis. In the setting of 3 weeks of fever with abnormal laboratory findings, trending the fevers without additional evaluation would be insufficient. Osteoarticular infections should be considered with prolonged fever, joint pain, and elevated inflammatory markers. However, such infections are unlikely to be bilateral; therefore, obtaining an MRI to evaluate for osteomyelitis would not be the best next step. *Bartonella* is often associated with solitary lymphadenopathy and unlikely in this patient with bilateral lymphadenopathy. This patient only has mild leukocytosis and anemia; therefore, a peripheral smear is unlikely to be helpful.

[ABP 1.O.5. Fever of unknown origin]

138. ANSWER: E

There are three first-line tests for Cushing syndrome: 24-hour urinary free cortisol excretion, late-night salivary cortisol, and overnight dexamethasone suppression test. Diagnosis requires abnormal results for at least two of these tests. An ACTH stimulation test is useful in the diagnosis of adrenal insufficiency but has no role in the diagnosis of Cushing syndrome.

Because cortisol is secreted in a diurnal pattern, with highest levels in the morning and lowest levels close to midnight, random cortisol values are not helpful. As in this case, iatrogenic Cushing syndrome may be seen in the setting of oral glucocorticoid use. Prednisone is the most likely causative agent.

[ABP 1.I.5. Adrenal disorders]

139. ANSWER: A

This patient has glomerulonephritis (GN) due to immunoglobulin (Ig) A nephropathy. There are many causes of gross hematuria, but more common causes such as nephrolithiasis and urine infection are less likely for this patient, who has no symptoms to suggest either diagnosis. This patient likely has bacterial pharyngitis, most likely from *Streptococcus*. The history of gross hematuria during an acute illness (sometimes called synpharyngitic hematuria) as well as similar symptoms with illness in the past is highly suggestive of IgA nephropathy. While postinfectious GN also has an association with infection (classically *Streptococcus* pharyngitis), the onset of GN is typically later in the illness course or after recovery from infection, and the history of prior episodes of hematuria would not be expected. As seen in the table below, postinfectious GN typically has low C3 and normal C4, while IgA nephropathy typically has normal complement levels. Low C3 and C4 is associated with lupus nephritis. Membranoproliferative glomerulonephritis is typically associated with low or normal C3 and a low C4.

	C3	C4
IgA nephropathy	Normal	Normal
Postinfectious GN	Low	Normal
Lupus nephritis	Low	Low
Membranoproliferative GN	Low/Normal	Low

[ABP 1.F.3. Glomerulonephritis]

140. ANSWER: E

Despite a presenting complaint of knee pain, this patient's stools, abdominal pain, weight loss, oral ulcers, and anemia (as suggested by her pallor) are suggestive of inflammatory bowel disease (IBD). The differential for arthritis is broad. Given her specific symptoms and findings, esophagogastroduodenoscopy (EGD) and colonoscopy would be diagnostic.

Of children with IBD, 25% present with extraintestinal manifestations (EIMs), including arthritis, arthralgias, fatigue, growth failure, erythema nodosum, or uveitis. Rarely, these EIMs may be the only findings present on initial presentation. EIMs most commonly occur within the first year of diagnosis and are associated with more severe disease. It is important to consider a broad differential diagnosis in patients with mono- or oligoarticular inflammatory arthritis, including

- Autoimmune conditions (Behçet disease, lupus, juvenile inflammatory arthritis)
- Infectious arthritis (bacterial, gonococcal, viral, fungal, Lyme)
- Oncologic causes (leukemia, lymphoma, osteosarcoma)
- Postinfectious arthritis (acute rheumatic fever, poststreptococcal arthritis, reactive arthritis)
- Trauma

This highlights the need for a thorough history and physical to provide a targeted diagnostic workup, which may include laboratory studies, imaging, or arthrocentesis.

[ABP 1.E.12. Inflammatory bowel disease, 1.H.2. Inflammatory arthritis]

REFERENCES

1. Shapiro JM, Subedi S, LeLeiko NS. Inflammatory bowel disease. *Pediatr Rev.* 2016;37(8):337–347.
2. John J, Chandran L. Arthritis in children and adolescents. *Pediatr Rev.* 2011;32(11):470–480.

141. ANSWER: D

The infant has PHACE (posterior fossa anomalies, hemangioma, arterial lesions, cardiac abnormalities/coarctation of the aorta, eye anomalies) syndrome, which is characterized by large infantile hemangiomas (IHs) of the face, neck, and scalp and developmental anomalies. She meets criteria due to the size and location of the IH, presence of a sternal pit, and VSD. Baseline evaluation for PHACE syndrome should include an echocardiogram and magnetic resonance imaging (MRI) and angiography (MRA) of the head, neck, and aortic arch.

The IHs that pose a high risk of disfigurement or disability, such as those in the periorbital region, should be treated medically with oral propranolol at a goal dose of 2–3 mg/kg/d. Propranolol reduces the size of IHs by an unclear mechanism. Side effects may include bradycardia, hypotension, gastroesophageal reflux, sleep disturbances, and hypoglycemia. The dose needs to be escalated while monitoring for side effects. For infants 8 weeks old or less, inpatient initiation and monitoring are recommended. Infants less than 4 weeks of age should not fast longer than 4 hours due to risk of hypoglycemia. Propranolol should be held if the child has an illness that limits oral intake or if oral intake is restricted. If propranolol is well tolerated in the hospital, further glucose, blood pressure, and heart rate monitoring are not needed at home.

[ABP 1.K.2. Dermatologic manifestations of systemic disease, ABP 3.B.8. Congenital anomalies]

REFERENCES

1. Garzon MC, Epstein LG, Heyer GL, et al. PHACE syndrome: consensus-derived diagnosis and care recommendations. *J Pediatr.* 2016;178:24–33.e2.
2. Drolet BA, Frommelt PC, Chamlin SL, et al. Initiation and use of propranolol for infantile hemangioma: report of a consensus conference. *Pediatrics.* 2013;131(1):128–140.

142. ANSWER: C

Fever, abdominal pain, and anorexia are common presenting symptoms for many illnesses. However, the most likely diagnosis in a patient with a history of SLE who presents with these symptoms is acute acalculous cholecystitis (AAC). AAC is more common in those with autoimmune diseases, particularly those with vasculitis. The underlying mechanism is thought to be systemic inflammation leading to inflammation of the gallbladder vasculature with subsequent ischemic injury. A RUQ ultrasound can help differentiate acalculous cholecystitis from cholecystitis due to gallstones. Primary sclerosing cholangitis (PSC) can be asymptomatic or can present with fatigue, pruritis, and jaundice. It is associated with inflammatory bowel disease, particularly ulcerative colitis, autoimmune hepatitis, and Langerhans cell histiocytosis. Cholangitis often presents with the Charcot triad of fever, abdominal pain, and jaundice. Laboratory findings include elevated aminotransferases, elevated γ-glutamyl transferase (GGT), elevated alkaline phosphatase, and increased conjugated bilirubin. Fitz-Hugh-Curtis syndrome is a perihepatitis associated with pelvic inflammatory disease. The RUQ pain often has a pleuritic component, and aminotransferases are usually normal. Hepatitis A presents with fever, nausea, vomiting, abdominal pain, and diarrhea. Many patients do not present until jaundice develops, often a week or so after initial symptoms develop. Laboratory test values show elevated aminotransferases and elevated bilirubin levels.

[ABP 1.E.2. Cholecystitis and cholangitis]

143. ANSWER: A

Vaso-occlusive stroke is a major cause of morbidity in patients with sickle cell disease. Approximately 10% of patients with hemoglobin (Hb) SS will have a primary stroke before age 20 years. Acute neurological findings, such as altered level of consciousness, abnormal speech, weakness, and seizure, require emergent evaluation with neuroimaging. Low baseline hemoglobin, preceding acute chest syndrome, hypertension, previous transient ischemic attack, and abnormal transcranial Doppler ultrasound are risk factors. Brain MRI with diffusion and T2-weighted fluid-attenuated inversion recovery (FLAIR) images is the gold standard and is more sensitive than head CT for acute ischemia. MRI also allows detection of acute hemorrhage and provides visualization of the posterior fossa. Head and neck CT angiography may be useful in older adults with risk factors for thromboembolism, but thromboembolic stroke is less common in pediatric patients with sickle cell disease. Patients with HbSS and HbS-β thalassemia should undergo regular screening via transcranial Doppler ultrasound, but this should not be used for stroke diagnosis. Lumbar puncture has no role in the diagnosis of stroke and should not be performed in patients when increased intracranial pressure is suspected.

[ABP 1.L.4. Sickle cell disease]

144. ANSWER: A

The patient in this case likely has a ductal-dependent left outflow tract obstruction causing cardiogenic shock after her ductus arteriosus has closed. Ductal-dependent lesions that lead to left outflow tract obstruction include aortic stenosis, hypoplastic left heart syndrome, and coarctation of the aorta. Tricuspid atresia, pulmonary atresia, and tetralogy of Fallot are ductal-dependent lesions that cause right outflow tract obstruction. These would not present with absent femoral pulses. Lesions that cause left-to-right shunts, such as ventricular septal defects or truncus

arteriosus also would not lead to absent femoral pulses and would worsen later than ductal-dependent lesions as pulmonary vascular resistance falls over the first 4–6 weeks of life. Myocardial contractility can be affected by conditions such as cardiomyopathies or myocarditis and lead to decreased cardiac output, but this patient's age at presentation is more consistent with a congenital heart defect. Cardiogenic shock can also occur due to pneumothoraces or cardiac tamponade, which cause decreased diastolic filling of the heart and decreased cardiac output. However, this patient does not have examination findings consistent with tension pneumothorax, such as asymmetric lung sounds, or with tamponade, such as muffled heart sounds.

[ABP 1.D.9 Shock (including septic, cardiogenic, hypovolemic)]

145. ANSWER: C

The Cushing triad is defined as the combination of increased systolic blood pressure with a widened pulse pressure, bradycardia, and irregular respirations. While the underlying pathology of the triad is not completely understood, it is seen in cases of increased intracranial pressure (ICP), which can result from intracranial hemorrhage. If there is concern for increased intracranial pressure, especially in the context of recent head trauma, it is important to obtain a noncontrast CT to evaluate for intracranial hemorrhage requiring emergent neurosurgical intervention.

This patient's bradycardia is more concerning for Cushing triad rather than a primary cardiac etiology, so an electrocardiogram or echocardiogram would not be indicated. A CT without contrast is more sensitive, specific, and faster than an MRI with contrast for intracranial hemorrhage. Sodium dysregulation in the form of cerebral salt wasting, diabetes insipidus, or syndrome of inappropriate antidiuretic hormone may be associated with head trauma. Therefore, a sodium level is important to obtain, but a CT head would be needed more urgently to exclude complications of increased ICP.

[ABP 1.N.5. Trauma (including head trauma)]

146. ANSWER: A

Respiratory syncytial virus (RSV) bronchiolitis is a common cause of hospitalization for infants. This is especially true of patients who are born prematurely given their poor lung development. These infants are more likely to have prolonged and complicated hospitalizations from RSV compared to term infants.

Palivizumab is a monoclonal antibody recommended by the American Academy of Pediatrics for prevention of RSV illness in certain infants. Indications include patients with a gestational age of less than 29 weeks and 0 days who are less than 12 months at the start of RSV season. Palivizumab is also considered in patients with chronic lung disease requiring oxygen who were born before 32 weeks' gestation and with congenital heart disease, anatomic pulmonary abnormalities, neuromuscular disorders, and immunodeficiency. Palivizumab is administered in monthly injections during the peak RSV season; however, if a patient becomes infected with RSV despite the vaccine, the injections should be discontinued. In the clinical vignette described above, this patient is not a candidate for the vaccine give her gestational age of late preterm (not less than 29 weeks and 0 days). The other answer choices are not contraindications for the vaccine.

[ABP 1.C.1. Bronchiolitis]

REFERENCE

1. American Academy of Pediatrics Committee on Infectious Diseases; American Academy of Pediatrics Bronchiolitis Guidelines Committee. Updated guidance for palivizumab prophylaxis among infants and young children at increased risk of hospitalization for respiratory syncytial virus infection. *Pediatrics.* 2014;*134*(2):415–420.

147. ANSWER: B

This patient likely has acute disseminated encephalomyelitis (ADEM). Symptoms of ADEM classically present 2 to 4 weeks following a viral infection or rarely following vaccination. Patients will have varied clinical presentations depending on the areas involved. Neurologic symptoms often include change in mental status; headache; pyramidal signs (e.g., spasticity, hyperreflexia, clonus); gait disturbance; ataxia; seizures; fever; and cranial nerve palsies. Other symptoms include vision changes, speech difficulties, and paresthesias. Classic MRI findings in ADEM are white matter lesions that are large, diffuse, and poorly demarcated. Of those listed, high-dose steroids are the best treatment option. Other treatment options include intravenous immunoglobulin and plasma exchange. There is limited evidence to support one treatment over the others.

Patients with ADEM can present with a clinical picture very similar to central nervous system infection (fever and encephalopathy), and initial evaluation of ADEM often includes CSF analysis and empiric antibiotics. CSF ultimately will be negative for infectious organisms. There are no CSF studies specific for ADEM, but often pleocytosis and elevated protein levels are seen. This patient's brain MRI is consistent with ADEM and not infection or acute ischemic stroke. Intravenous fluids may be necessary during hospitalization but would not treat the underlying condition. While patients with ADEM can present with seizures and may require antiepileptic therapy for symptom management, this would not be definitive treatment.

[ABP 1.A.8. Inflammatory neuropathies]

REFERENCE

1. Cole J, Evans E, Mwangi M, Mar S. Acute disseminated encephalomyelitis in children: an updated review based on current diagnostic criteria. *Pediatr Neurol.* 2019;*100*:26–34.

148. ANSWER: D

This patient's clinical picture is consistent with viral croup, of which the most common cause is parainfluenza virus. Viral croup, also known as viral laryngotracheitis, is a viral upper respiratory infection that leads to inflammation of the larynx and subglottic airway. This inflammation produces the classic inspiratory stridor due to narrowing of the airway. Other symptoms include a classic "barking" cough and hoarseness. Children are usually nontoxic appearing, although secondary bacterial infections can lead to worsening illness. The most common etiology is parainfluenza virus (types 1–3), accounting for more than 65% of cases. Other relatively common causes include respiratory syncytial virus (RSV) and adenovirus. Influenza virus is a less common cause of croup but can be associated with longer hospitalizations. Rhinoviruses can occasionally cause mild croup. Where present, measles is also known to be a cause of moderate-to-severe croup. Treatment consists of symptomatic management with cool mist or steam therapies, with additional consideration of racemic epinephrine and oral dexamethasone depending on symptom severity.

[ABP 1.B.1. Upper airway infections and conditions]

REFERENCE

1. Malhotra A, Krilov LR. Viral croup. *Pediatr Rev.* 2001;*22*(1):5–12.

149. ANSWER: B

This case demonstrates a classic presentation of chronic functional headache. Chronic pain syndromes are common in children, and nonpharmacological treatment options should be pursued whenever possible. Relaxation training with biobehavioral feedback is the preferred prophylactic treatment for recurrent headaches over any form of drug therapy. While acupuncture has been shown to be beneficial in adults for chronic pain, it is not well studied in children. Propranolol is used as a preventive medication for children with chronic headaches, but it should not be initiated prior to trialing nonpharmacological treatment options. Opioid therapy should never be considered first-line therapy for chronic pain in children. Acetaminophen and ibuprofen are generally good options for first-line acute pain in children, but this patient's headaches have proven to be refractory to these medications.

[ABP 1.O.8. Pain (acute and chronic)]

150. ANSWER: C

Hypoglycemia in the setting of low sodium and elevated potassium is concerning for adrenal insufficiency (AI). Diagnosis requires a corticotropin (ACTH) stimulation test. Stimulated cortisol levels should be low, and ACTH concentrations should be elevated in AI. A dexamethasone suppression test is used to diagnose Cushing syndrome but has no role in the diagnosis of AI. Renin, which is produced by the kidney in response to low sodium and triggers the conversion and activation of aldosterone, would be high rather than low in AI, a mineralocorticoid-deficient state. Ketogenesis is preserved in adrenal insufficiency; high rather than low serum ketones would be expected in a patient with hypoglycemia secondary to AI.

[ABP 1.I.5. Adrenal disorders]

151. ANSWER: C

This patient most likely has an infected nephrolithiasis. Her urinalysis is strongly suggestive of infection, most likely from a gram-negative organism given the positive nitrites. The colicky nature of her pain and the crystals in her urine suggest the presence of a renal stone. Of the stone types listed, struvite stones are the most likely to form staghorn calculi. Struvite stones often occur in the setting of infection with a urease-producing bacteria such as *Proteus* or *Klebsiella*. Such infections also increase the urine pH, as is seen with this patient. Bacteria are often present within the stone and create a local environment that promotes further stone formation. As such, medical therapy alone is rarely successful, and urologic intervention is almost always needed. Staghorn calculi not infrequently incorporate both struvite and calcium carbonate. Cystine can form staghorn calculi, but this is rare. Calcium oxalate and urate do not form staghorn calculi. Citrate is not a component of renal stones but rather helps prevent formation of certain types of stones.

[ABP 1.F.4. Nephrolithiasis]

152. ANSWER: D

Behçet disease (BD) is a systemic inflammatory disease affecting the eyes, skin, and mucosa of the mouth and genitals. The vasculitis of BD may affect vessels of all sizes, with the most common presenting symptoms including oral and genital ulcers and prolonged fever. BD most commonly presents in young adulthood. The diagnosis of pediatric BD requires three attacks per year that include three of the six following criteria:

- Oral aphthosis
- Genital ulceration (often scarring)
- Skin involvement (acneiform lesions, erythema nodosum, necrotic folliculitis)
- Ocular involvement (uveitis or retinal vasculitis)
- Neurologic signs
- Vascular signs (thrombosis, aneurysm)

This patient meets criteria for BD and will benefit from subspecialty evaluation by rheumatology and ophthalmology. Treatment varies based on disease severity and may include colchicine, steroids, azathioprine, and tumor necrosis factor α inhibitors. Young males have the worst prognosis, with more severe neurologic, vascular, and ocular involvement that often require a combination of steroids and immunosuppressive therapy.

[ABP 1.H. Rheumatologic/vasculitis, 1.K.2. Dermatologic manifestations of systemic disease]

REFERENCE

1. Koné-Paut I. Behçet's disease in children, an overview. *Pediatr Rheumatol Online J.* 2016;14(1):10.

153. ANSWER: D

The patient has tinea capitis with kerion. Tinea capitis is a cutaneous dermatophyte infection that often presents as scaly plaques of the scalp with overlying alopecia. The hair may have a broken off appearance. Itching is common. Kerion is an inflammatory variant of tinea capitis due to intense T-cell–mediated hypersensitivity to the pathogenic dermatophyte. Kerions often have overlying alopecia, pustules with purulent drainage, and superficial crusting. The lesion may be painful and is often mistaken for a bacterial infection. Fevers and painful regional lymphadenopathy are common. Tinea capitis can be confirmed with a potassium hydroxide wet-mount examination. Culture is the gold standard to diagnose dermatophyte infections but it can take 1–2 weeks to obtain a result.

Tinea capitis and kerion are treated with systemic antifungals. Oral griseofulvin, terbinafine, or fluconazole can be used, often for a 6-week total course. Oral or intralesional corticosteroids combined with antifungal therapy has not been shown to be superior to antifungal therapy alone. Bacterial superinfection has been reported and should be assessed with bacterial culture, if suspected. Antibiotics should be added only if bacterial superinfection is present. In this case, oral antifungal therapy can most likely be completed as an outpatient without need for hospitalization.

[ABP 1.K.1. Skin and soft tissue infections]

REFERENCE

1. John AM, Schwartz RA, Janniger CK. *The kerion: an angry tinea capitis. Int J Dermatol.* 2018;57(1):3–9.

154. ANSWER: D

Phenobarbital is used as both a diagnostic and therapeutic intervention for patients with Crigler-Najjar, type II. Crigler-Najjar syndrome is due to either absence or defect of the enzyme uridine diphosphate glucuronosyltransferase-1A1 (UGT1A1), which impairs bilirubin conjugation. Type I disease is more severe and results in higher elevations of unconjugated bilirubin levels due to absent UGT1A1 activity. Type II disease is characterized by less-severe elevations in bilirubin and is associated with decreased but still present UGT1A1 activity. Increasing feed volumes would not be expected to reduce bilirubin levels as the patient is taking appropriate volumes for age. Levothyroxine and exclusion of galactose from diet would be used in hypothyroidism and galactosemia, respectively, both of which can also cause unconjugated hyperbilirubinemia. This patient, however, does not demonstrate other signs of hypothyroidism or galactosemia. Red blood cell transfusions may be indicated for patients with severe hemolysis leading to hyperbilirubinemia but would not be expected to improve hyperbilirubinemia in this patient without evidence of hemolysis.

[ABP 1.E.9. Hyperbilirubinemia]

155. ANSWER: C

The patient has acute splenic sequestration, which has a mortality rate of 10%–15% in patients with sickle cell disease. Therefore, prompt identification and intervention are crucial. Children usually present between 6 months and 5 years of age. This patient's physical examination findings of weakness, pallor, tachycardia, tachypnea, and abdominal distension are typical. Splenic enlargement may be pronounced, such that the spleen tip is found in the right lower rather than the left upper quadrant. Sequestration occurs when the hypoxic environment of the spleen prompts acute sickling and accumulation of red blood cells, leading to a drop in hemoglobin of at least 2 g/dL below baseline. Acute correction of hypovolemia is critical before patients progress to shock. Intravenous crystalloid infusion is an appropriate initial intervention. Simple red blood cell transfusion rather than exchange transfusion would be appropriate if initiated in a timely fashion. Of note, improvement in the patient's volume status may result in release of trapped erythrocytes from the spleen, leading to a higher-than-expected increase in hemoglobin. Clinicians must consider this autotransfusion phenomenon when deciding on transfusion volume. Laparoscopic splenectomy is indicated for children requiring transfusion support, demonstrating persistent hypersplenism, or having multiple episodes of sequestration. Intravenous morphine is used in vaso-occlusive crises, and ceftriaxone is used in suspected sepsis in patients with sickle cell disease.

[ABP 1.L.4. Sickle cell disease]

156. ANSWER: B

The patient in this case meets criteria for sepsis with an elevated heart rate, temperature, respiratory rate, and white blood cell count for age, as well as a source of infection. His elevated heart rate but normal blood pressure suggest he is in compensated septic shock. The 2020 Surviving Sepsis Campaign International Guidelines provide differential recommendations for initial management of septic shock depending on whether the treating facility has access to intensive care services. For patients who are not hypotensive or demonstrating significantly compromised perfusion in facilities without intensive care facilities, maintenance fluids are recommended instead of fluid boluses. A bolus would be appropriate if the child was hypotensive, dehydrated, or had compromised perfusion with capillary refill greater than 3 seconds and weak pulses. There is no indication of hypoglycemia in this case that would warrant a dextrose bolus. Vasopressors may be appropriate if the child has hypotension or compromised perfusion despite multiple fluid boluses. Hydrocortisone may be appropriate if the shock is unresponsive to vasopressors.

[ABP 1.D.9. Shock (including septic, cardiogenic, hypovolemic)]

157. ANSWER: B

Cannabis intoxication differs based on the age of the patient. In children, cannabis overdose is much more likely than in adults, even with small doses. Patients present with lethargy and occasionally bradypnea, but otherwise normal vital signs.

Opiate overdose manifests similarly to cannabis overdose; however, patients with opiate intoxication also frequently have miosis, hypoactive bowel sounds, and vital sign abnormalities, including hypotension and bradycardia. Patients with PCP, cocaine, and amphetamine overdose are generally agitated with hypertension and tachycardia. PCP intoxication can also be associated with nystagmus. Cocaine intoxication is associated with mydriasis.

[ABP 1.N.1. Ingestions (intentional and unintentional)]

158. ANSWER: C

This patient's clinical picture is most consistent with acute viral bronchiolitis. Bronchiolitis is an inflammatory respiratory infection affecting the bronchioles. Of affected patients under 1 year of age, 2%–3% will require admission. RSV is one of the most common causes of bronchiolitis, though identifying the specific organism is not necessary. Higher-risk populations include preterm infants and patients with chronic lung disease, congenital heart disease, neurological disease, and immunodeficiencies. Although the risk of hospitalization is high in these patients, the rates of death are low.

In the clinical vignette above, this patient is at higher risk for being hospitalized and having more complications from bronchiolitis given her prematurity. The patient's acute work of breathing is most concerning, and this should be addressed first with oxygen therapy. Choices D and E are good options once she is stabilized from a respiratory standpoint. Choice B is not necessary at this point; an isolated elevated blood pressure does not require treatment except in cases of hypertensive urgency or emergency.

[ABP 1.C.1. Bronchiolitis]

REFERENCE

1. Smyth RL, Openshaw PJ. Bronchiolitis. *Lancet.* 2006;368(9532): 312–322.

159. ANSWER: E

One of the most common movement disorders in pediatrics is ataxia. Patients with ataxia will often present with difficulty ambulating or sitting upright, perceived clumsiness or poor coordination with movements, intention tremors when reaching for objects, dysmetria, nystagmus, or even speech impairment. When evaluating patients with ataxia, it is important to consider red flag symptoms such as altered levels of consciousness, focal neurological deficits, meningeal signs, or evidence of increased intracranial pressure.

In this scenario, the patient's acute onset of symptoms with a history of recent viral illness suggests a diagnosis of acute cerebellar ataxia. Acute cerebellar ataxia is a common movement disorder in pediatrics and the most common cause of childhood ataxia, usually occurring after an acute febrile illness. While it is considered a diagnosis of exclusion, it can often be reached with a detailed history and physical examination. Children typically have a good prognosis, with the vast majority having a complete recovery.

Intracranial processes, such as posterior fossa tumors, can also present with ataxia. These patients usually have a more insidious presentation combined with constitutional symptoms such as fevers, weight loss, chills, and night sweats. Ataxia can also be caused from ingestions of substances such as alcohols, cough syrups, benzodiazepines, and anticonvulsants. This patient has no history of an exploratory ingestion. Guillain-Barré syndrome is a peripheral nervous system disease that is characterized by ascending weakness and paresthesias. While meningitis should be considered, it is less likely in this vignette given the lack of fevers, meningeal signs, or other infectious systemic symptoms. Of note, cerebellar ataxia should be differentiated from sensory ataxia, which is related to a sensory neuropathy. These patients will often sway or fall over when asked to stand upright with their feet together and eyes closed (positive Romberg sign). In addition, patients with sensory ataxia often will have normal speech, and nystagmus will not be present.

[ABP 1.A.11. Other (eg, movement disorders, brain tumors)]

REFERENCE

1. Caffarelli M, Kimia AA, Torres AR. Acute ataxia in children: a review of the differential diagnosis and evaluation in the emergency department. *Pediatr Neurol.* 2016;65:14–30.

160. ANSWER: A

For any child with a prolonged febrile illness and neck mass not responding to antibiotics, the diagnosis of Kawasaki disease (KD) should be considered. KD is an immunoglobulin (Ig) E–mediated, medium-vessel vasculitis that can lead to coronary artery complications. Because no pathognomonic clinical or laboratory findings exist, diagnosis is based on the presence of four or more of the principle clinical features (Box 1.2) in the context of 5 or more days of fever. When fewer than four major criteria are present, the presence of three or more supplemental laboratory findings (Box 1.3) or abnormalities in echocardiography can support the diagnosis of incomplete Kawasaki disease (IKD). The prevalence of IKD is 15% to 36% of all KD cases. Features tend to present sequentially, and some features may resolve

---

Box 1.2 KAWASAKI DISEASE MAJOR CRITERIA[a]

Peripheral extremity changes

Bilateral nonexudative conjunctival injection

Unilateral cervical lymphadenopathy >1.5 cm diameter

Lip/oral mucosa changes

Polymorphous exanthematous rash

[a] Adapted from Reference 1.

Box 1.3 SUPPLEMENTAL LABORATORY CRITERIA FOR THE DIAGNOSIS OF INCOMPLETE KAWASAKI DISEASE[a]

Elevated ALT

Elevated white blood cell count ≥15,000/mm³

Elevated platelet count ≥450,000/mm³

Urine white blood cells ≥10/high-power field

Serum albumin ≤3.0 g/dL

Anemia for age

[a] Adapted from Reference 1.

---

early in the course of illness but still count toward the diagnosis. Treatment with high-dose intravenous immunoglobulin (IVIG) prior to the 10th day of fever has been shown to decrease the incidence of coronary artery aneurysms from 25% to under 5%. None of the other answer choices would aid in the diagnosis of Kawasaki disease and would delay prompt recognition and treatment.

[ABP 1.H.2. Kawasaki disease]

REFERENCE

1. Newburger JW, Takahashi M, Gerber MA, et al. Diagnosis, treatment, and long-term management of Kawasaki disease: a statement for health professionals from the Committee on Rheumatic Fever, Endocarditis, and Kawasaki Disease, Council on Cardiovascular Disease in the Young, American Heart Association. *Pediatrics*. 2004;*114*(6):1708–1733.

161. ANSWER: A

This patient has complex regional pain syndrome (CRPS), a chronic, intensified localized pain condition that can include allodynia, hyperalgesia, swelling, hyperhidrosis, and changes in skin color of the affected limb. Standard of care consists of a multidisciplinary approach with the implementation of intensive physical therapy in conjunction with psychological counseling. Gradually increasing aerobic activity is the gold standard of therapy for CRPS. Ketamine is an N-methyl-D-aspartate receptor antagonist with analgesic effect. There have been reports of ketamine infusions for CRPS, but the duration of effect can be limited, and it can cause psychotomimetic side effects; therefore, it would not be a first-line treatment option. A sympathetic nerve block is a treatment option utilized in CRPS, but there is weak evidence of its effectiveness in the pediatric population. Amitriptyline can be used in conjunction with other pharmacological medications such as gabapentin in an effort to facilitate physical therapy. Neither amitriptyline nor gabapentin alone would be the best choice for treatment in this patient.

In general, nonpharmacological treatment options should be pursued whenever possible for chronic pain syndromes in children.

[ABP 1.O.8. Pain (acute and chronic)]

162. ANSWER: A

Euthyroid sick syndrome is characterized by a period of low T_3 followed by low T_4. TSH is initially low and can then rise to well above the normal range as the patient recovers from their underlying illness. Binding proteins such as TBG and TTR are typically low, contributing to the low T_4 levels. A free T_4 index is an estimation of free T_4 and would be expected to be low in euthyroid sick syndrome. TSH initially falls then rises, sometimes to well over the normal range during the recovery phase of illness. Reverse T_3, the inactive form of thyroid hormone, is frequently high. TSI antibodies are elevated in Graves' disease, which is a hyperthyroid state, and would not support a diagnosis of euthyroid sick syndrome.

Thyroid function should be tested with caution in patients who are critically ill. Abnormal levels may lead to unnecessary and potentially harmful treatment, as the hypothyroid state may be part of the body's defense against excessive tissue catabolism in the setting of severe illness. There is no evidence that thyroid hormone replacement is of benefit in patients with euthyroid sick syndrome.

[ABP 1.I.3. Hypo and hyperthyroidism]

163. ANSWER: B

This patient most likely has ovarian torsion and requires emergent surgical intervention to prevent necrosis of the ovary. Sudden onset of severe pelvic or lower abdominal pain is a key symptom. Torsion may be precipitated by exercise or a sudden increase in abdominal pressure. Nausea and emesis are common associated symptoms, and fever may or may not be present. The ultrasound findings of an enlarged, edematous ovary, especially when compared to the contralateral ovary, are suggestive of torsion. In contrast to testicular torsion, Doppler ultrasound may show normal blood flow in ovarian torsion because the ovary has a dual blood supply. The most significant risk factor for ovarian torsion is the presence of an ovarian mass, the most common of which is an ovarian cyst. Many ovarian cysts respond to reproductive hormones, so pregnancy, polycystic ovarian syndrome, and ovulation induction treatments can all increase the risk of ovarian torsion. In general, the larger the mass, the greater the risk of torsion, although it is hypothesized that a very large mass might actually impede torsion. Factors that may lead to fixation of the ovary such as a tubo-ovarian abscess from pelvic inflammatory disease may actually decrease the risk of torsion. Endometriosis, prior abdominal surgery, and the use of an intrauterine device are not risk factors for ovarian torsion.

[ABP 1.F.8. Ovarian cysts and torsion]

164. ANSWER: C

This patient's cyclical fevers and oral ulcers are concerning for a periodic fever syndrome. Periodic fever, aphthous stomatitis, pharyngitis, and cervical adenitis (PFAPA) is an idiopathic periodic fever syndrome with onset before age 5. PFAPA occurs on a predictable cycle every 2–8 weeks and usually resolves by age 10. It is useful for families to keep a fever diary, as PFAPA is a clinical diagnosis with no specific confirmatory test. It is vital to rule out other etiologies, such as acute infections, oncologic processes, autoimmune disease, immunodeficiency, and other periodic fever syndromes. Consider pediatric rheumatology referral.

Corticosteroids may resolve PFAPA symptoms more quickly than the spontaneous resolution typically seen in 4–6 days, but they do not alter prognosis or prevent future episodes. Tonsillectomy may be considered for long-term management, but the risks of surgical and anesthetic intervention must be weighed and discussed on an individual basis, given the self-limited nature of PFAPA.

[ABP 1.O.5. Fever of unknown origin (prolonged/recurrent)]

165. ANSWER: C

The patient's presentation is highly suspicious for tuberous sclerosis complex (TSC) based on the presence of hypopigmented macules (ash leaf spots) and infantile spasms (ISs). ISs are characterized by sudden flexion or extension of predominantly proximal and axial muscles, with EEG often demonstrating hypsarrhythmia, as described for this patient. ISs are often difficult to treat and associated with developmental abnormalities. First-line treatment options for ISs include adrenocorticotropic hormone, corticosteroids, or vigabatrin.

Tuberous sclerosis complex is a multisystem genetic disorder that affects 1 in 6000 individuals and is diagnosed based on the presence of multiple clinical criteria. Hypopigmented macules, angiofibromas, retinal hamartomas, cortical dysplasia, cardiac rhabdomyomas, and renal cysts are among common clinical findings that comprise part of the diagnostic criteria. Genetic testing for TSC is available for the *TSC1* and *TSC2* genes and should be considered, but some individuals meet clinical criteria for TSC without an identified mutation. Baseline assessment for suspected TSC includes brain magnetic resonance imaging, echocardiogram, and renal ultrasound to help make the diagnosis and identify complications. Referral to a neurocutaneous disease specialist is recommended, as long-term surveillance for neurologic, renal, pulmonary, ophthalmologic, cardiac, and dermatologic complications is critical.

[ABP 1.A.2. Seizures, ABP 1.K.2. Dermatologic manifestations of systemic disease]

REFERENCES

1. In: Prose NS, Kristal L, eds. *Weinberg's Color of Pediatric Dermatology.* 5th ed. New York: McGraw-Hill; 2017.
2. Korf BR, Bebin EM. Neurocutaneous disorders in children. *Pediatr Rev.* 2017;38(3):119–128.

166. ANSWER: C

Magnets are a common household item, frequently used in children's toys, that represent an ingestion risk for young children. When more than one magnet is ingested, patients are at risk for serious intra-abdominal sequelae, including perforation, obstruction, and infection due to the magnets' propensity to attract across loops of bowel. Given this high risk, endoscopy for removal of magnets present in the esophagus or stomach is recommended. For magnets already in the small or large bowel, a more conservative approach of serial radiographs with or without total bowel clean-out to ensure passage may be appropriate. Sucralfate is not indicated for patients with a magnet ingestion. Given the risk of serious sequelae, the patient should not be discharged home until the magnets are removed.

[ABP 1.N.1. Ingestions (intentional and unintentional)]

167. ANSWER: E

The patient has autoimmune hemolytic anemia (AIHA). AIHA is classified as cold or warm based on the thermal reactivity of the autoantibodies. Diagnosis of cold agglutinin disease requires evidence of hemolytic anemia, such as high indirect bilirubin, high lactate dehydrogenase, and high plasma free hemoglobin. Diagnosis also requires a positive direct antiglobulin test. Note that in cold AIHA the direct antiglobulin test is positive for bound complement, whereas in warm AIHA the direct antiglobulin test is positive for immunoglobulin (Ig) G. Patients with cold agglutinin disease have intravascular hemolysis and resulting hemoglobinuria. They have grossly dark urine and urinalysis positive for blood, but urine microscopy will be negative for red blood cells. Alanine and aspartate aminotransferase are intrinsic liver enzymes and should be normal in AIHA. Leukocyte count should be normal in AIHA and, if abnormal, should prompt evaluation for other etiologies, such as leukemia or aplastic anemia.

Cold agglutinin disease is often caused by *Mycoplasma pneumoniae*, as in this vignette. For all types of AIHA, patients present with fatigue, shortness of breath, and pallor due to anemia, as well as icterus and jaundice due to hemolysis. Anemia may cause a high-output cardiac state, with associated tachycardia and a systolic flow murmur.

[ABP 1.L.1. Anemias]

168. ANSWER: C

As seen in Table 1.10, this patient's blood pressure can be classified as stage 2 hypertension (HTN). Clinicians should ensure blood pressures are measured properly by repeating measurement twice and obtaining it with a manual cuff. The initial history should focus on symptoms and signs of target organ damage, as well as possible etiologic origins. This patient with stage 2 HTN should have diagnostic evaluation and treatment initiated and/or follow-up with subspecialty care within 1 week. Evaluation should focus on secondary causes and target organ effects as guided by the history and

Table 1.10 BLOOD PRESSURE CATEGORIES AND STAGES OF HYPERTENSION

	AGE 1–13 YEARS	AGE 13 YEARS OR OLDER
Normal BP	<90th percentile	<120/<80 mm Hg
Elevated BP	≥90th percentile to <95th percentile or 120/80 mm Hg to <95th percentile[b]	120/<80 to 129/<80 mm Hg
Stage 1 HTN	≥95th percentile to <95th percentile + 12 mm Hg or 130/80 to 139/89 mm Hg[b]	130/80 to 139/89 mm Hg
Stage 2 HTN	≥95th percentile + 12 mm Hg or ≥140/90 mm Hg[b]	≥140/90 mm Hg

[a] Adapted from Reference 1.

[b] Whichever is lower; BP, blood pressure; HTN, hypertension.

physical examination. Symptomatic stage 2 HTN warrants expedited evaluation in an emergency department or inpatient setting. Acute severe hypertension is defined as a blood pressure 30 mm Hg or more above the 95th percentile or greater than 180/120 mm Hg in an adolescent. Severe hypertension with the presence of life-threatening symptoms or end-organ injury defines a hypertensive emergency, whereas a similar increase in blood pressure without evidence of acute target organ injury defines hypertensive urgency.

[ABP 1.D.7. Hypertension and hypertensive emergencies]

REFERENCE

1. Flynn JT, Kaelber DC, Baker-Smith CM, et al. Clinical practice guideline for screening and management of high blood pressure in children and adolescents. *Pediatrics*. 2017;*140*(3):e20171904.

169. ANSWER: C

While all of these complications can be caused by inhalant abuse, sudden sniffing death is the only one that can result from acute inhalant abuse. Sudden sniffing death refers to cardiovascular collapse resulting from catecholamine surge during inhalant abuse, especially when combined with exertion. This can occur in first-time users, making it especially important to mention to this occasional user. Subacute combined degeneration syndrome and megaloblastic anemia are complications from vitamin B_{12} deficiency from chronic exposure to nitrous oxide, which is a component found in some inhalants. Toxic leukoencephalopathy and peripheral neuropathy are neurologic complications of long-term inhalant use.

[ABP 1.N.1. Ingestions (intentional and unintentional)]

170. ANSWER: B

This patient is presenting with symptoms concerning for bacterial tracheitis. The next step would be to obtain a tracheal aspirate to further elucidate this diagnosis and tailor treatment appropriately.

Bacterial tracheitis involves bacterial superinfection of the tracheal (and sometimes laryngeal and bronchial) tissues, and presentation differs among patients with native or artificial airways. In previously healthy children without artificial airways, bacterial tracheitis occurs rarely and almost always in young children in the setting of a preceding viral respiratory infection. Symptoms include acute-onset respiratory distress, stridor, cough, and dyspnea. The most common isolate in these circumstances is *Staphylococcus aureus*.

For patients with artificial airways, the presentation may be along a spectrum of mild-to-severe illness, with possible symptoms including increased respiratory support, an increase or change in tracheal secretions, fever, and respiratory distress. The presentation may be difficult to distinguish from pneumonia, and imaging can be helpful. Obtaining a sample of tracheal aspirate can help to compare culture data to previous samples and to distinguish between colonization or new infection.

Given this patient's overall stable appearance, starting antibiotics before obtaining a tracheal sample for culture is unnecessary and may hinder future culture growth. Direct visualization can be helpful for diagnosis but is not prudent in this patient, who is not systemically ill. Chest physiotherapy is not likely to be helpful in this patient, who does not have a lower respiratory tract infection. While glycopyrrolate is used in the management of chronic secretions, it should not be used for acute changes in secretions that are suggestive of infection.

[ABP 1.C.7. Bacterial tracheitis]

REFERENCE

1. DeBlasio D, Real FJ. Tracheitis. *Pediatr Rev*. 2020;*41*(9):495–497.

171. ANSWER: A

The patient in this clinical vignette most likely has Prader-Willi syndrome (PWS). PWS is a genetic condition caused by the lack of expression of paternally active genes on chromosome 15. Patients with PWS can present prenatally with decreased fetal movement, polyhydramnios, and breech positioning. Polyhydramnios, resulting from impaired swallowing of amniotic fluid, may be evidence of hypotonia in utero. Hypotonia is the most common feature for PWS. Infants with PWS may also have almond-shaped eyes, a poor suck reflex, developmental delay, hypogonadism, and cryptorchidism. Later in life, children often present with excessive eating, central obesity, persistent hypotonia, and short stature.

When evaluating a patient with hypotonia, it is important to differentiate between central and peripheral hypotonia to help narrow the differential diagnosis (see table below). Central hypotonia is likely related to a central nervous system process such as trisomy 21, PWS, and cerebral palsy. Peripheral hypotonia is more likely caused by a neuromuscular disease, such as spinal muscular atrophy, infantile botulism, congenital myopathies, and muscular dystrophies.

CENTRAL HYPOTONIA	PERIPHERAL HYPOTONIA
Mild-to-moderate weakness (antigravity movement retained)	Significant weakness (absent/reduced antigravity movement)
Increased or decreased deep tendon reflexes	Absent deep tendon reflexes
Present neonatal reflexes	Absent neonatal reflexes
Antigravity movement retained	Absent/reduced antigravity movement

Patients with hypotonia who are placed supine will often have frog-like positioning with hips abducted. Vertical suspension is tested by the examiner placing their hands underneath the patient's arms. Infants with hypotonia will slip through the examiner's hands. Horizontal suspension is assessed by placing the infant in a prone position with a hand under his or her chest. Infants with low tone will form an inverted "U" position. Axial tone can be assessed by placing the patient supine and pulling to a sitting position; infants with hypotonia will have significant head lag. The "scarf sign" maneuver can be used to assess appendicular tone. While in a supine position, the infant's elbow is pulled across the chest; infants with low muscle tone will have their elbow extending beyond the body midline.

[ABP 1.A.7. Hypotonia]

REFERENCE

1. Peredo DE, Hannibal MC. The floppy infant: evaluation of hypotonia. *Pediatr Rev.* 2009;*30*(9):e66–e76.

172. ANSWER: D

Due to the abscess location at the angle of the mandible and presence of an enhancing fistula to the palatine tonsil on CT, the abscess likely represents an infected second branchial cleft anomaly (BCA). BCA can present as cysts, sinuses, or fistulas, with 70% arising from the second cleft. CT with contrast is the imaging modality of choice for second branchial cleft anomalies. Definitive diagnosis is by pathologic examination, and surgical excision is curative.

In the context of recurrent unilateral neck infection with hearing loss, renal ultrasound is indicated to evaluate for branchio-otorenal (BOR) syndrome. BOR syndrome is part of a spectrum of rare autosomal dominant disorders and is characterized by the presence of at least two of five features: BCAs, hearing loss, preauricular pits, pinna abnormalities, and renal malformations. Renal abnormalities range from mild to severe, potentially leading to the need for dialysis and transplantation.

While ectopic thyroid is on the differential diagnosis, most of these will present midline rather than near the angle of the mandible. Contrast-enhanced MRI is preferred for first branchial cleft anomalies due to the need to characterize facial nerve involvement; an MRI would not aid in the investigation of BOR syndrome. The patient's recurrent neck infections can be explained by the presence of a BCA and not a primary immunodeficiency or malignancy, so an immunoglobulin panel, uric acid, and LDH testing are not indicated.

[ABP 1.B.2 Neck masses and infections]

REFERENCE

1. Prosser JD, Myer CM 3rd. Branchial cleft anomalies and thymic cysts. *Otolaryngol Clin North Am.* 2015;*48*(1):1–14.

173. ANSWER: B

Infants with idiopathic hypertrophic pyloric stenosis (IHPS) will have normal electrolytes early in their presentation. However, with prolonged symptoms, infants will develop a hypokalemic hypochloremic metabolic alkalosis. This is due to the loss of hydrochloric acid with each emesis, leading to the hypochloremic alkalosis. In addition, the lack of hydrogen chloride reaching the duodenum results in a lack of stimulus to the pancreas to secrete bicarbonate. This adds to the alkalosis. To offset the rising alkalosis, hydrogen-potassium transporters move hydrogen out of the cells and shift potassium into the cells. This leads to the hypokalemia noted in the laboratory findings. Treatment for IHPS is initially fluid resuscitation and electrolyte stabilization followed by surgical correction. Most infants with IHPS are able to return to oral intake shortly after surgical repair.

[ABP 1.O.7. Acid/base disorders]

174. ANSWER: E

Patients with T1D are at increased risk for other autoimmune conditions, including autoimmune thyroid diseases (Graves' disease and Hashimoto thyroiditis); celiac disease; vitiligo, systemic lupus erythematosus; primary adrenal insufficiency (Addison disease); and inflammatory bowel disease. The presence of more than one autoimmune condition suggests a diagnosis of one of the autoimmune polyglandular syndromes (autoimmune polyendocrine syndrome [APS] 1 and APS 2). APS type 2 is characterized by Addison disease and an autoimmune thyroid disease with or without T1D.

This patient's lower insulin needs well outside of the honeymoon period are concerning for hypoglycemia. His symptoms of weight loss and fatigue are classic for adrenal insufficiency. Primary adrenal insufficiency results from loss of glucocorticoid and, typically, mineralocorticoid production in the adrenal gland. The ACTH level is markedly elevated, sodium levels are low, potassium levels are high, and cortisol and renin levels are low. Autoimmune thyroid disease is more commonly associated with T1D than is primary adrenal insufficiency, but this patient does not have symptoms consistent with hypothyroidism. His fatigue, low blood pressure, and hypoglycemia are much more concerning for adrenal disease. Tissue transglutaminase IgA is diagnostic of celiac disease. HLA-B27 typing is helpful in the workup of juvenile idiopathic arthritis (JIA). RF, ANA, and anti-dsDNA antibodies are used in the workup for lupus. None of these diagnoses is consistent with this patient's constellation of symptoms.

[ABP 1.I.5. Adrenal disorders]

175. ANSWER: D

This patient has abnormal uterine bleeding of unknown etiology. While a diagnostic workup is indicated, initial treatment must focus on stabilization of the patient by preserving hemodynamics and stopping the bleeding. This patient has significant anemia causing symptoms (tachycardia, dizziness, and fatigue); therefore, a transfusion with red blood cells is indicated. First-line treatment for uterine bleeding for most patients is estrogen in the form of combination oral contraceptives, given at high doses and tapered off. High doses of estrogen can cause significant nausea, and patients may require antiemetic medications. Intravenous estrogen therapy is typically reserved for patients who cannot tolerate medications by mouth. However, this patient has a history of migraines with aura, which is a contraindication to estrogen therapy by any route. Thus, progestin-only oral contraceptives are the best next choice for this patient. Tranexamic acid is typically reserved for patients whose bleeding is refractory to hormonal therapy or those with platelet disorders. Iron repletion for anemia due to uterine bleeding is recommended, but this will not address the acute need to stop the bleeding. Iron repletion is typically given by mouth for several months once the patient has been stabilized; intravenous iron infusion is reserved for patients who cannot tolerate or absorb oral iron.

[ABP 1.F.7. Dysfunctional uterine bleeding]

176. ANSWER: B

The mother most likely has undiagnosed juvenile Sjögren syndrome (SS). The most common manifestation of SS is parotitis. Patients may present with recurrent sialadenitis, dry eyes, xerostomia, renal disease, arthralgias/arthritis, corneal abrasions, and dental caries. Systemic symptoms (fever, fatigue, and malaise) may be present. Lymphoma is a rare but serious complication. SS may be primary or in association with another autoimmune disease, such as systemic lupus erythematosus (SLE). There are criteria for diagnosis of SS in adults, but these are not validated in children. The diagnosis is made based on clinical symptoms, histological findings, and supportive laboratory data. Anti-Ro (SSA) and anti-La (SSB) antibodies are associated with juvenile SS (20%–66%). Most patients have positive ANA, but this is less specific.

Neonatal lupus syndrome (NLS) may occur in infants born to mothers with SS or SLE with anti-Ro/La antibodies. Mothers may have other positive autoantibodies, but anti-Ro/La antibodies directly contribute to NLS by causing damage to cardiac Purkinje fibers. Findings may include heart block, rash, hepatitis, and thrombocytopenia. Most manifestations resolve as maternal autoantibodies clear, except for heart block, which may be permanent. In this case, positive anti-Ro/La antibodies help support diagnoses of baby and mother.

[ABP 1.H.4. Systemic lupus erythematosus, 1.K.2. Dermatologic manifestations of systemic disease]

REFERENCES

1. Silverman E, Jaeggi E, Barsalou J. Neonatal lupus erythematosis. In: Petty RE, Laxer RM, Lindsley CB, Wedderburn L, Fuhlbriggez RC, Mellins ED, eds. *Textbook of Pediatric Rheumatology.* 8th ed. Philadelphia: Saunders/Elsevier; 2020:346–359.
2. Tarvin SE, O'Neil KM. Systemic lupus erythematosus, Sjögren syndrome, and mixed connective tissue disease in children and adolescents. *Pediatr Clin North Am.* 2018;65(4):711–737.

177. ANSWER: C

This patient's birthmark, seizures, and developmental delays are concerning for Sturge-Weber syndrome (SWS). Features of SWS include

- Port wine stain birthmarks, vascular malformations typically present unilaterally on the face in a V1 and/or V2 distribution
- Seizures, which are often difficult to manage
- Leptomeningeal vascular malformations, typically ipsilateral to the vascular birthmark
- Developmental delay and intellectual disability
- Hemiparesis, typically contralateral to the intracranial lesion, which often first presents as seizures develop and

can be progressive, with resultant loss of motor function and decreased growth of the affected extremity
• Glaucoma and ocular vascular malformations, especially in patients with a dermatologic lesion

With the risk of glaucoma and other ocular problems, this patient should be evaluated by an ophthalmologist. Brain imaging to evaluate for intracranial vascular malformation and initiation of an antiepileptic drug regimen would also be warranted in this case.

[ABP 1.K.2. Dermatologic manifestations of systemic illnesses]

178. ANSWER: E

This patient's presentation is consistent with a Meckel diverticulum, which often presents as painless rectal bleeding. A Meckel diverticulum is a remnant of the omphalomesenteric duct found in approximately 2% of the overall population with a 2:1 male-to-female ratio. Meckel diverticula are most frequently diagnosed in children less than 10 years of age and are occasionally discovered incidentally. However, in addition to painless rectal bleeding or melena, patients may also present with Meckel diverticulitis with associated abdominal pain, intussusception, or symptoms mimicking appendicitis. The most appropriate test for diagnosis of a Meckel diverticulum is the technetium Tc 99m scan (Meckel scan). Colonoscopy would not readily identify a Meckel diverticulum given its typical location near the ileocecal valve. Stool culture and *H. pylori* antigen would be lower-yield tests in this patient given lack of other gastrointestinal or systemic symptoms. Abdominal ultrasound may be helpful if intussusception is suspected but would not be the optimal test for identifying a Meckel diverticulum.

[ABP 1.E.6. Gastrointestinal bleeding]

179. ANSWER: B

Hemophilia A and B are X-linked bleeding disorders due to congenital deficiencies in clotting factors. Hemarthroses affecting large joints as well as muscle bleeds are common. Timely clotting factor replacement is essential for management of acute bleeding. Patients with hemophilia A are deficient in factor VIII; therefore, administration of either plasma-derived or artificially produced factor VIII is the appropriate next step. Factor IX replacement would be appropriate for patients with hemophilia B. Fresh frozen plasma contains both factor VIII and factor IX, and cryoprecipitate contains factor VIII; these may be used as second-line treatment options if purified factors are unavailable. Supportive care, including rest, elevation of the affected limb, and pain management, is also essential in these cases. Desmopressin acetate may transiently increase factor

VIII levels but is not sufficient therapy for a severe musculoskeletal bleed. Likewise, the antifibrinolytic medications tranexamic acid and aminocaproic acid should be used only in cases of mild-to-moderate bleeding. Patients with muscle bleeding in the lower leg and forearm are at risk for compartment syndrome, which may require fasciotomy. However, the patient's physical examination with a warm and well-perfused extremity is not consistent with compartment syndrome.

[ABP 1.L.3. Bleeding disorders]

180. ANSWER: E

The patient's blood pressure is in the acute severe hypertension range, 30 mm Hg or more above the 95th percentile in a child or more than 180/120 mm Hg in an adolescent. This degree of elevation in blood pressure is classified as a hypertensive emergency if it leads to acute target organ effects, including encephalopathy, acute kidney injury, and congestive heart failure. This patient is presenting with central nervous system findings, which may include retinopathy, encephalopathy, seizure activity, hemiplegia, or facial palsies. Evaluation should focus on secondary causes and target organ effects as guided by the history and physical examination and may include urinalysis, electrolytes, blood urea nitrogen, creatinine, renal ultrasound, echocardiogram, and central nervous system imaging. Although workup is warranted, treatment should not be delayed, and transfer to the intensive care unit is often required. Children and adolescents who present with acute severe hypertension require immediate treatment with short-acting antihypertensive medications such as esmolol, hydralazine, labetalol, clonidine, or isradipine. Intravenous agents are indicated when oral therapy is not possible because of the patient's clinical status or when a severe complication has developed, requiring a more controlled blood pressure reduction. Blood pressure should be reduced by no more than 25% of the planned reduction over the first 8 hours, then gradually normalized over the next 24–48 hours. The ultimate short-term blood pressure goal should generally be around the 95th percentile.

[ABP 1.D.7. Hypertension and hypertensive emergencies]

181. ANSWER: E

This patient has a Glasgow Coma Scale (GCS) score of 7 as indicated by the underlined items in the (Table 1.11). Any patient with a score of 8 or less should be intubated for airway protection.

While this patient will need a CT head to rule out intracranial hemorrhage and she will likely have a central venous catheter placed for continued management, both steps should be taken after her airway is secured.

Laboratory work, including a urine pregnancy test and type and screen, may be pursued after the primary survey is complete and life-threatening conditions have been managed.

Table 1.11 GLASGOW COMA SCALE

SCORE	EYE OPENING	VERBAL RESPONSE	MOTOR RESPONSE
1	No response	No response	No response
2	Opens to pain	Incomprehensible sounds	Decerebrate posturing (abnormal extension)
3	Opens to command	Inappropriate words	Decorticate posturing (abnormal flexion)
4	Spontaneous opening	Confused	Withdraws from pain
5		Appropriate response	Localizes to pain
6			Obeys commands

ª Adapted from Reference 1.

[ABP 1.N.5. Trauma (including head trauma)]

REFERENCE

1. Teasdale G, Jennett B. Assessment and prognosis of coma after head injury. *Acta Neurochir (Wien).* 1976;34(1–4):45–55.

182. ANSWER: D

This is a patient with chronic lung disease of prematurity, or bronchopulmonary dysplasia (BPD), who is maintained on both fluids and full enteral feeds during his hospitalization for pneumonia. He has developed signs of pulmonary edema with wheezing and interstitial markings on chest radiograph. The next step in treatment is a trial of a diuretic like furosemide.

Bronchopulmonary dysplasia is generally diagnosed in premature infants who require oxygen therapy beyond 28 days of life, with various grades dependent on postnatal age and oxygen requirement. These infants can experience acute exacerbations for a variety of reasons, including bacterial and viral infections, irritants such as tobacco exposure, and pulmonary edema. Treatment varies depending on the cause.

Patients with BPD often require fluid restriction due to their risk of pulmonary edema. Caloric density of feeds may have to be increased in order to limit fluid volume while also supporting the infant's growth. Chronic diuretic use is not standard treatment, but it may be required in patients for whom fluid restriction is not successful, particularly those on chronic positive pressure ventilation.

Patients with BPD can have severely reactive airways that require inhaled bronchodilators; however, this patient's wheezing is due to edema rather than reactivity. Therefore, a trial of other nebulized medications, including ipratropium-albuterol and budesonide, would not be the first choice for treatment. His oxygenation is appropriate on his current supplemental oxygen, and increasing it would not improve his edema. Positive pressure support can be helpful in patients with significant pulmonary edema and respiratory distress; however, this patient's overall clinical picture appears stable. Given the patient improved initially and then worsened in the setting of increased volume status, it does not appear this is a decompensation due to infection, so broadening antibiotics is not necessary.

[ABP 1.C.5. Chronic respiratory conditions]

REFERENCE

1. Kair LR, Leonard DT, Anderson JM. Bronchopulmonary dysplasia. *Pediatr Rev.* 2012;33(6):255–264.

183. ANSWER: D

The patient in this question most likely has primary idiopathic intracranial hypertension (IIH). Headache is one of the most common symptoms and is frequently exacerbated by maneuvers that increase intracranial pressure, such as Valsalva or coughing. Additional symptoms include changes in vision, diplopia, transient visual obscurations, and pulsatile tinnitus. Physical examination will often reveal papilledema. In addition, patients with IIH may also be found to have visual field deficits and cranial nerve deficits, particularly abducens nerve (CN VI) palsy. IIH typically affects obese females but can also be observed in males. Several medications have been linked to IIH, including tetracyclines, excess vitamin A, corticosteroids, and growth hormone.

In patients with suspected IIH, medical evaluation should include neuroimaging to evaluate for secondary causes of increased intracranial hypertension. These secondary processes include, but are not limited to, brain abscesses, meningitis, malignancy, cerebral venous thrombosis, and pregnancy. After neuroimaging is completed, the patient should undergo lumbar puncture to assess opening pressure. Finally, formal ophthalmologic assessment is vital when diagnosing and treating a patient with idiopathic intracranial hypertension.

Acetazolamide is first-line treatment for IIH. Side effects include metabolic acidosis, transient paresthesias, and a metallic taste when drinking carbonated beverages. Furosemide is considered second-line treatment. Topiramate, a common treatment for migraines, is a weak carbonic anhydrase inhibitor and considered a potential second-line treatment for IIH. Surgical interventions, such as a lumboperitoneal shunt or optic nerve sheath fenestration, should be reserved for patients who have failed medical management. This patient does not have evidence of meningitis on CSF analysis, so empiric treatment with antibiotics is not indicated at this time.

[ABP 1.A.6. Headaches]

REFERENCE

1. Aylward SC, Reem RE. Pediatric intracranial hypertension. *Pediatr Neurol.* 2017;*66*:32–43.

184. ANSWER: A

This patient's dehydration in combination with left otitis media complicated by mastoiditis puts him at high risk for cerebral sinovenous thrombosis (CSVT). Acute mastoiditis (AM) classically presents with tenderness, erythema, edema, or fluctuance over the mastoid process. Common etiologies include *Streptococcus pneumoniae, Streptococcus pyogenes, Staphylococcus aureus,* and *Pseudomonas aeruginosa.* Recent recommendations to limit the use of antibiotics for AOM have led to an increased incidence of AM. Inadequate antibiotic treatment of AOM can lead to a low-grade persistent infection, which can in turn lead to subacute mastoiditis. Subacute mastoiditis, along with CRP greater than 72 mg/L, is associated with higher incidence of intracranial complications, such as meningitis, lateral sinus thrombosis, occipital osteomyelitis, and subdural/epidural abscess.

Clinical manifestations of CSVT can range from irritability and drowsiness to coma. The triad of altered mental status, headache, and vomiting should prompt neuroimaging with venography. Although seizure, vancomycin toxicity, gastritis, and renal injury could explain vomiting and worsening irritability in a dehydrated child, the most urgent concern is to evaluate for CSVT. While the role of surgery in mastoiditis-related CSVT remains unclear, antibiotics and anticoagulation, along with measures to address elevated intracranial pressure, are mainstays of treatment.

[ABP 1.B.4. Ear, eye, and sinus infections and complications]

REFERENCES

1. Dlamini N, Billinghurst L, Kirkham FJ. Cerebral venous sinus (sinovenous) thrombosis in children. *Neurosurg Clin N Am.* 2010;*21*(3):511–527.
2. Mierzwiński J, Tyra J, Haber K, et al. Therapeutic approach to pediatric acute mastoiditis—an update. *Braz J Otorhinolaryngol.* 2019;*85*(6):724–732.

185. ANSWER: A

Prescription Drug Monitoring Programs are electronic databases that track controlled substance prescriptions. The CDC requires states to develop these databases in an effort to reduce opioid misuse and abuse. While state requirements vary, the CDC recommends checking your state's PDMP every 3 months at a minimum for patients for whom you are writing a controlled substance prescription and prior to writing a new opioid prescription. This review of the PDMP is especially important for patients who have multiple providers and/or are on multiple controlled medications. If you find information in the PDMP that is concerning, you should assess for possible misuse or abuse and discuss your concerns with the patient with an emphasis on their safety as your primary interest. This practice should be standard and not performed only when opioid abuse is suspected or when a request is made by the pharmacy or the family.

[ABP 1.O.8. Pain (acute and chronic)]

186. ANSWER: B

This patient is presenting with diabetic ketoacidosis (DKA), the leading cause of mortality in patients with type 1 diabetes. In adolescence, DKA is most often due to omission of insulin and poor metabolic control. Despite the family's belief that he is adherent to the regimen, insulin nonadherence is the most likely cause of this patient's illness and should be discussed with the patient directly in order to assess adherence and potential barriers. While patients with type 1 diabetes are at increased risk for other autoimmune conditions, including celiac disease and primary adrenal insufficiency (Addison disease), these diagnoses would not increase this patient's risk for DKA. Rather, both conditions are associated with frequent episodes of hypoglycemia. While it is true that there are increased insulin requirements in puberty due to a transient physiologic increase in insulin resistance, puberty alone cannot lead to DKA. Acute illnesses can certainly trigger episodes of DKA, but nothing in this patient's history indicates a recent URI.

[ABP 1.I.6. Diabetes mellitus]

187. ANSWER: D

The "blue dot sign" on this patient's examination makes torsion of the appendix testis the most likely diagnosis. An appendix testis is a remnant of the Müllerian duct that can increase in size under hormonal stimulation in the preadolescent period. This increases the risk of twisting, which can decrease blood flow to the appendage. The blue dot sign seen in this patient is present early but may be obscured later by scrotal swelling. This condition typically self-resolves once the appendage infarcts and necroses. Treatment includes warm compresses, decreased activity, and nonsteroidal anti-inflammatory medications. Surgical resection of the ischemic appendage is indicated only in cases of persistent symptoms. Any patient with acute onset of testicular pain should be evaluated by scrotal ultrasound with Doppler to rule out testicular torsion; blood flow in a patient with torsion of the appendix testis would be normal.

Torsion of the appendix testis is a common mimicker of testicular torsion, a surgical emergency requiring surgical detorsion and fixation. Testicular torsion results from twisting of the spermatic cord and subsequent compromise of testicular blood flow. It is a true surgical emergency, with onset of significant ischemic damage occurring within 4–8 hours. Incidence peaks in the neonatal and adolescent periods, although it can occur at any age. The majority present during puberty, a period of increasing weight and vascularity of the testes. Scrotal ultrasound with Doppler is diagnostic and would show decreased or absent blood flow.

Manual detorsion is a reasonable intervention for patients with testicular torsion who are awaiting surgical repair. It involves rotating the involved testis one or two full 360° turns medial to lateral (outward toward the thigh); if no relief is provided, rotation in the opposite direction (lateral to medial) can be attempted. While manual detorsion may increase the likelihood of testicular salvage in cases of testicular torsion, it is not a substitute for surgical repair. Reassurance and discharge are inappropriate given this patient's persistent symptoms. Antibiotics would be indicated if testing was concerning for bacterial epididymitis, another mimicker of testicular torsion. The presentation and physical examination findings in this vignette make torsion of the appendix testis more likely.

[ABP 1.F.9. Testicular mass and torsion]

188. ANSWER: E

This girl has systemic lupus erythematosus (SLE), as suggested by discoid rash and nephritis. Mucocutaneous manifestations of SLE occur in 60%–85% of cases of juvenile SLE. Malar rash (44%–85%) and generalized lupus rash (30%) are the most common forms of acute cutaneous lupus erythematosus. Discoid rash is more chronic and occurs in less than 10% of cases of juvenile SLE. It can occur without systemic symptoms in discoid lupus. These lesions are often scarring purplish lesions that expand into "coin-shaped" atrophic lesions on the head and face. Oral ulcers may be seen.

Hydroxychloroquine is often used to treat pediatric SLE. Treatment of mucocutaneous lesions of SLE may include topical steroids and/or calcineurin inhibitors. Severe skin lesions or systemic disease flares are often treated with systemic steroids and other immunomodulators. Sunscreen use is important.

Management of SLE often requires a multidisciplinary approach. Consultation with rheumatology is warranted for further workup and treatment. Dermatology and nephrology consultations are indicated, given her mucocutaneous lesions and nephritis. Given her severe presentation with nephritis, her evaluation and treatment are best completed in the inpatient setting.

[ABP 1.H.4. Systemic lupus erythematosus, 1.K.2. Dermatologic manifestations of systemic disease]

REFERENCE

1. Paller A, Mancini A. Discoid lupus erythematosus. In: *Hurwitz Clinical Pediatric Dermatology*. 5th ed. Philadelphia: Elsevier; 2015:509–539.e8.
2. Chiewchengchol D, Murphy R, Edwards SW, Beresford MW. Mucocutaneous manifestations in juvenile-onset systemic lupus erythematosus: a review of literature. *Pediatr Rheumatol Online J*. 2015;*13*:1.

189. ANSWER: D

This boy has Stevens-Johnson syndrome (SJS). SJS and toxic epidermal necrolysis (TEN) are immunologically mediated reactions with rash and mucous membrane involvement that occur as part of a clinical spectrum. Detachment of less than 10% of the total body surface area (BSA) defines SJS, while greater than 30% defines TEN. Cases with 10%–30% BSA involvement are called SJS/TEN overlap. Rash may start as atypical targetoid or painful, erythematous lesions that progress to blistering and skin sloughing. In contrast to the acral distribution seen with many other rashes, SJS/TEN is more widespread, and the full-thickness denudation can lead to issues with thermoregulation, secondary infection, and fluid losses. Triggers may include medications or infections. The most common medication triggers for SJS/TEN include sulfonamides and antiepileptics. Additional inciting medications may include nonsteroidal anti-inflammatory drugs and acetaminophen.

Management includes hospitalization for management of fluids, electrolytes, wound care, and close monitoring for signs of infection and sepsis. Depending on the severity of illness, patients may require transfer to a burn center.

[ABP 1.K.2. Dermatologic manifestations of systemic illness; ABP 1.K.3. Erythema multiforme and Stevens-Johnson syndrome]

190. ANSWER: B

This patient's presentation is consistent with hepatitis A virus (HAV) infection. HAV is a single-stranded RNA virus that is transmitted via the fecal-oral route. Infection with HAV typically results in a self-limited illness that includes fever, abdominal pain, nausea, vomiting, and diarrhea. Patients may develop jaundice approximately 1 week following onset of symptoms and can also present with hepatomegaly. Liver enzymes and conjugated bilirubin can be significantly elevated but typically return to normal within several months. Acute liver failure is very rare in HAV infections, occurring in less than 1% of all cases. HAV is diagnosed by the presence of immunoglobulin (Ig) M antibodies. Autoimmune hepatitis, hepatitis B infection, cholelithiasis, and primary sclerosing cholangitis are all less likely in the patient given the acute onset of symptoms as well as lack of past medical and family history and normal imaging findings.

[ABP 1.E.7. Hepatitis]

191. ANSWER: C

Catheter-related venous thrombi have become an increasing problem among hospitalized children and may contribute to patient morbidity, hospitalization cost, and length of stay. Patients may be asymptomatic or demonstrate extremity edema, phlebitis, or emboli. If a central catheter is placed, the hospitalist should be aware of factors that confer additional risk for thrombosis.

Factor V Leiden is an inherited thrombotic disorder that places patients at risk of both catheter and non–catheter-related thrombosis. Affected patients have a variant of human factor V that prevents binding of the anticoagulant protein C, creating a hypercoagulable state. Glanzmann thrombasthenia is a genetic platelet disorder that predisposes to bleeding rather than thrombosis. Characteristics of the catheter itself also contribute to clotting risk. Larger catheter size relative to a vein will prevent blood flowing freely and predispose to stagnation; accordingly, large-diameter and multilumen catheters carry increased risk of thrombosis. Peripherally inserted catheters have higher rates of thrombosis than centrally inserted catheters, again likely due to their placement in smaller blood vessels.

[ABP 1.L.2. Deep venous thrombosis/pulmonary embolism/hypercoagulable states]

192. ANSWER: B

This patient's syncopal episode has several features concerning for a cardiac cause, including its occurrence during exercise, lack of prodromal symptoms, rapid return to baseline, and absence of abnormal movements and incontinence during the event. Thus, a workup including an ECG, echocardiogram, and cardiac monitoring is warranted to evaluate for cardiac causes of syncope, such as structural heart disease, arrythmias, or myocardial dysfunction. An ECG may demonstrate baseline abnormalities, including a delta wave in Wolff-Parkinson-White, which is associated with supraventricular tachycardia or prolonged QT intervals. Episodes associated with chest pain or palpitations are also concerning for a cardiac etiology, but these symptoms are not always present. There may be an associated family history of sudden cardiac death in relatives under 50 years of

age or congenital deafness, which can be associated with prolonged QT syndrome. An EEG would not be helpful as this patient did not have abnormal or tonic-clonic movements, a postictal period, prolonged altered mental status, incontinence, or other features suggestive of a neurologic etiology. Psychogenic syncope is rare in patients less than 10 years of age and often presents with prolonged syncope from 20 to 60 minutes. An expanded social history would be warranted in a workup of psychogenic syncope. Organic causes of syncope must be ruled out before considering psychogenic etiologies. Dehydration, hypoglycemia, anemia, and electrolyte abnormalities can all cause syncope, but the patient is unlikely to improve to baseline without intervention.

[ABP 1.D.6. Syncope]

193. ANSWER: A

This patient with a lower extremity long-bone fracture, now with an external cast, is at high risk for compartment syndrome. The first sign of compartment syndrome is pain out of proportion to the injury, which in this case is noted by an acute increase in his pain level. Although his toes are warm and well perfused, the other Ps of compartment syndrome (poikilothermy, pallor, paresthesia, paralysis, and pulselessness) are all late signs and poor prognostic indicators. Therefore, the best next step would be to remove the cast and measure compartment pressures while awaiting orthopedic surgery consultation for possible fasciotomy. Reassuring the patient without further evaluating him for compartment syndrome would not be appropriate at this stage. Increasing the patient's pain medications or prescribing an anxiolytic would not address his underlying compartment syndrome. Rather, it may mask his symptoms and cause adverse effects, such as respiratory depression. While computed tomography of his leg may show evidence of compartment syndrome, x-rays in this postoperative patient would not be helpful.

[ABP 1.N.5. Trauma (including head trauma)]

194. ANSWER: B

Viruses can destroy the respiratory epithelium, thus impairing mucociliary clearance and setting the stage for bacterial superinfection, as in this patient with uncomplicated community-acquired pneumonia (CAP). Methicillin-resistant *Staphylococcus aureus* (MRSA) infections are increasing, while vaccination has decreased the incidence of pneumonia due to *Hemophilus influenzae type B*. For previously healthy, fully immunized children with CAP, narrow-spectrum antibiotics are recommended. Because *Streptococcus pneumoniae* is the most likely etiology in this fully immunized child, and higher serum concentration levels can be achieved with parenteral antibiotics than with oral amoxicillin, ampicillin is the best initial choice for this patient unless local antibiograms indicate high-level penicillin resistance among isolates. If no clinical improvement is seen within 48–72 hours, consideration should be given to additional diagnostic testing and broadening antibacterial coverage. In the absence of severe disease and negative influenza testing, *Staphylococcus aureus* coverage is not indicated. Likewise, attempts should be made to obtain a high-quality sputum culture, reserving BAL for patients with severe disease if initial testing is nondiagnostic. Azithromycin should be considered for treatment of CAP with characteristics consistent with *Mycoplasma pneumoniae* in school-age children, but its effects as an anti-inflammatory and immunomodulating agent lack sufficient data to recommend use. Urinary antigen testing for pneumococcal pneumonia is not routinely recommended due to the high false-positive rate.

[ABP 1.C.3. Pneumonia]

REFERENCE

1. Bradley JS, Byington CL, Shah SS, et al. The management of community-acquired pneumonia in infants and children older than 3 months of age: clinical practice guidelines by the Pediatric Infectious Diseases Society and the Infectious Diseases Society of America. *Clin Infect Dis.* 2011;53(7):e25–e76.

195. ANSWER: A

This patient most likely has Duchenne muscular dystrophy (DMD). DMD is inherited in an X-linked recessive manner and causes a defect in the production of dystrophin. Given this pattern of inheritance, males are predominantly affected. Patients usually present with chronic weakness starting around 2–3 years of age. Weakness preferentially affects proximal muscles as manifested in this patient's use of hand support to transition to an upright position (known as the Gower sign). Serum creatine kinase will usually be elevated in DMD. Children with DMD will have gradual motor function decline, ultimately resulting in being wheelchair bound by the age of 13 years. Long-term complications include the risk for dilated cardiomyopathy and chronic respiratory failure. Examples of the other modes of inheritance include Marfan syndrome (autosomal dominant), cystic fibrosis and sickle cell disease (autosomal recessive), Leigh syndrome (mitochondrial), and fragile X syndrome (X-linked dominant).

[ABP 1.A.11. Other (weakness)]

196. ANSWER: E

Prompt diagnosis of orbital cellulitis is imperative to avoid serious complications, including vision loss, intracranial extension, and thrombosis. In patients with periorbital edema and erythema, differentiating between preseptal and orbital cellulitis involves exclusion of orbital involvement signs (Table 1.12). Contrast-enhanced computed tomography may be helpful when physical examination is equivocal or concern exists for neurologic involvement. Sinusitis, particularly ethmoiditis, is a common predisposing factor for orbital cellulitis in children under 6 years. Routine blood cultures have been shown to be low yield without evidence of systemic involvement, but ocular and surgical site cultures should be obtained as indicated. For uncomplicated patients, antibacterial coverage targeting *Staphylococcus* and *Streptococcus* species is sufficient as these organisms cause 75% of disease. If hematogenous seeding or odontogenic etiology is suspected, coverage should be broadened to include gram-negative and anaerobic organisms. CRP and WBC count are more likely to be elevated in orbital cellulitis versus preseptal. While corticosteroid use is not routinely currently recommended, recent data suggest that corticosteroid use is safe and effective and can significantly decrease length of hospitalization. Surgical intervention targets draining abscesses, releasing pressure on the orbit, and obtaining cultures; however, patients with small medial subperiosteal abscess, non–frontal sinus involvement, and age less than 9 years may be safely and effectively managed with antibiotics alone.

Table 1.12 DIFFERENTIATING BETWEEN PRESEPTAL AND ORBITAL CELLULITIS

	PRESEPTAL	ORBITAL
Predisposing factor(s)	Trauma/local skin infection	Rhinosinusitis (ethmoiditis)
Fever at admission	Less frequent	Frequent
Periorbital edema	Yes	Yes
Periorbital erythema	Yes	Yes
Chemosis	Rare	Frequent
Ophthalmoplegia	Rare	Frequent
Ocular pain	Less frequent	Frequent
Proptosis	Rare	Frequent
Photophobia	Less frequent	Frequent
Painful extraocular motion	Less frequent	Frequent
Visual impairment	Rare	Frequent
Elevated WBC and CRP	Less frequent	Frequent

CRP, C-reactive protein; WBC, white blood cell.

[ABP 1.B.4. Ear, eye, and sinus infections and complications]

REFERENCE

1. Chen L, Silverman N, Wu A, Shinder R. Intravenous steroids with antibiotics on admission for children with orbital cellulitis. *Ophthalmic Plast Reconstr Surg.* 2018;34(3):205–208.

197. ANSWER: B

The Centers for Disease Control and Prevention asks providers to calculate MME for patients on opioids in an effort to improve patient safety by identifying patients who may benefit from closer monitoring, reduction or tapering of opioids, prescribing of naloxone, or other measures to reduce risk of overdose. Table 1.13 showing how to calculate MMEs for different medications:

Table 1.13 CALCULATING MORPHINE MILLIGRAM EQUIVALENTS (MMES)

OPIOID	CONVERSION FACTOR
Codeine (mg/d)	0.15
Fentanyl transdermal (μg/h)	2.4
Hydrocodone (mg/d)	1
Hydromorphone (mg/d)	4
Methadone 1–20 (mg/d)	4
Methadone 21–40 (mg/d)	8
Methadone 41–60 (mg/d)	10
Methadone ≥61–80 (mg/d)	12
Morphine (mg/d)	1
Oxycodone (mg/d)	1.5
Oxymorphone (mg/d)	3

ᵃ Adapted from Reference 1.

[ABP 1.O.8. Pain (acute and chronic)]

REFERENCE

1. Module 6: dosing and titration of opioids: how much, how long, and how and when to stop? Centers for Disease Control and Prevention. Updated August 7, 2020. Accessed June 1, 2021. https://www.cdc.gov/drugoverdose/training/dosing/accessible/index.html.

198. ANSWER: D

This patient has diabetic ketoacidosis (DKA), evidenced by the hyperglycemia, anion-gap metabolic acidosis, and ketones in the urine. Gastroenteritis is a risk factor for the development of DKA as it leads to release of stress hormones that increase glucose output. Hyperventilation is a classic symptom as the patient attempts to breathe off the excess acid in the form of carbon dioxide. Children with DKA are typically dehydrated on presentation, often due to underlying illness as well as polyuria from hyperglycemia. The first step in management is to perform isotonic volume resuscitation with 10 to 20 mL/kg of normal saline. The remaining fluid deficit should be corrected slowly over the next 24–48 hours.

Hyponatremia is common in DKA as hyperglycemia increases plasma osmolality and leads to fluid shifts that dilute the sodium concentration proportionately. The degree of hyponatremia can be predicted by a reduction in the serum sodium by 1.6 mmol/L for every 100 mg/dL increase in glucose over 100 mg/dL. Serum hyperkalemia is also common due to potassium shifts into the extracellular space in the setting of acidosis; however, patients should be presumed to have low total-body potassium levels. While dangerously high potassium levels may require calcium gluconate infusion to prevent cardiotoxicity, this patient's hyperkalemia is not high enough to require it. Most children in DKA will have some degree of cerebral edema; imaging is generally not helpful in patients who have a normal neurologic examination as detection of mild cerebral edema will not change management. An insulin infusion is necessary for this patient, but volume resuscitation is the most important first step. Bicarbonate should not be given to patients in DKA; its administration has been associated with worse outcomes, including cerebral injury.

[ABP 1.I.6. Diabetes mellitus]

REFERENCE

1. Kuppermann N, Ghetti S, Schunk JE, et al. Clinical trial of fluid infusion rates for pediatric diabetic ketoacidosis. *N Engl J Med.* 2018;378(24):2275–2287.

199. ANSWER: B

This patient is presenting with symptoms of nephrolithiasis. The most sensitive test for detecting renal stones is CT without contrast, which can detect radio-opaque and radiolucent stones, as well as those that are small or in harder to visualize locations, such as the renal calyces or ureters. Contrast is not needed and may decrease the sensitivity for detecting smaller stones. Ultrasonography, when done by an experienced technician, is an appropriate initial imaging study in patients with suspected nephrolithiasis as it can detect radiolucent and radio-opaque stones without radiation. However, ultrasound may miss small stones as well as those in harder-to-visualize locations. Plain radiographs may miss radiolucent stones, such as urate stones. MRI is not typically used to identify renal stones.

[ABP 1.F.4. Nephrolithiasis]

200. ANSWER: C

This patient has classic KD, which is diagnosed in the setting of 5 days of fever with at least four out of five of the following clinical criteria: enlarged cervical lymph node greater than 1.5 cm; bilateral conjunctival injection; polymorphous rash; mucous membrane changes (e.g., fissured lips, strawberry tongue); and extremity changes (e.g., edema, erythema, desquamation). IVIG is the recommended treatment and reduces the risk of development of coronary artery ectasias and aneurysms. It is common for patients to continue to have fevers in the first 24 hours after treatment; patients are only considered refractory if they continue to have fevers 36 hours after completion of the first dose of IVIG. At this time, acetaminophen is the best choice for symptomatic treatment of the fever. Of note, ibuprofen should be avoided as nonsteroidal anti-inflammatory drugs should not be given to children receiving aspirin.

For refractory KD, both a second dose of IVIG and infliximab have been found to be effective in resolving the disease; the decision between these two agents is typically based on local expert consensus and is an area currently under further study. Neither is indicated unless the fevers continue 36 hours after completion of IVIG. The data on the benefits of corticosteroids is conflicting; some populations at particularly high risk of refractory KD may benefit from corticosteroids, but there is not currently a role for them in the standard management. An echocardiogram is recommended on diagnosis in order to describe the coronary arteries at baseline; repeat studies are recommended at approximately 2 and 6 weeks posttreatment to monitor for development of coronary artery changes. There is no benefit to repeating an echocardiogram at this time.

[ABP 1.H.2. Kawasaki disease]

201. ANSWER: D

The boy has cellulitis of the right lower extremity and failed empiric outpatient antibiotics. He meets sepsis criteria given the presence of systemic inflammatory response syndrome (SIRS) and documented infection. He requires admission for IV antibiotics with activity against streptococci and staphylococci per Infectious Disease Society of America (IDSA) guidelines. For patients with penetrating trauma-associated cellulitis, evidence of colonization or methicillin-resistant *Streptococcus aureus* (MRSA) infection elsewhere, injectable drug use, or SIRS, vancomycin or another antimicrobial effective against both MRSA and streptococci is recommended. Expanding coverage to include MRSA is also advisable given treatment failure of a non–MRSA-active drug. The local antibiogram should be considered. The recommended duration of antimicrobial therapy is 5 days but should be extended if the infection is not resolved. There is no evidence of abscess or necrotizing infection necessitating surgical consultation at this time.

[ABP 1.K.1. Skin and soft tissue infections]

202. ANSWER: A

The patient's presentation is concerning for primary sclerosing cholangitis (PSC), a progressive disease characterized by inflammation and fibrosis of the ducts of the intra- and extrahepatic biliary tree. An overwhelming majority of patients with PSC also have ulcerative colitis, although less than 10% of patients with ulcerative colitis will develop PSC. Patients with PSC are often asymptomatic, receiving a diagnosis following abnormal laboratory tests, including elevated alkaline phosphatase and bilirubin. Symptomatic patients most frequently experience fatigue and pruritis. The most specific histologic findings of PSC on liver biopsy include fibrous obliteration of small bile ducts with concentric replacement by connective tissue. Steatosis is most consistent with nonalcoholic fatty liver disease. A finding of portal mononuclear cell infiltrates surrounding the portal triad is characteristic of autoimmune hepatitis. Proliferation of hyperplastic hepatocytes surrounding a central stellate scar is seen with focal nodular hyperplasia. Lobular inflammation with focal necrosis can indicate drug injury with agents such as acetaminophen.

[ABP 1.E.2. Cholecystitis and cholangitis]

203. ANSWER: B

This vignette is most consistent with vasovagal syncope. Typical features of vasovagal events include (1) a preceding event, such as prolonged standing or heat exposure; (2) a brief prodrome of symptoms, including dizziness, lightheadedness, or flushing; (3) full recovery with no prolonged confusion; and (4) loss of consciousness of less than 1 minute. Vasovagal syncope can include myoclonic jerks. The mechanism involves a series of events leading to increased parasympathetic activity, bradycardia, vasodilation, hypotension, and subsequent decreased cerebral perfusion and loss of consciousness. Orthostatic hypotension is a decrease in blood pressure due to inadequate vasoconstriction of the vessels and can be caused by chronic illness, autonomic dysfunction, and hypovolemia. It usually occurs when moving from a seated or supine position into a standing position rather than from remaining in a standing position for a prolonged period of time. The episode was not consistent with cardiogenic syncope from an AV conduction abnormality or seizures from an area of abnormal brain activity. An episode of psychogenic syncope, in which emotions are manifested through physical symptoms, typically lasts longer (up to 20–60 minutes) than in this case. Furthermore, this child has no known risk factors for psychogenic syncope.

[ABP 1.D.6. Syncope]

204. ANSWER: B

Tetanus prophylaxis should be considered for any wound. If a patient has not yet received three doses of a tetanus toxoid-containing vaccine, they should receive a dose of the vaccine for all wounds. Tetanus immune globulin is only indicated in incompletely vaccinated patients if the wound cannot be classified as both clean and minor. In patients who have received at least three doses of a tetanus toxoid–containing vaccine, they should receive a booster if the most recent vaccine was more than 10 years ago for clean, minor wounds or if the most recent tetanus toxoid vaccine was more than 5 years ago in other cases. Animal bites are not considered clean. Given that this patient received her last tetanus vaccine more than 5 years ago, she should receive a booster at this time.

Postexposure prophylaxis (PEP) for rabies involves administration of rabies vaccine and rabies immune globulin. For high-risk animals, including those suspected of having rabies and wild animals such as bats, skunks, raccoons, foxes, and coyotes, the patient should be given PEP. For domesticated animals that can be observed for 10 days, PEP only needs to be given if the animal develops symptoms of rabies during this time.

[ABP 1.N.2. Insect and animal bites]

205. ANSWER: E

Pneumonia is one of the most frequent healthcare-associated infections and a leading cause of mortality. Hospital-acquired pneumonia (HAP), including the subtype ventilator-associated pneumonia, can be bacterial, viral, fungal, and polymicrobial and is generally characterized by the development of pneumonia after more than 48 hours of hospitalization. Risk factors for HAP development in this patient include neurological impairment, high aspiration risk, frequent airway suctioning, malnutrition, antibiotic exposure in the past 90 days, gastric tube feeding, and increasing age. Other risk factors include immunosuppression or deficiency, trauma, and recent blood product transfusion. Risk factors for development of multidrug resistant (MDR) organisms, particularly *Pseudomonas aeruginosa*, Enterobacteriaceae, and *Staphylococcus aureus*, include hospitalization longer than 2 days in the past 90 days and current hospitalization of 5 or more days. The risk of MDR pathogens should guide decision-making in initial empiric therapy. While PPIs have been associated with *Clostridium difficile* infections in children, currently there are no large population studies assessing the risk of HAP in pediatric patients on short- or long-term PPI therapy. In fact, recent prospective data suggest the use of PPIs and noninvasive ventilation were associated with protection from developing HAP. While scoliosis, homelessness, and recent travel may be associated with other pulmonary diseases, they are not specifically a risk factor for hospital-acquired pneumonia.

[ABP 1.C.3. Pneumonia]

REFERENCE

1. Stark CM, Nylund CM. Side effects and complications of proton pump inhibitors: a pediatric perspective. *J Pediatr.* 2016;*168*:16–22.

206. ANSWER: D

The first step in the management of a seizure is stabilizing the patient and addressing immediate concerns impairing airway, breathing, or circulation. This patient is experiencing hypoxia because of her seizure activity, and supplemental oxygen should be started immediately. Seizures can be life threatening, and seizures of longer duration are associated with higher morbidity and mortality. Benzodiazepines are the initial therapy of choice in the treatment of seizures lasting longer than 5 minutes. Acceptable first-line treatments include IV lorazepam and IV diazepam. Studies do not demonstrate superiority of one medication over another. Rectal diazepam and intranasal midazolam are also effective. The patient may require additional head imaging or initiation of a daily antiseizure drug, but these would not be an appropriate first step.

[ABP 1.A.2. Seizures]

REFERENCE

1. Glauser T, Shinnar S, Gloss D, et al. Evidence-based guideline: treatment of convulsive status epilepticus in children and adults: report of the Guideline Committee of the American Epilepsy Society. *Epilepsy Curr.* 2016;*16*(1):48–61.

207. ANSWER: A

Frontal sinuses appear by age 7 years and are pneumatized in adolescence. Common predisposing factors for frontal sinusitis include viral upper respiratory infection and allergic rhinitis. A Pott puffy tumor (PPT) is an osteomyelitis of the frontal bone in the setting of frontal sinusitis that presents with forehead swelling and tenderness. PPT is often associated with sinogenic intracranial extension (SIE). The association of epidural abscess with PPT is well documented. The most common bacterial etiologies include *Streptococcus pneumoniae*, *Haemophilus influenzae*, and *Moraxella catarrhalis*, although most complications are polymicrobial. Contrast-enhanced head and sinus CT provides the best delineation of bone and sinus detail; however, MRI with contrast remains the gold standard for diagnosing SIE, as is suspected in this patient. Lumbar puncture can be helpful in diagnosing associated meningitis, and a low threshold for obtaining EEG should be maintained given the high incidence of seizures in SIE, but neither procedure should delay necessary diagnostic imaging. Management consists of targeted antibacterial therapy with adequate central nervous system penetration and surgical drainage. After obtaining appropriate imaging, evaluating the need for sinus surgery and debridement by a pediatric otolaryngologist will be necessary. Consultation with a pediatric neurosurgeon is critical for addressing drainage of any intracranial fluid collections visualized on MRI. Supportive care may include anticonvulsants, analgesics, and intracranial pressure-reducing agents as indicated.

[ABP 1.B.4. Ear, eye, and sinus infections and complications]

REFERENCES

1. Anfuso A, Ramadan H, Terrell A, et al. Sinus and adenoid inflammation in children with chronic rhinosinusitis and asthma. *Ann Allergy Asthma Immunol.* 2015;*114*(2):103–110.
2. Patel NA, Garber D, Hu S, Kamat A. Systematic review and case report: intracranial complications of pediatric sinusitis. *Int J Pediatr Otorhinolaryngol.* 2016;*86*:200–212.

208. ANSWER: B

This infant is presenting with a metabolic acidosis with hyperkalemia and hyponatremia consistent with congenital adrenal hyperplasia (CAH). Patients with CAH are often noted on newborn screening; however, a newborn born at home may not be screened appropriately. While females with CAH often present with ambiguous genitalia, males with CAH may have little to no genitourinary abnormalities on examination. There may be subtle findings, such as hyperpigmentation of the scrotal area or enlargement of the phallus.

Patients with the salt-wasting form of CAH present routinely around 7–14 days of life with dehydration, hypotension, vomiting, diarrhea, and/or lethargy. Electrolyte abnormalities, including a metabolic acidosis and hyperkalemia with or without hyponatremia, should prompt the consideration of adrenal crisis. The mainstay of therapy for adrenal crisis is high-dose corticosteroids. While the patient does have a metabolic acidosis that could be improved with sodium bicarbonate, this would not address the underlying disease process. Similarly, while the infant is in a high-risk age group for infection, history and laboratory findings do not support a diagnosis of infection. While empiric antibiotics and dextrose-containing intravenous fluids may be warranted, they would not treat the underlying disease process in this patient.

[ABP 1.O.7. Acid/base disorders]

209. ANSWER: E

Hyponatremia is common in hospitalized children. This patient has hyponatremia due to the syndrome of inappropriate antidiuretic hormone secretion (SIADH). Antidiuretic hormone (ADH) is secreted by the posterior pituitary primarily in response to increases in serum osmolality, resulting in increased retention of free water by the kidneys and a more concentrated urine. In SIADH, the patient retains free water even though the serum osmolality is not elevated. As this patient's hyponatremia is mild and she is asymptomatic, the mainstay of management is fluid restriction.

Causes of SIADH include central nervous system disturbances (e.g., trauma or infection); drugs; pulmonary diseases (e.g., pneumonia and asthma); pain; psychosis; tumors; and more. SIADH should be suspected in patients who appear well hydrated but have a hypoosmolar hyponatremia and concentrated urine. A urine sodium greater than 40 mEq/L is also consistent with the diagnosis. Patients with mild hyponatremia may have symptoms such as irritability and fatigue; more severe hyponatremia (particularly below 125 mmol/L) can cause lethargy and headache, progressing to seizures and coma. Symptoms tend to be more dramatic with an acute decrease in sodium rather than chronic changes. Care should be taken not to correct sodium too quickly in chronic hyponatremia as osmotic demyelination can result. It is unclear whether this patient's hyponatremia is acute or chronic, so her hyponatremia must be presumed chronic. Given this and her lack of symptoms, there is no reason to rapidly correct her sodium level. Hypertonic saline should be reserved for children with severe symptoms. A 20-mL/kg normal saline bolus would be recommended if the patient's hyponatremia were due to dehydration; dehydration is unlikely as the patient is well hydrated on examination, and a urine sodium of less than 20 mEq/L would be expected. Desmopressin is a synthetic form of ADH used either for patients who do not make sufficient ADH (e.g., diabetes insipidus) or in circumstances where a more concentrated urine is desired (e.g., a slumber party for a child with urinary incontinence). This patient has the opposite problem—too much ADH effect rather than too little. Certain drugs can cause SIADH, such as certain anticonvulsants and opiates, but ampicillin does not.

Given the high rate of hyponatremia in the hospitalized patient population, including due to SIADH, recent guidelines recommend use of isotonic maintenance fluids for inpatients in order to avoid iatrogenic hyponatremia.

[ABP 1.I.2. Syndrome of inappropriate diuretic hormone secretion]

REFERENCE

1. Feld LG, Neuspiel DR, Foster BA, et al. Clinical practice guideline: maintenance intravenous fluids in children. *Pediatrics.* 2018;*142*(6):e20183083.

210. ANSWER: B

Most patients with urinary tract infections improve on therapy within 24–48 hours. The lack of expected response may indicate the presence of a renal or perirenal abscess, pyonephrosis, or an anatomic abnormality that can be detected using RBUS. Parenchymal scarring is associated with pyelonephritis, particularly if there is delayed initiation of treatment. However, identifying renal scarring with a Tc 99m DMSA scan would not change management at this time. The rates of bacteremia have not been found to be significantly different in patients who remain febrile for more than 48 hours compared to those who do not, so a blood culture would not be indicated. A VCUG may be helpful to look for vesicoureteral reflux if the RBUS is abnormal; however, it would not be the best next step. An abdominal CT scan may also reveal abscesses or anatomic abnormalities; however, a RBUS is the preferred next step to avoid radiation.

[ABP 1.F.10. Pyelonephritis/urinary tract infections]

211. ANSWER: B

The patient's presentation is concerning for infantile hypertrophic pyloric stenosis (IHPS). Most commonly impacting infants between 3-6 weeks of age, IHPS is characterized by hypertrophy of the pylorus, which can cause persistent vomiting due to partial or complete obstruction. It is more common in males, with a 4:1 male-to-female ratio. These patients often have hypochloremic, hypokalemic metabolic alkalosis given the increased loss of gastric contents. Increased white blood cell count and conjugated bilirubin levels are not associated with IHPS, though some cases are associated with an unconjugated hyperbilirubinemia. Patients more commonly present with metabolic alkalosis with associated elevated bicarbonate level. This patient does not show signs of significant clinical dehydration, which could contribute to a lactic acidosis and obscure the typical findings.

[ABP 1.E.8. Obstruction]

212. ANSWER: D

The child in this case presents with hyperkalemia resulting in ventricular fibrillation and cardiopulmonary arrest. The Pediatric Advanced Life Support (PALS) cardiac arrest algorithm recommends administering a shock as soon as a defibrillator is available for patients in cardiac arrest with a shockable rhythm, including ventricular tachycardia and ventricular fibrillation. Delivering a shock takes precedence over treating reversible causes, even if the cause of the arrest is clear, as it is in this case. The appropriate initial dose for the first

shock is 2 J/kg and for the second is 4 J/kg. Epinephrine 0.01 mg/kg should be given after two shocks have been delivered. Insulin will treat the patient's hyperkalemia, and calcium gluconate can antagonize the hyperkalemia-induced depolarization of cardiac myocytes; both should be given after shock delivery.

[ABP 1.D.8. Cardiac arrest]

213. ANSWER: B

This child has failure to thrive and a non–anion gap metabolic acidosis. Non–anion gap metabolic acidosis is generally due to the excess loss of bicarbonate from the gastrointestinal tract (i.e., as diarrhea) or in the urine due to RTA. Given this patient's growth concerns and lack of history of diarrhea, RTA is the most likely diagnosis.

Renal tubular acidosis can be either genetic or acquired (often due to medications). There are three types (Table 1.14): Type 1 is due to pathology in the distal tubule, type 2 is due to pathology in the proximal tubule, and type 4 is due to aldosterone insufficiency or resistance. All forms can be associated with failure to thrive. Some forms, particularly type 2, may be mild and resolve within several years. The treatment varies by etiology, but typically includes bicarbonate administration. Diabetes mellitus causes a high anion gap metabolic acidosis due to accumulation of keto acids. Organic acidemia causes a high anion gap metabolic acidosis due to the accumulation of organic acids. Some mitochondrial disorders cause a high anion gap metabolic acidosis due to the accumulation of lactic acid. While hypoaldosteronism causes type 4 RTA, aldosterone excess does not cause acidosis.

Table 1.14 TYPES OF RENAL TUBULAR ACIDOSIS (RTA)

	ASSOCIATIONS	URINE PH	SERUM POTASSIUM
Type 1 RTA (distal)	Nephrocalcinosis, deafness	>5.3	Low
Type 2 RTA (proximal)	Fanconi syndrome	<5.3	Low/normal
Type 4 (hypoaldosteronism)	—	>5.3	High

[ABP 1.O.2. Failure to thrive, ABP 1.O.7. Acid/base disorders]

214. ANSWER: D

Deep wounds from an animal bite, especially cat bites, and bites near a joint should receive antibiotic prophylaxis with an agent that has good activity against anaerobes and skin flora, as well as specifically *Pasteurella multocida*. The preferred agent in this case is amoxicillin-clavulanate; however, doxycycline or a combination of trimethoprim-sulfamethoxazole and clindamycin are appropriate alternative regimens for patients with penicillin allergies. Cephalexin is inappropriate as it does not provide adequate coverage for anaerobic bacteria. Azithromycin has shown in vitro activity against organisms responsible for bite wound infections, but there is insufficient data to recommend azithromycin over the regimens listed. Azithromycin can be used for *Bartonella henselae* infections such as in cat scratch disease. However, these patients would present with a cutaneous lesion at the site of the bite, regional lymphadenopathy, prolonged fever, neurologic manifestations, or occasionally solid-organ lesions.

[ABP 1.N.2. Insect and animal bites]

215. ANSWER: A

Increased lipid content in alveolar macrophages of BAL fluid is a useful indicator of recurrent pulmonary aspiration. Children with neurologic impairment and technology dependence are at high risk of aspiration with resulting respiratory failure. Children with aspiration pneumonia are more likely to have complex chronic conditions, prolonged and repeated hospitalizations, and need for intensive care. Oropharyngeal dysphagia, esophageal motility disorders, and enteral tube feeding are also risk factors for recurrent aspiration. Recurrent pneumonia is defined as two or more episodes in 1 year or three or more episodes in a lifetime with intervening radiographic resolution. Recurrent pneumonia requires further investigation in the presence of certain risk factors, including onset in the first months of life, severe symptoms, serious complications, unusual causative pathogens, and a family history of genetic respiratory disorders. In addition to chest radiography, diagnostic modalities include flexible bronchoscopy with BAL and high-resolution computed tomography, with characteristic findings and etiologies detailed in the Table 1.15.

Persistent opacification in the same area on chest radiography suggests recurrent aspiration (classically right middle lobe), persistent pathogens (tuberculosis and fungal infections), or focal anatomic abnormalities. Repeat chest imaging 6–8 weeks after clinical resolution is indicated to evaluate for an underlying structural abnormality with recurrent pneumonia in a specific location. Infiltrates that recur in different areas have a broad differential diagnosis, so a targeted diagnostic approach based on clinical suspicion is recommended.

Table 1.15 CHARACTERISTIC BRONCHOALVEOLAR LAVAGE ANALYSIS AND CHEST HIGH-RESOLUTION COMPUTED TOMOGRAPHY FINDINGS IN CHILDREN WITH RECURRENT PNEUMONIA

DIAGNOSTIC MODALITY	FINDING(S)	SUGGESTED DIAGNOSIS
Flexible bronchoscopy with bronchoalveolar lavage	Pathogen culture, cytology	Infection: bacterial (majority), fungal (patients with immune dysfunction)
	Dynamic compression/collapse	Tracheo-/bronchomalacia
	Intraluminal obstruction	Bronchogenic cysts/malformations, foreign body, mucus plugs, blood clots
	Lipid-laden macrophages	Recurrent aspiration
Chest high-resolution computed tomography	Airway bronchiectasis, cystic changes	Cystic fibrosis, primary ciliary dyskinesia, immunodeficiency, foreign body, recurrent aspiration
	Airway compression	Lymph node, tumor, vascular ring/sling, cardiomyopathy
	Consolidation, cavitary abscesses, pleural effusions with loculations	Infection, eosinophilc pneumonia, hemorrhage

[ABP 1.C.3. Pneumonia]

REFERENCE

1. Montella S, Corcione A, Santamaria F. Recurrent pneumonia in children: a reasoned diagnostic approach and a single centre experience. *Int J Mol Sci*. 2017;18(2):296.

216. ANSWER: C

The patient in this clinical vignette is displaying signs and symptoms most consistent with serotonin syndrome. His symptoms are likely due to fluoxetine, a selective serotonin reuptake inhibitor (SSRI) with a long drug half-life, and the recent addition of an over-the-counter cough medicine. The active ingredient in many cough suppressants is dextromethorphan, a medication known to impair serotonin reuptake. Symptoms of serotonin syndrome include altered mental status (disorientation, agitation, delirium); neuromuscular abnormalities (tremors, hyperreflexia, rigidity, clonus, bilateral Babinski sign); and autonomic hyperactivity (tachycardia, hypertension, hyperthermia, flushed skin, diaphoresis, vomiting, diarrhea). Management involves discontinuation of all precipitating serotonergic agents and supportive care as needed with intravenous fluids and supplemental oxygen. Benzodiazepines can also be utilized to control agitation.

Intoxication with LSD can also present with hyperthermia, hypertension, and diaphoresis; however, there is usually a predominance of neuropsychiatric symptoms, such as auditory or visual hallucinations, altered time perception, and feelings of euphoria. While infective meningitis should be considered in patients presenting with fever and confusion, the patient's other symptoms could not be attributed to this diagnosis. Neuroleptic malignant syndrome (NMS) is a severe reaction typically in response to antipsychotic medications. Symptoms of NMS include hyperthermia, tachycardia, diaphoresis, altered mental status, and "lead-pipe" muscle rigidity. Patients with NMS typically will not present with hyperreflexia or clonus. Malignant hyperthermia is a rare, potentially life-threatening reaction that can occur after a patient is exposed to a volatile anesthetic or succinylcholine.

[ABP 1.A.1. Altered mental status]

REFERENCE

1. Boyer EW, Shannon M. The serotonin syndrome. *N Engl J Med.* 2005;*352*(11):1112–1120.

217. ANSWER: C

This patient presents with acute onset of epiglottitis, which first requires emergent airway stabilization. Addressing the underlying infectious cause requires initiation of antibiotics with a third-generation cephalosporin and an antistaphylococcal agent. The antistaphylococcal agent should be chosen based on community prevalence of methicillin-resistant *Staphylococcus aureus* (MRSA) and its susceptibilities. Obtaining epiglottic cultures in intubated patients prior to the start of antibiotics can help guide antibiotic management. While *Haemophilus influenzae* type B has become less common, other bacterial culprits include *Streptococcus pneumoniae*, group A *Streptococcus*, and *S. aureus* (including MRSA). Thus, antibiotic treatment should be initiated with a third-generation cephalosporin as well as an antistaphylococcal agent and later narrowed based on culture results.

[ABP 1.B.1. Upper airway infections and conditions]

REFERENCE

1. Shah RK, Roberson DW, Jones DT. Epiglottitis in the *Hemophilus influenzae* type B vaccine era: changing trends. *Laryngoscope.* 2004;*114*(3):557–560.

218. ANSWER: B

The patient has fever in the setting of severe neutropenia likely caused by the methotrexate needed to treat his dermatomyositis. Patients with severe neutropenia as defined by an ANC below 500 are at risk for serious bacterial infection. In addition to fluid resuscitation, prompt initiation of broad-spectrum intravenous (IV) antibiotics with an antipseudomonal β-lactam, a fourth-generation cephalosporin such as cefepime, or a carbapenem within the first hour of presentation is the most appropriate next step. The coverage provided by IV ampicillin is too narrow. While hydrocortisone may be indicated in septic patients with adrenal insufficiency due to chronic steroid use, high-dose methylprednisolone would not be advisable in a septic patient, as it has been shown to increase the risk of secondary infection. Antifungal medications such as amphotericin would not be indicated unless the patient is at high risk of developing invasive fungal disease, has persistent fever for more than 4 days despite broad-spectrum antibacterial administration, and no other source has been identified. G-CSF is not routinely used in the acute management of patients with febrile neutropenia.

[ABP 1.L.6. Fever and neutropenia]

219. ANSWER: A

Salicylates stimulate the respiratory center in the brain, leading to tachypnea. The increased respiratory rate leads to a decrease in carbon dioxide, resulting in a primary respiratory alkalosis. Salicylates also cause a primary gap metabolic acidosis as a result of accumulation of organic acids such as lactic acid and keto acid. The severity of salicylate intoxication is determined by aspirin blood levels, acid-base status, and clinical examination findings. Serial salicylate levels, electrolyte panels, and blood gases should be monitored every 2–4 hours. Additional studies to consider include coagulation and hepatic transaminases to monitor hepatic function and a chest x-ray to monitor for pulmonary edema.

[ABP 1.O.7. Acid/base disorders]

220. ANSWER: A

Galactosemia is an autosomal recessive disease caused by deficiency of one of several enzymes required for metabolism of galactose (found in human and cow's milk). Patients with classic galactosemia generally present within the first few days of life; the hallmarks of the disease are liver dysfunction (including jaundice and hepatosplenomegaly), failure to thrive, cataracts, and propensity for serious infections. The most common cause of infection in these patients is *Escherichia coli* (76% of sepsis cases). In all 50 states in the United States, galactosemia testing is a part of the newborn screen; however, patients may require medical attention before newborn screening results are available. Laboratory testing will demonstrate metabolic acidosis, and urine testing will be positive for reducing substances due to galactosuria. Patients with suspected galactosemia should be switched to a soy-based formula while confirmatory testing is done. Neutropenia, arrhythmias, acute renal failure, and hearing loss would not be typical for this condition.

[ABP 1.I.8. Inborn errors of metabolism]

221. ANSWER: B

Poststreptococcal glomerulonephritis (PSGN) is by far the most common glomerulonephritis in children. Patients with PSGN typically present with the classic triad of hematuria, peripheral edema, and hypertension. A preceding history of pharyngitis or impetigo in the weeks before presentation along with antibodies against streptococcal antigens such as DNase B help to confirm the diagnosis of PSGN. Antistreptolysin (ASO) titers may also be helpful; however, there are limitations to this test as serial measurements are needed to show a rise in levels, and streptococcal skin infections do not typically lead to a rise in ASO titers. Nephritic symptoms and infection with *Escherichia coli* O157:H7 indicate hemolytic uremic syndrome. Patients with nephrolithiasis may have gross hematuria and hypercalciuria. Patients with lupus nephritis may have hypocomplementemia and elevated anti-dsDNA titers. However, this patient's presentation is not consistent with these diagnoses.

[ABP 1.F.3. Glomerulonephritis]

222. ANSWER: C

The patient's presentation is consistent with superior mesenteric artery syndrome (SMAS). SMAS results from compression of the third segment of the duodenum between the aorta and the superior mesenteric artery due to loss of the mesenteric fat pad in that space. While many cases of SMAS are due to rapid, acute weight loss, other causes (including scoliosis corrective surgery) have been reported. Clinical manifestations are consistent with proximal small bowel obstruction and include abdominal pain, vomiting, and anorexia. Of the listed options, MRA is the study most likely to reveal the patient's diagnosis. While abdominal radiograph, ultrasound, upper endoscopy, and MRCP

may show findings associated with SMAS, they would not be preferred studies. Conventional arteriography was traditionally the gold standard evaluation method prior to advances in MR technology.

[ABP 1.E.8. Obstruction]

223. ANSWER: C

In general, pediatric cardiac arrest is a rare event that is associated with high morbidity and mortality. In-hospital arrests are associated with better outcomes than out-of-hospital arrests. Factors associated with higher survival from out-of-hospital arrests include witnessed arrests, early high-quality CPR, use of an AED, shockable rhythms, shorter duration of compressions, fewer doses of epinephrine, events occurring on weekdays rather than weekends, and compressions not required at hospital arrival. Infants less than 1 year old and children 5–12 years old are at higher risk of mortality than children aged 1–4 or more than 12 years of age.

[ABP 1.D.8. Cardiac arrest]

224. ANSWER: A

Nonfatal drowning events can result in hypothermia. Hypothermia can cause decreased heart rate, blood pressure, and respiratory rate. Many thermometers may not give an accurate reading of lower body temperatures, which is likely the case in this patient given his other vital signs. Treatment of hypothermia involves passive and active warming. The core should be warmed first rather than the extremities; and in moderate-to-extreme hypothermia, internal warming should be performed rather than active external warming. Administering warmed parenteral fluids is an active internal warming method that will help limit a further drop in core temperature. Additional active internal warming measures should be also taken, for example, warmed gastric lavage. The ideal temperature for warmed fluids is 40°C–45°C.

Although similar vital signs may be seen in opiate overdoses, this patient's history is more consistent with hypothermia. Therefore, naloxone would not be the best next step. Dantrolene is used for malignant hyperthermia, not hypothermia.

[ABP 1.N.3. Drowning, ABP 1.N.4. Hypo—and hyperthermia]

225. ANSWER: E

Complications of CAP include parapneumonic effusions, empyema, pulmonary abscesses, bronchopleural fistulas, necrotizing pneumonia, sepsis, and respiratory failure. Parapneumonic effusions begin as simple exudative fluid collections, then become fibrinopurulent before organizing over 10 to 14 days into an empyema with fibrin deposition, septation, and stiffened pleural membranes. Surgical intervention is generally based on effusion size and duration along with the degree of respiratory compromise and illness severity. There is not strong evidence to support drainage of small- to moderate-size effusions or abscesses to improve outcomes over medical therapy alone. Two to four weeks of antibiotic therapy targeting *Streptococcus pneumoniae* is generally recommended for empyema, with additional coverage of *Streptococcus pyogenes* and *Staphylococcus aureus* in very ill patients or those with influenza. Intravenous-to-oral antibiotic conversion is determined by clinical course and response to therapy. For pleural effusions that persist despite appropriate antibiotics and chest tube drainage, options include chest tube instillation of fibrinolytics, such as tissue plasminogen activator, and video-assisted thoracoscopic surgery (VATS). Although equivalent in terms of length of hospitalization, fibrinolytic instillation has been shown to be cheaper, while early VATS decreases the need for additional drainage procedures. Children with complicated pneumonia are significantly more likely to have bacteremia than children with uncomplicated pneumonia. CXR may show blunting of the costophrenic angle and a rim of fluid ascending the lateral chest wall (positive meniscus sign). Chest US has lower cost and equal sensitivity and specificity to CT for pleural space evaluation.

[ABP 1.C.3. Pneumonia]

REFERENCE

1. de Benedictis FM, Kerem E, Chang AB, Colin AA, Zar HJ, Bush A. Complicated pneumonia in children. *Lancet.* 2020;396(10253):786–798.

226. ANSWER: D

This patient is at increased risk for reversible posterior leukoencephalopathy syndrome (RPLS), also known as posterior reversible encephalopathy syndrome (PRES). The best next step in management is advanced neuroimaging not only to confirm the diagnosis of RPLS but also to evaluate for other serious possible etiologies, such as cerebrovascular accident or intracranial hemorrhage. MRI is the gold standard imaging modality when evaluating for RPLS. Children with RPLS will often have bilateral white matter edema involving the posterior cerebral hemispheres.

Several medical conditions have been associated with RPLS, including hypertension and use of immunosuppressive medications, such as cyclosporine and tacrolimus. RPLS is also a known complication after HSCT and solid-organ transplantation. Moderate-to-severe hypertension is documented in approximately 75% of patients with RPLS.

Lumbar puncture would not be immediately indicated unless there were concerns for meningitis or encephalitis.

Neurosurgery consultation is not required in the initial diagnosis and management of RPLS. Electrocardiogram is not warranted at this time. This patient does not meet criteria for status epilepticus and is no longer having clinical seizure activity. Fosphenytoin is one of several medications considered a second-line treatment option for status epilepticus. Benzodiazepines are the preferred first-line therapy for children in status epilepticus.

[ABP 1.A.11. Other (encephalopathy)]

REFERENCE

1. Bartynski WS. Posterior reversible encephalopathy syndrome, part 1: fundamental imaging and clinical features. *AJNR Am J Neuroradiol.* 2008;29(6):1036–1042.

227. ANSWER: B

This patient is presenting with symptoms of viral croup, also called laryngotracheitis. This is an upper respiratory infection that leads to inflammation of the larynx and subglottic airway. This inflammation produces the classic inspiratory stridor due to narrowing of the airway. Other symptoms include a "barking" cough and hoarseness; there is usually no drooling or dysphagia. Racemic epinephrine can help decrease subglottic inflammation, leading to improvement in stridor. Glucocorticoids, preferably dexamethasone, are also recommended to decrease airway inflammation.

Epiglottitis is inflammation of the epiglottis and surrounding supraglottic structures, often secondary to bacterial infection. Both epiglottitis and bacterial tracheitis may present with stridor, but patients with epiglottitis often have a short, if any, prodrome, sudden onset of severe symptoms, absence of cough, dysphagia, and drooling. Bacterial tracheitis is an infection of the trachea that leads to edema and purulence, seen rarely in children without artificial airways, in whom infection generally follows a prior mucosal injury of the trachea, such as viral infection, tonsillectomy, or trauma. Patients with bacterial tracheitis may present with fevers, cough, drooling, and dysphagia and do not respond to racemic epinephrine. Bronchoconstriction, seen in patients with acute asthma and bronchiolitis, presents with expiratory wheezing and not stridor. Alveolar filling and consolidation due to bacterial invasion is descriptive of pneumonia. While cough may be present, stridor (an upper airway problem) is not.

[ABP 1.B.1. Upper airway infections and conditions]

228. ANSWER: D

Herpes simplex virus should be considered in febrile neonates, especially those who present with ill appearance, altered mental status, seizures, or a vesicular rash. Recurrent HSV has a lower risk of transmission compared to primary, but the risk is not zero, even when on suppressive therapy during pregnancy. Other risk factors include chorioamnionitis, peripartum fever, preterm/prolonged rupture of membranes, scalp electrodes, and risky sexual behaviors. Neonatal HSV is seen in the form of skin, eye, or mouth (SEM) disease, central nervous system (CNS) disease, and disseminated disease. Laboratory tests may show transaminitis, leukopenia, thrombocytopenia, coagulopathy, and CSF pleocytosis. HSV testing is obtained as a PCR from the blood and CSF and viral culture from the conjunctivae, nasopharynx, mouth, anus, and skin lesions. This patient's positive CSF HSV PCR indicates that he has either CNS or disseminated disease. Both of these are treated with acyclovir IV 60 mg/kg/d divided three times daily for a minimum of 21 days, with discontinuation following a negative CSF HSV PCR. Localized SEM disease is treated for 14 days. Ocular disease requires a topical ophthalmic medication. All patients then receive 6 months of oral acyclovir suppression three times daily. While on oral suppression, it is important to monitor for neutropenia.

[ABP 1.O.4. Fever in infants less than 60 days]

229. ANSWER: C

Reversing catabolism is of critical importance when managing a metabolic crisis and should take priority over other interventions. This patient should receive dextrose-containing fluids that will deliver 8 mg/kg/min of dextrose, which can usually be achieved by running 10% dextrose at 1.5 times the maintenance rate. Intravenous carnitine is given to patients with organic acidemias (e.g., MMA, propionic acidemia, or isovaleric acidemia) when they are in metabolic crises, as carnitine binds to the toxic metabolites produced in these disorders and causes these patients to be carnitine deficient. Carnitine is vital to the functioning of mitochondria, but supplementation with IV carnitine should not take priority over reversing catabolism. While this patient is hypoglycemic, 25% dextrose should not be delivered through a peripheral IV line due to the high risk of burns should the fluid extravasate. While fluid resuscitation is important, a normal saline bolus will not arrest this patient's metabolic crisis. Finally, sodium phenylacetate–sodium benzoate is an ammonia scavenger that may well be required if this patient's ammonia is elevated. However, it should be given through a central line and should not take priority over giving dextrose-containing fluids.

[ABP 1.I.8. Inborn errors of metabolism]

230. ANSWER: C

Eczema herpeticum is a complication of atopic dermatitis that results from the infection of eczematous skin with herpes simplex virus (HSV). Patients present with punched-out erosions, crusts, and/or vesicles that can be painful or itchy. It can be difficult to distinguish this presentation from severe underlying atopic dermatitis and/or bacterial superinfection. HSV PCR of the lesions can help confirm the diagnosis. It is important to start expedited treatment of eczema herpeticum with an antiviral agent such as acyclovir. When the diagnosis is suspected, treatment should be started while awaiting laboratory results since the disease can quickly spread, leading to systemic illness complicated by organ dysfunction and death.

While bacterial superinfection can occur concurrently with eczema herpeticum and may require antibiotic treatment, amoxicillin/clavulanate is broad spectrum and would not be an appropriate first-line antibiotic for this indication. First-line therapy should focus on coverage for *Staphylococcus aureus* and *Streptococcus pyogenes*, such as clindamycin or nafcillin, depending on local sensitivities. Increasing the potency of her topical steroid may eventually be needed for long-term eczema management but is not the most important next step in acute management.

[ABP 1.K.1. Skin and soft tissue infections, ABP 1.K.4. Complicated eczema]

231. ANSWER: D

The patient's presentation is concerning for intestinal malrotation, resulting in small bowel obstruction. An upper GI series remains the gold standard for diagnosis of intestinal malrotation. HIDA scans are used to visualize the hepatobiliary tract and can aid in the diagnosis of cholecystitis or biliary atresia but would not be helpful in this case. While abdominal CT and MRI can assist in diagnosis of intestinal malrotation, they are not recommended as part of the standard evaluation. Barium enema is not indicated in evaluation of intestinal malrotation. Intestinal malrotation is most commonly found in children less than 1 year of age and is frequently associated with underlying congenital diseases, including omphalocele, congenital diaphragmatic hernia, and intestinal atresias. Presenting symptoms often include bilious emesis, abdominal distension, abdominal rigidity, and shock. However, it should be noted that the absence of bilious emesis does not exclude intestinal malrotation as a potential diagnosis. Hemodynamically unstable patients should be immediately resuscitated and taken to the operating room for treatment.

[ABP 1.E.8. Obstruction]

232. ANSWER: B

This patient meets one major criterion of two separate positive blood cultures with a HACEK (*H. parainfluenzae, Haemophilus aphrophilus, Haemophilus paraphrophilus, Actinobacillus actinomycetemcomitans, Cardiobacterium hominis, Eikenella corrodens,* or *Kingella* species) organism (Table 1.16), and three minor criteria of fever, vascular phenomenon (Janeway lesions), and immunologic phenomenon (glomerulonephritis). He meets criteria for diagnosis of infective endocarditis even though he has normal echocardiographic findings.

Table 1.16 MODIFIED DUKE CRITERIA FOR DIAGNOSIS OF INFECTIVE ENDOCARDITIS

Major criteria	1. Two separate positive blood cultures for a typical endocarditis microorganism, such as *Streptococcus viridans* or a HACEK organism (*H. parainfluenzae, H. aphrophilus, H. paraphrophilus, Actinobacillus actinomycetemcomitans, Cardiobacterium hominis, Eikenella corrodens,* or *Kingella* species); persistently positive blood cultures; or evidence of infection with a *Coxiella* organism 2. Positive echocardiographic findings
Minor criteria	1. Predisposing heart condition or intravenous drug use 2. Fever with a temperature more than or equal to 38°C 3. Vascular phenomenon (arterial emboli, septic pulmonary infarcts, mycotic aneurysm, intracranial hemorrhages, conjunctival hemorrhages, Janeway lesions) 4. Immunologic phenomena (glomerulonephritis, Osler nodes, Roth spots, rheumatoid factor) 5. Positive blood culture that does not meet major criteria
Criteria for diagnosis	1. 2 major criteria, OR 2. 1 major and 3 minor criteria, OR 3. 5 minor criteria

ᵃ Adapted from Reference 1.

[ABP 1.D.5. Endocarditis, myocarditis, and pericarditis]

REFERENCE

1. Durack DT, Lukes AS, Bright DK. New criteria for diagnosis of infective endocarditis: utilization of specific echocardiographic findings. Duke Endocarditis Service. *Am J Med.* 1994;96(3):200–209.

233. ANSWER: E

Submersion duration greater than 5 minutes is a strong predictor of poor outcomes. An initial blood gas with a pH less than 7.1 and resuscitation time of more than 25 minutes are also poor prognostic factors. Age has generally not been shown to be a significant predictor of mortality or morbidity, although in some studies patients younger than 5 years have done better. Although low water temperatures and hypothermia can theoretically be protective, large-scale studies have not shown this to be the case.

[ABP 1.N.3. Drowning]

234. ANSWER: A

The infant has acute hypoxemic respiratory failure (RF) due to viral bronchiolitis, which would cause respiratory alkalosis, hypoxemia, and a low $PaCO_2$. While choice C shows hypoxemia,

the normal pH and $PaCO_2$ indicate chronic hypoxemia, which would be unexpected in this acutely ill, otherwise healthy infant. Choices B, D, and E reflect normal arterial oxygen content.

Respiratory failure is divided into type 1 (hypoxemic) and type 2 (hypercapnic). Hypoxemic RF is impaired gas exchange due to lung failure, resulting in ventilation-perfusion (V/Q) mismatch and a fall in arterial oxygen partial pressure to less than 60 mm Hg. Common etiologies include infection, trauma, and inhalation injury. Infants are more susceptible to respiratory compromise due to lower metabolic reserve, increased airway resistance, decreased lung volume, and decreased efficiency and endurance of respiratory muscles. Additionally, fear and anxiety worsen dynamic expiratory collapse.

Respiratory failure can be acute or chronic. ABG analysis is critical in distinguishing between the various forms of respiratory failure (Table 1.17). Mood changes, disorientation, pallor, hypertension, ataxia, and fatigue can signal impending respiratory arrest requiring immediate respiratory support. Early recognition and ability to efficiently manage the upper airway are crucial in the initial stabilization of acute RF, using techniques that include jaw thrust, chin lift, and bag-mask ventilation.

Table 1.17 CHARACTERISTIC ARTERIAL BLOOD GAS ANALYSIS FEATURES IN THE DIFFERENT TYPES OF RESPIRATORY FAILURE

	PH	PO₂ (MM HG)	PCO₂ (MM HG)	BICARBONATE (MEQ/L)
Normal	7.38–7.42	80–100	35–45	22–26
Acute hypoxemic RF	High	Low	Low	Low or normal
Chronic hypoxemic RF	Normal	Low	Low or normal	Low or normal
Acute hypercapnic RF	Low	Low or normal	High	Low or normal
Chronic hypercapnic RF	Slightly low or normal	Low or normal	High	High

[ABP 1.C.4. Acute respiratory distress and failure]

REFERENCE

1. Friedman ML, Nitu ME. Acute respiratory failure in children. *Pediatr Ann.* 2018;47(7):e268–e273.

235. ANSWER: A

This patient has a presentation and findings consistent with Guillain-Barré syndrome (GBS). Patients classically have an infectious exposure causing upper respiratory or gastroenteritis symptoms approximately 4 weeks prior to the development of neurologic symptoms. Infectious triggers include *Campylobacter jejuni* (most common), influenza, *Haemophilis influenzae*, cytomegalovirus, human immunodeficiency virus, and *Mycoplasma pneumoniae*. Rarely, GBS can follow immunizations or transplantation and can be seen in the setting of lupus and lymphoma. As in this case, the cerebrospinal fluid analysis in patients with GBS may demonstrate an elevated protein level but a normal white blood cell count, a finding known as albuminocytologic dissociation. In *C. jejuni* infection, molecular mimicry between microbial glycans and axonal surface molecules is responsible for the autoantibodies that cause nerve damage. Autoantibodies against acetylcholine receptors cause myasthenia gravis. Various genetic mutations have been linked to spinal muscular dystrophy. Infection of the central nervous system with poliovirus is rare in countries with vaccination and prior eradication. Tick-borne paralysis is often misdiagnosed as GBS and occurs 3–7 days after tick attachment, depending on the species. Removal of the tick causes symptoms to resolve.

[ABP 1.A.8. Inflammatory neuropathies]

REFERENCE

1. Willison HJ, Jacobs BC, van Doorn PA. Guillain-Barré syndrome. *Lancet*. 2016;*388*(10045):717–727.

236. ANSWER: C

Suppurative odontogenic infections are often polymicrobial in nature. Common isolates from dental abscesses include *Bacteroides*, *Streptococcus*, *Peptostreptococcus*, *Actinomyces*, and *Fusobacterium*. The remaining answer choices are uncommon in previously healthy patients. Prompt treatment with antibiotics such as ampicillin-sulbactam, which includes coverage of anaerobic organisms, is important to avoid complications. These complications include extension into orofacial and deep neck spaces (e.g., retropharyngeal, parapharyngeal), osteomyelitis of the jaw, and hematogenous spread. If no complications arise, antibiotics may be transitioned to oral therapy and continued for a total course of 7–14 days until evidence of inflammation has resolved.

[ABP 1.B.3. Oropharyngeal infections]

237. ANSWER: E

Bacterial organisms to consider in this age group include *Escherichia coli*, group B *Streptococcus*, and *Listeria monocytogenes*, though *Listeria* is not commonly seen in term infants. In older infants, *Haemophilus influenzae* type b, *Staphylococcus aureus*, *Streptococcus pneumoniae*, and *Neisseria meningitidis* should also be considered. This patient's urinalysis suggests a urinary tract infection, most commonly caused by *E. coli* in the neonatal period, but meningitis cannot be ruled out due to the CSF WBC count. When there is low concern for meningitis, ampicillin and gentamicin provide appropriate coverage. However, if CSF studies are abnormal, a third- or fourth-generation cephalosporin should be used instead of gentamicin for improved blood-brain barrier penetration. A cephalosporin alone would be adequate empiric coverage in infants between 29 and 60 days of age given the low risk of *Listeria*, making the addition of ampicillin unnecessary. Vancomycin is usually not used as monotherapy, but may be added if there is concern for resistant organisms, severe sepsis, or meningitis in infants older than 28 days.

[ABP 1.O.4. Fever in infants less than 60 days]

REFERENCE

1. Pantell RH, Roberts KB, Adams WG, et al. Evaluation and management of well-appearing febrile infants 8 to 60 days old. *Pediatrics*. 2021;*148*(2):e2021052228.

238. ANSWER: B

Newborns born to mothers with a history of Grave's disease can have significant morbidity and mortality and require careful monitoring. While removal of the thyroid tissue either surgically or with radiation can lead to hypothyroidism in the mother, thyroid-stimulating autoantibodies do not always disappear and can then cross the placenta during pregnancy. This can lead to a transient but clinically significant thyroid storm in the newborn. It is recommended to test mothers with a history of Grave's disease for thyroid-stimulating hormone (TSH) receptor antibodies (TRAb) in the second or third trimester. If negative, no additional monitoring of the newborn is necessary. If maternal antibodies are positive or unknown, it is recommended to send the infant's serum for TRAb, TSH, and free thyroxine (T_4) levels at more than 48 hours of life (after the TSH surge), again at 10–14 days of life, and then clinically follow for 2–3 months. It is important to note that the newborn screen in most states screens for hypothyroidism but not hyperthyroidism.

It is good practice to directly ask mothers who are currently hypothyroid about a past history of Grave's disease, especially when they are on a high dose of levothyroxine. Levothyroxine is safe to take during pregnancy without additional monitoring, does not require a wean for the infant, and is compatible with breastfeeding.

[ABP 1.I.3. Hypo and hyperthyroidism]

REFERENCE

1. van der Kaay DC, Wasserman JD, Palmert MR. Management of neonates born to mothers with Graves' disease. *Pediatrics*. 2016;*137*(4):e20151878.

239. ANSWER: B

This patient's presentation is concerning for eosinophilic esophagitis (EoE) with esophageal narrowing or strictures contributing to his symptoms. Presentation of EoE varies depending on age. Young children often have feeding dysfunction; school-age children may have vomiting and abdominal pain; older children often present with dysphagia and food impaction. A history of atopy is common. Diagnosis is based on symptoms, esophageal appearance on endoscopy, and histologic findings; therefore, an endoscopy is the most appropriate study to obtain at this time. An upper GI series may also be helpful to characterize esophageal abnormalities such as segmental narrowing or proximal strictures; however, a small bowel follow-through is not necessary. An abdominal ultrasound does not evaluate the esophagus. A urea breath test is a noninvasive test for *Helicobacter pylori* (*H. pylori*) in children over 6 years of age. Noninvasive testing is not recommended for the initial diagnosis of *H. pylori* in children as current evidence indicates that *H. pylori* infection does not cause symptoms in the absence of peptic ulcer disease. Therefore, performing a noninvasive test to detect infection and treat if the test is positive is not warranted. Allergy testing may be warranted in cases of EoE, especially if there is concern for environmental triggers. However, this would not be the appropriate study to obtain at this point.

[ABP 1.E.8. Obstruction]

240. ANSWER: D

A diagnosis of complete or typical Kawasaki disease (KD) requires fever 5 days or longer plus 4 or more of the following clinical symptoms: nonspecific rash, nonexudative conjunctivitis, erythema of lips/tongue, cervical lymphadenopathy 1.5 cm or larger, and extremity changes. KD is an acute vasculitis of childhood, and coronary artery aneurysm or ectasia can develop in 15%–20% of untreated patients. The patient in this vignette meets criteria for typical KD and should be treated; the most important treatment is prompt initiation of IVIG, which has been found to reduce the risk of coronary artery aneurysms to less than 5% if given within the first 10 days of fever onset. Aspirin is also recommended as a part of the treatment plan for KD and may have benefits such as reduced fever duration in addition to its antiplatelet activity, but there is no clear evidence that it prevents long-term complications. The evidence for corticosteroids is mixed; it may have a role in treatment of a subset of patients at particular risk for

developing aneurysms, but the evidence is not as robust as for IVIG. Normal saline may be indicated for this patient given his decreased oral intake, but it does not prevent long-term complications of KD. Ibuprofen is not a specific part of the treatment of KD.

[ABP 1.H.2. Kawasaki disease]

REFERENCE

1. McCrindle BW, Rowley AH, Newburger JW, et al. Diagnosis, treatment, and long-term management of Kawasaki disease: a scientific statement for health professionals from the American Heart Association. *Circulation*. 2017;*135*(17):e927–e999.

241. ANSWER: A

Mitral valve prolapse (MVP) is when one or more leaflets of the mitral valve prolapse into the left atrium. Although it is typically a congenital lesion, symptoms may not present until adolescence. Symptoms can include chest pain, exertional dyspnea, palpitations, and syncope. The classic examination findings for MVP are a mid-to-late systolic click with a high-pitched late systolic murmur. The classic murmur for hypertrophic cardiomyopathy is a systolic ejection crescendo-decrescendo murmur that increases with the Valsalva maneuver. Both atrial and pulmonary stenosis present with systolic ejection murmurs. Myocarditis does not typically present with a murmur.

[ABP 1.D.2. Congenital heart disease]

242. ANSWER: A

Cyanide poisoning and carbon monoxide poisoning should be suspected in any smoke inhalation injury, including house fires. This girl likely is suffering from both. Cyanide impairs mitochondrial oxidative phosphorylation resulting in cells being unable to utilize oxygen. The classic sign of "cherry red" flushed skin is present in only about 10% of patients with cyanide toxicity. Other nonspecific signs include vomiting and tachycardia, tachypnea, and hypertension as a reflex response to decreased oxygen utilization. Treatment includes a combination of hydroxocobalamin, a precursor to vitamin B_{12}, and sodium thiosulfate. Be aware that hydroxocobalamin may cause reddish discoloration of urine. Carbon monoxide competitively inhibits the oxygen-binding capability of hemoglobin but cannot be distinguished from oxygen by a pulse oximeter. Thus, carbon monoxide levels must be measured to definitively diagnose carbon monoxide poisoning. Signs of carbon monoxide poisoning include changes to mental status, malaise, and vomiting. Treatment includes administration of 100% oxygen via a nonrebreather face mask.

Methylene blue is used to treat methemoglobinemia. Sodium nitroprusside can precipitate cyanide ion formation and subsequently worsen cyanide toxicity. Naloxone is used in opioid toxicity, which can result in impaired consciousness but would also be associated with depressed vital signs and constricted pupils. Physostigmine would be used in anticholinergic toxicity, which can present with impaired mental status, hypertension, and tachycardia, but given this patient's vomiting and history of smoke exposure, cyanide poisoning is more likely.

[ABP 1.N.6. Burns]

243. ANSWER: E

The patient's ABG will demonstrate acidosis due to elevated $PaCO_2$ despite having an elevated serum bicarbonate level, reflecting an acute-on-chronic hypercapnic respiratory failure (RF), most likely due to the sedative effects of valproic acid. Due to underlying neuromuscular weakness, this patient is at high risk of chronic hypercapnic RF with decreased ability to compensate for acute respiratory illness. While the bicarbonate level is elevated in choice D, the normal pH reflects metabolic compensation for chronic hypercapnic RF without an acute component. Choices A, B, and C show low or normal $PaCO_2$ levels, which would not be expected in this patient with weakness and respiratory depression.

Hypercapnic RF results from impaired gas exchange due to respiratory pump failure, leading to ventilation-perfusion (V/Q) mismatch and an increase in arterial carbon dioxide ($PaCO_2$) to greater than 50 mm Hg. In patients with neuromuscular weakness, total lung capacity is decreased, leading to chronic hypercapnia and reliance on the hypoxic respiratory drive to compensate when ill. Patients may be too weak to display increased work of breathing or accessory muscles use. A GCS score of less than 8 indicates severe neurologic compromise with loss of airway protective reflexes and should prompt emergent endotracheal intubation. In chronic hypercapnic RF, any degree of respiratory acidosis or increase in $PaCO_2$ of greater than 20 mm Hg above baseline represents acute-on-chronic hypercapnic RF. Early hospital admission to provide supportive care with aggressive airway clearance, judicious use of supplemental oxygen, and noninvasive or invasive ventilation is often necessary.

[ABP 1.C.4. Acute respiratory distress and failure]

REFERENCE

1. Vo P, Kharasch VS. Respiratory failure. *Pediatr Rev.* 2014;35(11):476–486.

244. ANSWER: D

This patient is likely suffering from an acute dystonic reaction (ADR) due to haloperidol administration. ADR is characterized by abrupt onset of involuntary muscle contractions that result in abnormal movements or postures. Patients may exhibit tongue protrusion, torticollis or retrocollis, trismus, dysphagia, dysarthria, blepharospasm, or back arching. Mental status and vital signs remain normal. Rarely, life-threatening laryngeal dystonia can occur. ADR is distressing to the patient and typically occurs following initiation or titration of medications that block dopamine function. In pediatrics, the most commonly implicated medications include antiemetics, such as metoclopramide and prochlorperazine, and antipsychotics. First-generation antipsychotics, such as haloperidol and thioridazine, are associated with a higher risk for ADRs than second-generation medications. History of exposure to these medications will help in distinguishing ADRs from focal seizures, motor tics, and tetanus. First-line therapy includes intravenous benztropine or diphenhydramine. ADRs will respond quickly to treatment. This patient does not have tetanus and therefore does not require human tetanus immune globulin. Lorazepam can be used for treatment of ADRs but is not considered first-line therapy. Fosphenytoin is a second-line therapy for status epilepticus. Dantrolene can be used for treatment of neuroleptic malignant syndrome, which is characterized by fever, altered mental status, abnormal vitals, and muscle rigidity, in addition to extrapyramidal movements.

[ABP 1.A.11. Other (movement disorders)]

245. ANSWER: D

Refeeding syndrome occurs when a patient with malnourishment develops electrolyte abnormalities on initiation of feeds. The three most worrisome electrolyte disturbances that may be seen during refeeding in the setting of severe malnutrition are hypokalemia, hypophosphatemia, and hypomagnesemia. These electrolyte changes are the result of insulin secretion causing intracellular shifts as the body moves to carbohydrate breakdown for energy. Additionally, as carbohydrates are broken down, adenosine triphosphate is created from free phosphate joining with adenosine diphosphate, further worsening the hypophosphatemia. Due to these electrolyte fluctuations, close monitoring and replacement of electrolytes are warranted. Hyponatremia is not typically seen in refeeding syndrome; however, hypernatremia may be noted—this is the body's effort to maintain positive ion homeostasis. Hypoglycemia or hyperglycemia have not been associated with morbidity during refeeding.

[ABP 1.O.6. Electrolyte abnormalities]

REFERENCE

1. Pulcini CD, Zettle S, Srinath A. Refeeding syndrome. *Pediatr Rev.* 2016;37(12):516–523.

246. ANSWER: B

This patient's presentation is consistent with OTC deficiency, which is a urea cycle disorder (UCD). Most UCDs have an autosomal recessive inheritance pattern; however, OTC deficiency is X linked and seen more often and more severely in male infants. UCDs and organic acidemias such as propionic acidemia often present within the first several days of life as the infant is exposed to proteins in breastmilk or formula, often before the newborn screen has resulted. Patients with urea cycle disorders typically have significant hyperammonemia with a respiratory alkalosis. This is in contrast to patients with organic acidemias who have significant metabolic acidosis as well as hyperammonemia that is often less pronounced than patients with UCDs. Mitochondrial disorders lead to an inability for cells to perform oxidative phosphorylation, impacting the function of organs such as muscle that depend on aerobic metabolism. Patients often present with lactic acidosis; hyperammonemia is not seen. Fructosemia is a disorder of carbohydrate metabolism that typically presents with hypoglycemia after introduction of fructose in solid foods at about 4–6 months of age. MCADD is a disorder of fatty acid oxidation that may also present with hypoglycemia; it can be distinguished from disorders of carbohydrate metabolism by the absence of ketones.

[ABP 1.I.8. Inborn errors of metabolism]

247. ANSWER: C

Children with nephrotic syndrome are at increased risk of infections, especially those caused by encapsulated bacteria. In part, this is due to the natural medium that ascites and pleural fluid provide for bacteria to grow, but also due to potential reduction in immune function due to the loss of immunoglobulins in the urine protein. This patient's symptoms and physical examination findings are most concerning for bacterial peritonitis. Pneumonia and urinary tract infections are possible but do not fit the clinical picture. Myocarditis can present with nonspecific symptoms; however, children often have some evidence of heart failure as well. Patients with nephrotic syndrome are at increased risk of thromboembolism due to the loss of proteins involved in coagulation; while tachycardia and fevers can be seen in the setting of emboli, her abdominal symptoms make peritonitis more likely.

[ABP 1.E.11. Peritonitis]

248. ANSWER: D

Postural orthostatic tachycardia syndrome (POTS) is a clinical syndrome of orthostatic intolerance lasting at least 6 months characterized by a heart rate increase of 30 beats per minute or more, often with standing, and in the absence of orthostatic hypotension. A diagnosis of orthostatic hypotension requires a minimum 20-point drop in systolic blood pressure or a 10-point drop in diastolic blood pressure within 3 minutes of standing.

Other symptoms often coexist with standing and include lightheadedness, palpitations, tremulousness, generalized weakness, blurred vision, exercise intolerance, fatigue, presyncope, and syncope. Postconcussive syndrome and migraine are frequently described comorbidities in POTS patients. However, the described elevation in heart rate accompanying a change in position from sitting to standing is a defining feature of POTS. An elevated heart rate in inappropriate sinus tachycardia persists independent of body position. While dehydration can present with tachycardia, there is no indication by history or examination that this patient is dehydrated.

[ABP 1.D.6. Syncope]

249. ANSWER: C

Fluid resuscitation after a burn injury is important given the increased losses through the damaged skin. The Parkland formula can be used to estimate the amount of fluid that needs to be given during the first 24 hours as (Percentage body surface area involved) × (Patient's weight) × (4). Half of this fluid should be given over the first 8 hours, with the remainder given over the next 16 hours. Fluids should be titrated to a goal urine output of 1–2 mL/kg/h.

The rule of nines is generally used to estimate the percentage of body surface area involved. In adults, the head is 9%, each arm is 9%, each leg is 18%, and the anterior and posterior thorax are each 18%. In infants, the head is a much larger proportion of the patient's body, so for young pediatric patients, a better estimate is 18% for the head, 18% each for the anterior and posterior thorax, 9% for each arm, and 14% for each leg. Superficial burns should not be included. For this patient with half of her head and her back involved, this is 18 + 9 = 27%, which gives 27 × 4 × 12 = 1296 mL IV fluid over the first 24 hours, with 648 mL given over the first 8 hours.

For extensive burns, patients will need to be kept nil per os in case of surgical intervention or if they need to be intubated for inhalational injuries, so the patient's maintenance fluid rate will need to be included. This patient's maintenance fluids would be 44 mL/h, or 352 mL over 8 hours. This gives a total of 352 + 648 = 1000 mL over the first 8 hours.

[ABP 1.N.6. Burns]

250. ANSWER: C

The ABG demonstrates significant hypoxemia despite delivery of 100% fraction of inspired oxygen (FiO_2) at a maximally high flow rate through a nonrebreather face mask. He is receiving the highest recommended dose of continuous albuterol for his age and weight. Because his pH and $PaCO_2$ remain normal and he is not showing signs of fatigue, the next most reasonable step in management is to initiate noninvasive ventilation.

Noninvasive ventilation (NIV), including high-flow nasal cannula (HFNC), pressure support (PS), continuous positive airway pressure (CPAP), and bilevel positive airway pressure (BiPAP), is first-line treatment in managing both acute and chronic respiratory failure. In the treatment of acute asthma exacerbation, NIV improves work of breathing and asthma severity scores, lessening the need for invasive ventilation. Similar to mechanical ventilation, the goal of NIV is to decrease work of breathing to improve gas exchange in a spontaneously breathing patient with preserved airway protective reflexes.

Noninvasive ventilation should be initiated for children of any age prior to the development of severe acidosis. The degree of tachypnea, dyspnea, and accessory muscle use is an important determinant. NIV is contraindicated in patients with altered mental status, uncontrolled vomiting, facial trauma, or cardiac instability. Blood gas analysis should be performed 1 to 4 hours after initiation and 1 hour after each setting change. Complications include noncompliance from improper device fit, patient-ventilator asynchrony, pressure skin injury, eye irritation, dry mucous membranes, and thickened secretions.

[ABP 1.C.4. Acute respiratory distress and failure]

251. ANSWER: C

Children with failure to thrive need additional caloric intake on top of their baseline energy needs (Table 1.18) to allow for catch-up weight gain. The following formula can be used to calculate the needed caloric intake:

Estimated Calories for Catch-up Growth = (IBW * Estimated Caloric Intake for Age)/Current Weight

Table 1.18 ESTIMATED ENERGY NEEDS BY AGE[a]

AGE	ESTIMATED ENERGY NEEDS
0–2 months	100–110 kcal/kg/d
3–5 months	85–95 kcal/kg/d
6–8 months	80–85 kcal/kg/d
9–11 months	80 kcal/kg/d
12–24 months	80–83 kcal/kg/d

[a] Adapted from Reference 1.

For this patient, the estimated catch-up needs are calculated below:

Estimated Calories for Catch-up Weight = (10 kg × 80 kcal/kg/d)/8 kg = 100 kcal/kg/d

[ABP 1.O.2. Failure to thrive]

REFERENCE

1. Motil KJ, Duryea TK. Poor weight gain in children younger than two years in resource-abundant countries: management. Updated Nov 12, 2019. Accessed June 1, 2021. https://www.uptodate.com/contents/poor-weight-gain-in-children-younger-than-two-years-in-resource-abundant-countries-management.

252. ANSWER: D

Oral rehydration therapy (ORT) is the preferred management of mild-to-moderate dehydration in the setting of acute gastroenteritis. Mild-to-moderate volume loss should be repleted with 50–100 mL/kg of an oral rehydration solution over a 4-hour period, with additional fluid supplied for any ongoing losses. If this is tolerated in a medical setting, the patient can be discharged to home after the family has been provided guidance on additional ORT for home. ORT with 5 mL every 15 minutes is not enough to make up the volume losses in this child and may contribute to further dehydration. Until a child has proven he can tolerate ORT, the family should not be discharged home. Intravenous fluid may be needed for children with severe dehydration or in those who cannot tolerate enteral fluids (either orally or via a nasogastric tube); however, this child presents with mild-to-moderate dehydration and should be given the chance to tolerate ORT first. Normal saline boluses are preferred to replace the volume loss and if dextrose is needed, maintenance fluids can be started after the normal saline has been given.

[ABP 1.E.4. Gastroenteritis]

253. ANSWER: B

Drowning is defined as any respiratory impairment as a result of submersion or immersion in liquid. It is a common cause of injury and accidental death in children. Children ages 1–5 years and 15–25 years are at highest risk, with a strong predilection for male gender. Initial prehospital management of drowning victims includes prompt provision of cardiopulmonary resuscitation if appropriate.

Hospital care should focus on evaluation and treatment for common complications, such as respiratory compromise, hypoxic ischemic encephalopathy, and cardiovascular impairment. Patients who are asymptomatic at presentation, as in this vignette, can be discharged home if they remain asymptomatic with normal vital signs, respiratory status, and neurologic status following an observation period of 4–8 hours. Most children who go on to develop symptoms will do so within this time frame, at which point disposition to the pediatric ward versus intensive care unit may be determined based on the severity of their symptoms. Immediate discharge home with strict return precautions would be premature, as symptoms may not be apparent and could develop following the initial presentation. While laboratory tests and imaging studies are a part of the evaluation of a patient following a drowning event, patients with a normal workup should still be observed.

[ABP 1.N.3. Drowning]

254. ANSWER: A

This patient has developed a pulmonary embolism (PE) with hypoxemia due to ventilation-perfusion (V/Q) mismatch. Because of pulmonary vascular autoregulation, blood is shunted to non-embolized regions of the lung, resulting in overperfusion of these areas and subsequent hypoxemia. Additionally, cardiac output is decreased, leading to a lower level of mixed venous blood oxygen and further hypoxemia. While this scenario could be explained by pneumonia and subsequent physiologic right-to-left shunting leading to hypoxemia, the presence of hypertension, right heart strain on ECG, improvement with supplemental oxygen, and lack of distinct infiltrate on CXR is highly suspicious for PE.

Hypoxemia is a fall in the partial pressure of oxygen (PaO_2) below 60 mm Hg due to V/Q mismatch, hypoventilation, right-to-left shunt, diffusion impairment, or a low fraction of inspired oxygen (FiO_2) (Table 1.19). V/Q mismatch is the most common cause. Right-to-left shunting occurs when deoxygenated blood enters the arterial circulation without participating in gas exchange, either via anatomic or physiologic shunts. Impaired oxygen diffusion across the alveoli can be seen in interstitial edema or inflammation.

[ABP 1.C.4. Acute respiratory distress and failure]

REFERENCE

1. Bhutta BS, Alghoula F, Berim I. Hypoxia. In: *StatPearls*. Treasure Island, FL: StatPearls Publishing. Updated May 7, 2021. Accessed May 31, 2021. https://www.ncbi.nlm.nih.gov/books/NBK482316/.

255. ANSWER: C

Ideal body weight can be identified using multiple methods, but there is no clear consensus on the best method to use. The McLaren, Moore, and body mass index (BMI) are commonly used and provide very similar results in children under the age of 8 years. The McLaren method uses growth charts to identify the IBW. To do so, first plot the height for the patient on the chart. Next, from the plotted height, move horizontally on the chart to the 50th percentile line for height. Using this point, move vertically down the chart to the 50th percentile for weight. This is the child's ideal body weight (see Figure 1.16):

Table 1.19 CAUSES OF HYPOXEMIA[a]

	EXAMPLES	RESPONSE TO SUPPLEMENTAL OXYGEN	PACO$_2$
V/Q mismatch	Asthma, cystic fibrosis, sickle cell disease, pulmonary embolism, pulmonary hypertension	Improvement	Normal or low
Right-to-left shunt	1. Anatomic shunts: intracardiac, pulmonary arteriovenous malformations 2. Physiologic shunts: pneumonia, pulmonary edema, atelectasis, acute respiratory distress syndrome	No change	Normal
Diffusion impairment	Emphysema, interstitial lung disease/inflammation/edema	Improvement	Normal
Reduced FiO$_2$	High altitude/decreased atmospheric pressure	Resolution	Normal
Hypoventilation	Impaired central drive, Guillain-Barré syndrome, myopathy	Improvement	High

[a] Adapted from Reference 1.

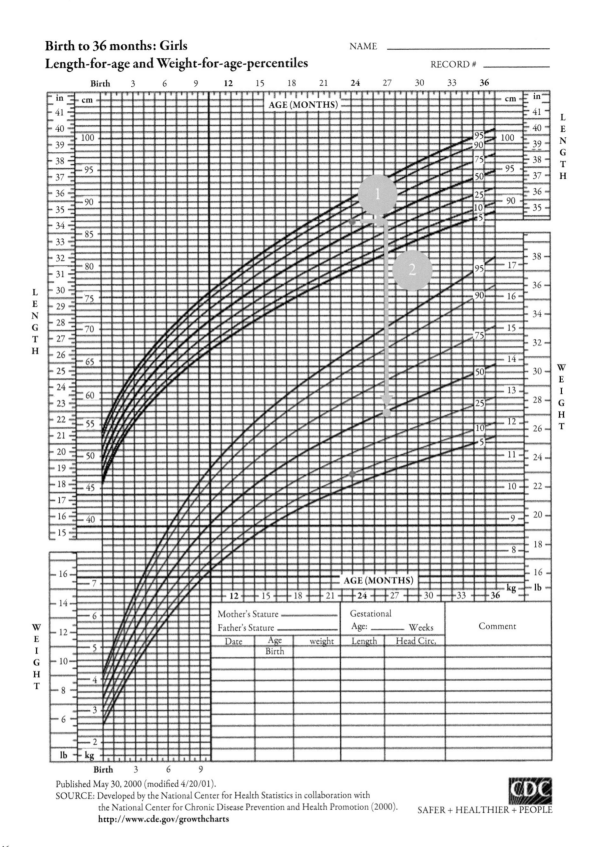

Birth to 36 months: Girls
Length-for-age and Weight-for-age-percentiles

NAME _____

RECORD # _____

Published May 30, 2000 (modified 4/20/01).
SOURCE: Developed by the National Center for Health Statistics in collaboration with
the National Center for Chronic Disease Prevention and Health Promotion (2000).
http://www.cdc.gov/growthcharts

SAFER + HEALTHIER + PEOPLE

Figure 1.16

Using the McLaren method, the IBW for this patient is approximately 12.4 kg.

The Moore method uses percentiles on the growth charts to identify IBW. To do this, identify the percentile for height for age for the child. In this case, the height is just below the 75th percentile. Then, identify the weight for age at the same percentile. In this case, weight for age just below the 75th percentile for a 23-month-old is approximately 12.8 kg.

Finally, the BMI method calculates IBW as [BMI at the 50th Percentile for Age × (Height in Meters)^2].

[ABP 1.O.2. Failure to thrive]

REFERENCES

1. Centers for Disease Control and Prevention. Clinical growth charts. Published June 16, 2017. Accessed June 1, 2021. https://www.cdc.gov/growthcharts/clinical_charts.htm.
2. Phillips S, Edlbeck A, Kirby M, Goday P. Ideal body weight in children. *Nutr Clin Pract.* 2007;22(2):240–245.

256. ANSWER: B

This child's presentation is concerning for acute cholangitis, a serious and potentially life-threatening infection of the biliary tract. Patients who have undergone a hepatoportoenterostomy are at increased risk of cholangitis due to the postsurgical changes in anatomy that lead to stasis and bacterial growth. Most of these children will have at least one episode in early childhood, and it is not uncommon for patients to have multiple episodes. The most common organisms isolated include *Escherichia coli* and other gram-negative bacteria, *Enterococcus*, and anaerobes such as *Bacteroides*. Piperacillin/tazobactam is one effective empiric regimen for cholangitis; it is the best choice of the options listed.

The combination of ceftriaxone and vancomycin is a standard regimen for the treatment of presumed sepsis; however, this regimen lacks adequate coverage for enteric anerobic organisms. Recurrent cholangitis may hasten cirrhosis and lead to early liver transplantation; in order to reduce the risk of cholangitis, antibiotic prophylaxis is generally recommended for patients who have undergone a hepatoportoenterostomy. TMP/SMX is an effective prophylactic antibiotic, but it would not be recommended for treatment. While linezolid and meropenem would cover the relevant organisms, it is an unnecessarily broad antibiotic regimen as the primary concern is coverage for the common causes of cholangitis. Cefepime does cover most gram-negative organisms, but it lacks adequate coverage for enteric anaerobes.

[ABP 1.E.2. Cholecystitis and cholangitis]

257. ANSWER: E

Antibiotic treatment for dog bites is indicated for wounds that show signs of clinical infection. Prophylaxis is indicated for bites with risk factors for infection such as deep puncture wounds; wounds involving the hands, face, or genitalia; those in close proximity to bony structures or joints; or wounds that are associated with crush injuries. Due to the risk of meningitis or brain abscess from bites to the head with associated skull fractures, ceftriaxone and metronidazole would be the preferred regimen for this patient.

Ampicillin-sulbactam would be an appropriate choice in a hospitalized child with a dog bite located in other areas of the body. First-generation cephalosporins do not have sufficient coverage for common pathogens implicated in infections following dog bites, most notably *Pasteurella multocida*, and should not be used. Observation without antibiotics may be sufficient for wounds lacking the risk factors listed above or those that are left open to heal by secondary intention.

[ABP 1.N.2. Insect and animal bites]

258. ANSWER: D

This patient presents with subacute hypercarbic respiratory failure with metabolic compensation. His history of congenital myopathy along with worsening fatigue, inability to lay flat, and low lung volumes on imaging are concerning for hypoventilation due to muscle failure. His symptoms are most likely to improve with NIPPV (e.g., bilevel positive airway pressure, or BiPAP) to help with lung recruitment and gas exchange.

Myopathies and neuromuscular diseases can lead to muscle weakness and respiratory failure due to hypoventilation. Ascertaining the underlying cause is important to discern if there are treatments available. Congenital myopathies are generally not curable, and treatment of respiratory failure includes supportive care (noninvasive or invasive ventilation). This patient's metabolic alkalosis is a compensatory mechanism for his primary respiratory acidosis. IV fluids will not reverse his respiratory acidosis or improve his respiratory symptoms. High-flow oxygen delivery is less helpful in patients whose oxygenation is limited by their low lung volumes, as high flow will not significantly improve alveolar recruitment. IVIG may be helpful in patients with Guillain-Barré syndrome, but this patient's presentation is not consistent with this disease. There is no role here for inhaled corticosteroids, which are reserved for patients with small airways disease such as asthma.

[ABP 1.C.5. Chronic respiratory conditions]

259. ANSWER: B

A brief resolved unexplained event (BRUE) is defined as an event occurring in an infant younger than 1 year, when the observer reports a sudden, brief, and now resolved episode of one or more of the following: (1) cyanosis or pallor; (2) absence, decreased, or irregular breathing; (3) marked change in tone (hyper- or hypotonia); and (4) altered level of responsiveness. In infants, pertussis infection can cause color change followed by respiratory pause several days before the development of fever, cough, or lower respiratory symptoms. Thus, the guidelines state clinicians may consider pertussis testing in lower risk infants, particularly those who are underimmunized with possible exposures, as you may identify a potentially treatable infection. The guidelines do not recommend CXR, EEG, echocardiogram, or respiratory viral testing in low-risk infants.

[ABP 1.O.1. Brief resolved unexplained event (BRUE)]

REFERENCE

1. Tieder JS, Bonkowsky JL, Etzel RA, et al. Brief resolved unexplained events (formerly apparent life-threatening events) and evaluation of lower-risk infants. *Pediatrics.* 2016;*137*(5):e20160590.

260. ANSWER: D

Severe abdominal distension is an alarm sign for obstructive gastrointestinal diseases such as Hirschsprung disease or pseudo-obstruction. Other alarm signs for underlying diseases in patients presenting with constipation are outlined in the Table 1.20.

Table 1.20 ALARM SIGNS FOR UNDERLYING DISEASE IN PATIENTS WITH CONSTIPATION[a]

History	No passage of meconium the first 2 days of life
	Constipation in the first month of life
	Ribbon stools
	Bloody stools in the absence of anal fissures
	Bilious emesis
	Family history of Hirschsprung disease
Examination	Fever
	Failure to thrive
	Severe abdominal distension
	Decreased lower extremity strength, tone, or reflexes
	Tuft of hair on spine
	Sacral dimple
	Gluteal cleft deviation
	Extreme fear during anal inspection
	Abnormal position of the anus
	Absent anal or cremasteric reflex
	Anal scars
	Perianal fistula
Laboratory tests	Abnormal thyroid studies

[a] Adapted from Reference 1.

Children who present with an alarm sign should receive a digital rectal examination (DRE) and further workup as indicated by the history to rule out conditions such as Hirschsprung disease, celiac disease, hypothyroidism, botulism, cystic fibrosis, anatomic malformations, and tethered cord, among others.

Children without any alarm signs for organic pathology meet the criteria for functional constipation if any two of the following criteria are met: two or fewer defecations per week, one or more episodes of incontinence per week (in patients with toileting skills), a history of excessive stool retention in children under 4 years of age (or retentive posturing or excessive volitional tool retention in children over 4 years of age), a history of painful or hard bowel movements, the presence of a large fecal mass in the rectum, or a history of large-diameter stools that may obstruct the toilet. Children with functional constipation should not undergo extensive testing. Abdominal radiographs are not indicated. Polyethylene glycol (PEG) is the treatment of choice for functional constipation.

The child in the vignette does not meet criteria for functional constipation due to her severe distension. Further workup, including a DRE, is recommended.

[ABP 1.E.3. Constipation]

REFERENCE

1. Tabbers MM, DiLorenzo C, Berger MY, et al. Evaluation and treatment of functional constipation in infants and children: evidence-based recommendations from ESPGHAN and NASPGHAN. *J Pediatr Gastroenterol Nutr.* 2014;58(2):258–274.

261. ANSWER: E

The child in this vignette is suffering from envenomation from a black widow spider, which can be found throughout North America, most often in the Southeast and Western portions of the United States. Widow spider venom is neurotoxic and can cause a variety of symptoms with varying degrees of severity. As these bites do not contain cytotoxins, local tissue damage at the bite site is typically not seen, but "target" lesions can be present, as in the example above. Muscle cramping, rigidity, and tenderness in the affected limb are the hallmark of black widow spider bites, with potential for these symptoms to spread to the chest, back, and abdomen. Children may be irritable or agitated, and autonomic symptoms such as diaphoresis, tachycardia, hypertension, nausea, and vomiting may be seen.

First-line treatment is appropriate analgesia, often with opioid medications. Benzodiazepines are considered adjunctive therapies and may be utilized if symptoms are not adequately managed with first-line analgesics. Antivenom is an effective treatment but is often not readily available and is typically reserved for patients with severe envenomation who are unresponsive to initial treatment. Ice and elevation of the extremity have not proven to be effective therapies. Antibiotics are rarely indicated as these bites typically do not become secondarily infected.

[ABP 1.N.2. Insect and animal bites]

262. ANSWER: C

This patient with severe asthma, elevated IgE levels, and multiple exacerbations despite maximum outpatient therapies may benefit from immunomodulator therapy to help improve his asthma control and reduce hospital admissions.

Patients who should be considered for immunomodulators include those with severe asthma with frequent exacerbations despite consistent and appropriate use of medium- or high-dose inhaled corticosteroids (ICSs), long-acting β-agonists (LABAs), and leukotriene receptor antagonists (LTRAs). Immunomodulators can benefit patients with asthma who also have elevated IgE or eosinophilia and have been shown to reduce emergency department visits and hospitalizations significantly.

Switching the type of ICS and LABA would not be expected to significantly change this patient's clinical trajectory. When used appropriately, treatments with nebulizers versus MDIs are similar in efficacy. Pulmonary function tests are not routinely obtained during an asthma exacerbation as they do not guide further therapy. Prolonged steroid therapy is not necessary in this patient who is improving from his acute exacerbation, and extended steroid courses have not been proven to reduce readmission.

[ABP 1.C.2. Asthma]

REFERENCE

1. Boulet LP, Godbout K. Oral corticosteroids tapering in severe asthma. *Am J Respir Crit Care Med.* 2021;203(7):795–796.

263. ANSWER: A

Neuropathic pain is caused by a lesion or dysfunction of the somatosensory system. Alternatively, nociceptive pain is caused by damage or potential damage to tissue. It is important to differentiate these as medical management for the two pain types differs. Neuropathic pain is characterized by sharp, shooting, "electric-like," stabbing pain, which commonly radiates distally. It can also be associated with numbness, tingling, temperature, and color changes, as well as allodynia and hyperalgesia. Nociceptive pain is often described as throbbing, aching, and pressure-like, with proximal radiation. It often lacks sensory deficits, vasomotor signs, hypersensitivity, or allodynia. Exacerbations of neuropathic pain are common and unpredictable, while exacerbations of nociceptive pain are often associated with activity. Neuropathic pain is often poorly responsive to opiates.

[ABP 1.O.8. Pain (acute and chronic)]

264. ANSWER: C

This child most likely has hypercalcemia secondary to prolonged immobilization, which can cause increased bone resorption. This patient's PTH is appropriately suppressed. In hyperparathyroidism, either primary or secondary, the PTH would be elevated. Hypoparathyroidism is associated with hypocalcemia, not hypercalcemia. Severe vitamin D deficiency can lower calcium and phosphorus levels but would not be associated with hypercalcemia. Tumors that cause hypercalcemia due to secretion of a PTH-related protein are extremely rare in children.

[ABP 1.I.4. Hypo and hypercalcemia]

265. ANSWER: A

The combination of bradycardia and hypotension is concerning for β-blocker toxicity. Other clinical findings may include mental status changes, such as delirium, seizures, and coma. Respiratory depression has been noted in certain cases, as well as acute bronchospasm. Hypoglycemia is another common complication from this condition. Initial treatment of β-blocker toxicity is focused on maintaining an adequate airway, breathing, and circulation. In this patient with hypotension and significant bradycardia, treatment with boluses of isotonic fluid and atropine are indicated. Frequently, these interventions alone are sufficient; however, repeat administration may be required. Patients who are refractory to initial therapies may require intravenous glucagon and epinephrine.

[ABP 1.N.1. Ingestions (intentional and unintentional)]

266. ANSWER: C

Hemoptysis is a common occurrence among patients with CF and may be one of the first clinical signs of an acute exacerbation. For this reason, it is important to start and continue appropriate antimicrobials to cover for infection when patients present with bloody sputum. Treatment also includes the cessation of offending medications, including nonsteroidal anti-inflammatory drugs and aerosolized therapies that may provoke bleeding. This patient was recently started on hypertonic saline nebulizers, which likely incited his hemoptysis.

This patient's sputum culture does not include methicillin-resistant *Staphylococcus aureus*, and adding vancomycin is not likely to be of clinical benefit. While evidence is lacking for the benefit of double coverage of *Pseudomonas*, expert consensus guidelines continue to recommend this until data can show that single-coverage therapy is not inferior. Therefore, stopping ciprofloxacin is not appropriate, and doing so would not provide direct relief of his hemoptysis. Inhaled dornase alfa can also cause irritation of the airways and promote bleeding, and therefore is often stopped temporarily alongside hypertonic saline in patients who develop hemoptysis. One should consider obtaining a CT with contrast if a patient has massive hemoptysis that may require embolization. However, the patient's hemoptysis was moderate and has already resolved, so a CT scan is not yet warranted.

[ABP 1.C.5. Chronic respiratory conditions]

REFERENCE

1. Flume PA, Mogayzel PJ Jr, Robinson KA, et al. Cystic fibrosis pulmonary guidelines: treatment of pulmonary exacerbations. *Am J Respir Crit Care Med.* 2009;*180*(9):802–808.

267. ANSWER: E

In children and adolescents, hypercalcemia in the setting of hyperparathyroidism is most commonly sporadic and due to a parathyroid adenoma. Most patients are symptomatic, and kidney stones, acute pancreatitis, and bony involvement are the most common end-organ findings. Primary hyperparathyroidism is seen in multiple endocrine neoplasia (MEN) type 1 and is the most common presentation of this autosomal dominant syndrome. Less often, primary hyperparathyroidism can be seen with a parathyroid carcinoma or in MEN type 2. The normal albumin level rules out pseudohypercalcemia. The elevated PTH, low phosphorus, and normal vitamin D rules out nonparathyroid causes of hypercalcemia, such as malignancy, disuse osteoporosis or immobilization, vitamin D intoxication, infection, and granulomatous disease. The fractional excretion of calcium (FeCa) can be used to help evaluate for FHH.

FeCa = (Urine Ca × Serum Creatinine)/(Serum Ca × Urine Creatinine) = 0.019 in this case

A FeCa greater than 0.01 makes FHH unlikely (see Table 1.21).

Treatment of hypercalcemia depends on the underlying cause, but the initial goal is to increase calcium excretion with fluids and furosemide, and in some cases, bisphosphonates are considered.

[ABP 1.0.6. Electrolyte abnormalities]

REFERENCE

1. Lietman SA, Germain-Lee EL, Levine MA. Hypercalcemia in children and adolescents. *Curr Opin Pediatr.* 2010;*22*(4):508–515.

268. ANSWER: D

Activated charcoal provides gastrointestinal decontamination of acute ingestions by adsorbing chemicals within the gastrointestinal tract, thereby preventing systemic absorption. Thus, it is most effective if given within 1 hour of ingestion, prior to passage of the chemical into the intestines. Ingestion of extended-release medications or chemicals with extensive enterohepatic recirculation may benefit from repeated doses of activated charcoal to prevent continued absorption over time. Some agents are not well adsorbed by activated charcoal, including heavy metals (e.g., iron, lead); lithium; alcohols; and caustic agents such as bleach. Additionally, caustic ingestions require urgent endoscopy to evaluate the degree of esophageal damage, and activated charcoal may obscure the view. Substances that are particularly damaging if aspirated, such as hydrocarbons, should not be treated with charcoal as it may induce vomiting. Patients who are at risk for aspiration (including those who are too lethargic to protect their airway) or with evidence of bowel obstruction should also not receive activated charcoal.

[ABP 1.N.1. Ingestions (intentional and unintentional)]

269. ANSWER: C

This patient likely has syndrome of inappropriate secretion of antidiuretic hormone (SIADH) secondary to his new antiepileptic medication. Drug-induced SIADH can most commonly be traced back to five different types of medications: antiepileptics, antidepressants, antipsychotics, cytotoxic drugs, and some pain medications. Inappropriately increased secretion of antidiuretic hormone (ADH) leads to renal tubular changes and water retention, resulting in euvolemic hyponatremia, low plasma osmolality (Posm), and high urine osmolality secondary to low free water excretion as seen in this patient.

Posm = 2[Na] + [BUN]/2.8 + [Glucose]/18 = 248 + 8.9 + 4.4 = 261.3 (normal range 280–295)

Pseudohyponatremia would result in normal Posm and can be seen in hyperlipidemia or high-protein states.

Table 1.21 LABORATORY VALUES IN CAUSES OF HYPERCALCEMIA (N = NORMAL)[a]

	CALCIUM	PHOSPHOROUS	FECA	PTH	PTHRP	25(OH)D
Primary hyperparathyroidism	High	Low	>0.01	High	Low	N
Malignancy	High	N/high/low	High	Low	High	N
FHH	High	N or low	<0.01	N or high	Low	N
Immobilization	High	High	High	Low	Low	N

[a] Adapted from Reference 1.

Hypertonic hyponatremia would result in high Posm and can be seen in high-glucose states. This is considered factitious hypernatremia, as the sodium level can be corrected for a high-glucose level. Hypovolemic hyponatremia usually occurs secondary to renal or extrarenal (e.g., gastrointestinal) losses. Hypervolemic hyponatremia is seen in nephrotic syndrome, liver failure, renal failure, and other edema-forming conditions. In addition to SIADH, water intoxication may cause euvolemic hyponatremia; however, the UNa would not be elevated as seen in this case.

[ABP 1.0.6. Electrolyte abnormalities]

270. ANSWER: B

This patient presents with a severe, acute asthma exacerbation. Her symptoms are only mildly improved after nebulizer treatments, and she warrants further interventions prior to consideration of admission to the hospital. IV magnesium causes bronchial smooth muscle relaxation and has shown benefit and decreased hospitalization rates when used among children with moderate-to-severe asthma exacerbations. Early administration of a systemic corticosteroid within 1 hour of arrival to an emergency department has been shown to reduce admission rates. There is also evidence that treatment with two or three doses of inhaled ipratropium in combination with an inhaled β-agonist such as albuterol can reduce hospitalization more than use of an inhaled β-agonist alone; the addition of continuous albuterol in this patient would not be expected to provide added protection against hospitalization.

There is no evidence to suggest that temporary supplemental oxygen improves hospitalization rates. While LABAs and LTRAs may be part of a long-term preventative strategy for patients with moderate to severe asthma, often in combination with an inhaled corticosteroid, they have not been shown to prevent hospitalization in the acute setting.

[ABP 1.C.2. Asthma]

REFERENCE

1. Cheuk DK, Chau TC, Lee SL. A meta-analysis on intravenous magnesium sulphate for treating acute asthma. *Arch Dis Child.* 2005;*90*(1):74–77.

271. ANSWER: D

Acute rheumatic fever (ARF), a postinfectious sequela of group A streptococcal (GAS) infection, usually develops 2–3 weeks after acute GAS pharyngitis. Diagnosis is based on the Jones criteria (see Table 1.22) and requires either two major or one major and two minor criteria, plus evidence of prior GAS infection, which can include positive rapid strep test, nucleic acid amplification test, throat culture, or

Table 1.22 DIAGNOSTIC CRITERIA FOR ACUTE RHEUMATIC FEVER[a]

MAJOR CRITERIA	MINOR CRITERIA
1. Carditis	1. Fever (>38.5°C)
2. Migratory polyarthritis	2. Polyarthralgia
3. Chorea[b]	3. Prolonged PR interval (in the absence of carditis)
4. Erythema marginatum	4. Elevated acute-phase reactants (C-reactive protein >3 mg/dL and erythrocyte sedimentation rate >60 mm/h)
5. Subcutaneous nodules	

[a] Adapted from Reference 1.

[b] In the presence of chorea, no evidence of prior GAS infection is required.

elevated titers of anti-DNase B or anti–streptolysin O. This patient has two major criteria (erythema marginatum and migratory polyarthritis) and one minor criteria (fever), and an ASO titer may help establish evidence of GAS infection to make the diagnosis of ARF.

Carditis occurs more commonly in children than adults with ARF. An electrocardiogram may show first-degree heart block or cardiomegaly, and an echocardiogram may demonstrate regurgitation at the mitral and/or aortic valves. Treatment of ARF includes antibiotic therapy for the eradication of GAS, acute symptomatic management, and long-term antibiotic prophylaxis due to risk of recurrence of ARF.

Creatine kinase is useful as a marker of muscle injury and would be elevated in the setting of muscle injury. It is a nonspecific test and would not be helpful in clarifying this child's diagnosis. Blood cultures would also not be helpful for confirming a diagnosis of ARF. The annular rash of Lyme disease is a target-like rash with central clearing; the rash described above is more consistent with erythema marginatum. Anti–double-stranded DNA titers are useful for managing systemic lupus erythematosus (SLE).

[ABP 1.H.2. Inflammatory arthritis, 1.K.2. Dermatologic manifestations of systemic disease]

REFERENCE

1. Gewitz MH, Baltimore RS, Tani LY, et al. Revision of the Jones criteria for the diagnosis of acute rheumatic fever in the era of Doppler echocardiography: a scientific statement from the American Heart Association. *Circulation.* 2015;*131*(20):1806–1818.

272. ANSWER: A

This patient is displaying signs of central diabetes insipidus (CDI), which results from decreased production or release of ADH. ADH regulates water balance in the body by increasing water reabsorption in the renal tubules and stimulating thirst. It is produced in the hypothalamus, stored in the pituitary gland, and secreted into circulation with increased plasma osmolality. It then binds to vasopressin V2 in the kidneys to allow for water movement across the osmotic gradient to decrease plasma osmolality. With decreased ADH, the patient develops polyuria, leading to increased plasma osmolality, including hypernatremia. CDI occurs secondary to genetic defects in the ADH gene or processes that affect the hypothalamus or pituitary gland, including trauma, infections, neoplasms, autoimmune diseases, or anatomical defects. Treatment includes desmopressin, which is a synthetic ADH replacement. Nephrogenic diabetes insipidus (NDI) is related to renal resistance to ADH or mutations and deficiency of vasopressin V2, leading to polyuria, increased plasma osmolality, and hypernatremia. Increased vasopressin V2 response would lead to oliguria and hyponatremia. Syndrome of inappropriate ADH results from increased production of ADH and also leads to oliguria and hyponatremia.

[ABP 1.0.6. Electrolyte abnormalities]

273. ANSWER: A

Supracondylar fractures are the most common elbow fractures in children. Children with these fractures are at increased risk of acute compartment syndrome (ACS). Agitation and increased need for analgesia may be early signs of ACS in preverbal children. The presence of some or all of the "5 Ps" (pain, paresthesia, paralysis, pallor, and pulselessness) should further raise suspicion. Other than emergent orthopedic consultation, early management of ACS includes removal of any constrictive dressings or splints. The limb should not be elevated as this can diminish distal arterial flow and further exacerbate ischemia. Since the compromised vascular flow is a result of high compartment pressure and not a thrombus, heparin would not be helpful. Measurement of compartment pressure should be done after removal of the constrictive dressing, ideally by the operating surgeon. Unnecessary imaging that may delay management such as a venous Doppler ultrasound should be avoided when suspicion for ACS is high as it is in this case.

[ABP 1.G.1. Fractures]

274. ANSWER: E

This patient's clinical picture is most concerning for bacterial tracheitis. He arrived at the emergency room in respiratory distress without improvement with nebulized epinephrine or oxygen via nasal cannula. Before further workup can be done or medications given, it is imperative to secure the patient's airway as he is at risk for further severe decompensation. Bacterial tracheitis involves bacterial superinfection of the tracheal (and sometimes laryngeal and bronchial) tissues. In previously healthy children without artificial airways, bacterial tracheitis occurs rarely and almost always occurs in young children in the setting of a preceding viral respiratory infection. Symptoms include acute-onset respiratory distress with stridor, cough, and dyspnea. Drooling is less likely; more often this is a symptom of epiglottitis. Given the overlap in presentation with viral croup, trials of nebulized epinephrine are warranted but often have incomplete or no response. Diagnosis is initially made clinically; definitive diagnosis is made by direct visualization of the trachea via laryngoscopy or bronchoscopy along with microbial cultures. The most common bacterial culprit is *Staphylococcus aureus*, a small subset of which are methicillin resistant. Other common microbes include *Streptococcus pneumoniae*, group A *Streptococcus*, *Moraxella catarrhalis*, and *Haemophilus influenzae*. Gram-negative infections are rare. Broad-spectrum antibiotics should be initiated early and should include coverage for methicillin-resistant *S. aureus*. Laboratory tests are generally nonspecific, with variable white blood cell count and inflammatory markers. Radiographs may show irregular tracheal borders and a hazy tracheal column. They may also show a "steeple sign" with subglottic tracheal narrowing, but this is nonspecific and can also be seen in viral croup. Dexamethasone is generally not recommended for initial therapy when bacterial tracheitis is highly suspected.

[ABP 1.C.7. Bacterial tracheitis]

REFERENCE

1. Kuo CY, Parikh SR. Bacterial tracheitis. *Pediatr Rev.* 2014;35(11): 497–499.

275. ANSWER: C

This presentation is most consistent staphylococcal scalded skin syndrome (SSSS). SSSS is caused by an exfoliative toxin produced by certain strains of *S. aureus* that cleave the protein desmoglein-1, which is responsible for epidermal cell-cell adhesion. When the toxin is hematogenously spread, it can lead to diffuse cleavage of the protein and resultant sloughing of superficial skin layers. The source of staphylococcal infection may be apparent but is often occult.

Patients may initially present with fussiness, pain, and diffuse erythroderma, which can progress to flaccid bullae, erosions, and diffuse skin sloughing. Flexural and perioral surfaces are often most affected. SSSS mostly affects infants and younger children, possibly due to absence of antibody to the toxin and/or slow renal clearance of the toxin. Because only superficial skin layers are involved, the lesions typically heal without scarring. Treatment includes systemic antibiotics directed at *S. aureus* (such as nafcillin), pain control, and skin-protective measures such as emollients. There is no role for corticosteroids. IVIG is not routinely indicated.

[ABP 1.K.1. Skin and soft tissue infections]

REFERENCE

1. Cutaneous Bacterial Infections. In: Kane SM, Nambydiri VE, Stratigoes AJ, eds. *Color Atlas & Synopsis of Pediatric Dermatology.* 3rd ed. New York: McGraw-Hill; 2016.

276. ANSWER: A

The patient has evidence of isolated thrombocytopenia. While a platelet count of 32 is concerning, the most appropriate next step is to repeat the CBC with a peripheral smear to confirm the value is not a laboratory error given that it is inconsistent with the clinical picture. If confirmed, more extensive workup, such as a bone marrow biopsy may be considered. Since there is no evidence of bleeding or apparent clinical sequelae on examination, a CT scan or platelet transfusion is not indicated at this time.

[ABP 1.L.5. Isolated thrombocytopenia]

277. ANSWER: D

This patient's presentation is concerning for pertussis. *Bordetella pertussis* is a vaccine-preventable illness spread through respiratory droplets. Macrolide antibiotics such as azithromycin should be given as soon as possible; antibiotics given within the first 7 days of illness may shorten the duration of symptoms and help prevent transmission.

Pertussis classically presents initially with the catarrhal phase of mild cough and rhinorrhea, followed by the paroxysmal phase of severe coughing fits characterized by post-tussive vomiting and the classic "whoop," and finally the convalescent phase of weeks to months of gradually improving cough. Young infants are at risk for a more severe presentation complicated by apnea, gagging, cyanosis, seizures, and shock. Marked leukocytosis with lymphocyte predominance is common; very high WBC counts greater than 50,000/μL are associated with a higher rate of complications. Pertussis can also occur in vaccinated children, but the presentation is generally mild.

Pertussis is primarily a clinical diagnosis. While it may be useful to send PCR testing, it should not delay the initiation of treatment in a high-risk patient. Young infants generally warrant hospitalization; observation in the ED would not be sufficient. Racemic epinephrine is useful for the treatment of croup; it has no utility for this patient. A chest radiograph may be normal or may demonstrate nonspecific findings such as peribronchial cuffing; it is more important to initiate prompt treatment.

[ABP 1.C.4. Acute respiratory distress and failure]

278. ANSWER: A

The evaluation of a patient with a nongap metabolic acidosis includes the calculation of a UAG:

UAG = Urine Sodium + Urine Potassium – Urine Chloride

A normal UAG is positive; it varies by diet but is in the range of 20–90 for most healthy individuals. With GI losses, sodium, potassium, and bicarbonate are lost in the stool, while chloride levels are maintained. In an effort to compensate for the stool loss of sodium and potassium, there is reduced urinary excretion of sodium and potassium. This leads to a negative UAG (-20 to -50). In renal losses, there is bicarbonate loss without associated changes in sodium, potassium, or chloride excretion. This results in a positive UAG consistent with the patient's baseline. A neutral UAG (-20 to 20) cannot be interpreted.

[ABP 1.O.7. Acid/base disorders]

2.

SPECIALIZED SERVICES AND CORE SKILLS

QUESTIONS

1. A 39-week infant was born to a mother with diet-controlled gestational diabetes. The mother breastfed immediately after delivery. The infant's plasma glucose level 30 minutes after this first feed is 24 mg/dL. The physical examination is unremarkable. What should be done next for the management of this baby?

A. Start dextrose 10% in water intravenously at 5 to 8 mg/kg per minute
B. Start dextrose 10% in water intravenously at 10 to 13 mg/kg per minute
C. Feed the infant again now and check a blood glucose level 30 minutes after the feeding
D. Feed the infant again now and check a blood glucose level 1 hour after the feeding
E. Feed the infant within 2–3 hours and check a preprandial glucose level

2. An 8-month-old female born at 28 weeks' gestation with short-gut syndrome due to necrotizing enterocolitis is noted to have increased abdominal distension, foul-smelling stools, and difficulty advancing enteral feeds. She is currently receiving 70% of her calories enterally, and the remainder are given via total parenteral nutrition (TPN). Her digestive tract is in continuity, and she is thought to have approximately 60 cm of small bowel and no ileocecal valve. On physical examination, she is well appearing with normal vital signs. Her abdomen is noted to be moderately distended but soft and nontender. This patient is at risk for developing which of the following complications?

A. D-Lactic acidosis
B. Nephrolithiasis
C. Meningitis
D. Anemia
E. Thrombocytopenia

3. You are called to the delivery of an infant born at 36 weeks' gestation. The infant transitions well, requires no resuscitation beyond routine drying and stimulation,

and has no signs of respiratory distress, so the infant is placed skin to skin on the mother's chest. The first set of vital signs is notable for an axillary temperature of 36.2°C, which is confirmed by a rectal temperature. Which of the following best explains the reason for the hypothermia?

A. A thermal mattress was not used immediately after birth
B. The infant has excess brown adipose tissue
C. There was excessive heat loss because of a high ratio of the infant's body surface area to weight
D. Skin to skin contact was initiated too early
E. This temperature is considered normal for age

4. You are evaluating a 1-year-old girl with a history of necrotizing enterocolitis with large resections of jejunum and ileum who is admitted for malnutrition and poor growth for the last 6 months. Despite overnight enteral tube feeding, the patient continues to lose weight, and gastroenterology is interested in starting her on daily parenteral nutrition. Which of the following would you recommend for this patient?

A. No line placement; continue optimizing enteral nutrition
B. Implanted port
C. Double-lumen tunneled catheter
D. Single-lumen tunneled catheter
E. Peripherally inserted central catheter (PICC)

5. A mother who has opiate use disorder (OUD), under good control on maintenance methadone therapy, presents in labor at term. She is otherwise healthy, and routine prenatal laboratory tests for human immunodeficiency virus (HIV), syphilis, group B streptococcus, and hepatitis B and C are negative. The mother asks whether she should breastfeed her infant. Which of the following is most accurate?

A. Breastfeeding has been shown to decrease length of hospital stay for infants at risk for opioid withdrawal syndrome

B. Methadone is not excreted into human milk
C. Breastfeeding may increase clinical signs of neonatal opioid withdrawal in this scenario
D. Mothers with OUD have higher rates of breastfeeding initiation and duration than other mothers
E. Breastfeeding is contraindicated in this scenario

6. A 14-year-old male with febrile infection-related epilepsy syndrome (FIRES) controlled on multiple antiepileptic drugs, chronic encephalopathy, and tracheostomy presents with fever, thick malodorous secretions, and increased need for airway suctioning. The chest radiograph shows no opacity. Respiratory Gram stain shows gram-negative rods with 2+ poly-morphonuclear leukocytes (PMNs). The patient and his family just moved to the area, and you do not have his medical records, but the mother reports that the patient has had multiple admissions in the past for "the same thing," most recently 6 weeks ago. The patient is admitted after receiving ceftriaxone and clindamycin. Which of the following changes in the antimicrobial regimen is most appropriate?

A. Add azithromycin
B. Discontinue ceftriaxone and add cefepime
C. Discontinue ceftriaxone and clindamycin
D. Add isoniazid
E. Discontinue ceftriaxone and clindamycin and add ampicillin

7. You admit a 2-year-old with trisomy 21 following an adenoidectomy. His mother is distraught because he is being physically aggressive with the staff, repeatedly hitting nurses. She tells you that at home he has been hitting himself frequently. She is concerned he may have an underlying psychiatric disorder. Which of the following statements is true regarding aggressive behaviors in children?

A. Physical aggression is most common in adolescence
B. Aggressive behavior in childhood is not related to risk of mental health problems as an adult
C. Children with Down syndrome have high rates of aggressive behaviors
D. Aggressive behavior is developmentally normal between 2 and 3 years of age
E. Cognitive behavioral therapy is not effective in the management of aggression due to mental illness

8. An infant is born by uncomplicated spontaneous vaginal delivery at 37 weeks' gestation and is admitted to the well-baby nursery. The infant is exclusively breastfed and is currently 6% below birth weight. Maternal blood type is A+. The newborn's blood type is A+, and the newborn's direct antibody test (DAT) is negative. An older sibling required phototherapy. At 30 hours of life, the infant's total serum bilirubin (TSB) is 9 mg/dL, and phototherapy is initiated. At 42 hours of life, repeat TSB is 8.5 mg/dL. Based on the Figure 2.1, what is your next step in management?

A. Continue phototherapy and investigate for signs of ongoing hemolysis
B. Continue phototherapy and instruct the mother to feed formula instead of breastmilk
C. Continue phototherapy until the TSB has fallen by 1–2 mg/dL
D. Discontinue phototherapy and discharge home; treatment was not clearly indicated
E. Discontinue phototherapy and check a rebound TSB in 8 hours

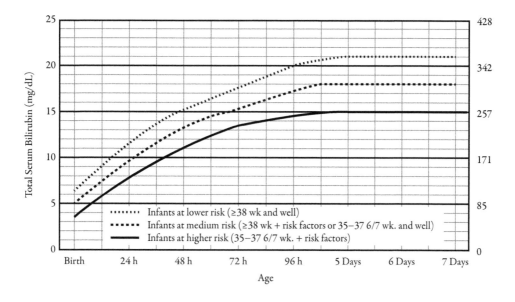

Figure 2.1.

9. A 2-year-old male with a history of herpes enceph-alitis with ongoing severe encephalopathy, epilepsy, and dystonia presents to the clinic with increased oral secretions. The mother reports that she is suctioning thin saliva pooled in the back of his mouth every hour because he starts to cough and choke. She reports self-resolved pauses in breathing lasting greater than 20 seconds with some of these choking episodes. The patient is admitted to the hospital and is started on glycopyrrolate. Which of the following is a known side effect of this medication?

A. Increased intraocular pressure
B. Myelosuppression
C. Bronchoconstriction
D. Tendonitis
E. Hepatotoxicity

10. A parent asks for your advice on elective newborn circumcision. Prenatal ultrasounds demonstrated some kidney swelling, and they are interested in a circumci-sion to reduce any risks of infection. Which of the fol-lowing statements about circumcision is true?

A. Neonates with urinary tract abnormalities have a higher risk of bleeding
B. Neonates with urinary tract abnormalities should not have circumcision performed
C. A urologist should complete the circumcision
D. Renal ultrasound should be completed prior to circumcision
E. Circumcision leads to a 10-fold reduction of urinary tract infection (UTI) risk in boys with urinary tract abnormalities

11. An infant is born to a mother with human immuno-deficiency virus (HIV). What information is needed to determine the type of antiretroviral therapy (ART) that is needed for the infant?

A. Mode of delivery
B. Maternal hepatitis C serology results
C. Maternal ART history
D. Results of HIV polymerase chain reaction (PCR) from cord blood
E. Mother's intended feeding plans

12. You are called to the emergency department (ED) to see a 9-year-old boy whose parents brought him in after he was physically aggressive with his sister. His mother reports that he has a diagnosis of oppo-sitional defiant disorder (ODD) but has never been violent until today. After a thorough review of his his-tory, you believe this child may have conduct disorder (CD). Which of the following statements is true re-garding CD?

A. Diagnosis before age 10 is associated with milder symptoms
B. CD typically resolves by adulthood
C. Comorbid conditions are rare
D. ODD is a common antecedent to CD
E. Diagnosis requires two incidents in the last 12 months

13. The obstetric team calls the delivery response team for the anticipated vaginal delivery of a term newborn through meconium-stained amniotic fluid. What per-sonnel should be present at the delivery to attend to the newborn?

A. One qualified person, and this person may also be responsible for the care of the mother
B. One qualified person, but this person's only responsibility should be for the care of the newborn
C. At least two qualified people should be solely responsible for the newborn
D. No specific personnel need to be present for the delivery as long as a delivery response team is able to arrive within 10 minutes of birth
E. The full delivery response team with at least four providers solely responsible for the newborn

14. A 14-month-old male with a history of tracheo-esophageal fistula status post repair, gastrostomy tube dependence, tracheomalacia, and chronic lung disease is admitted with viral lower respiratory tract infection. At home, the patient receives ipratropium bromide and budesonide twice daily with manual chest physio-therapy. On admission, according to the pulmonologist, the patient is placed on his "pulmonary sick plan" of albuterol and ipratropium alternating every 4 hours, budesonide four times daily, and manual chest phys-iotherapy every 4 hours. The parents report that he is constantly coughing and unable to bring up the phlegm into his throat. You observe that he has a weak cough, and he has audible crackles on chest auscultation. This patient would likely benefit most from which of the fol-lowing therapies?

A. Guaifenesin
B. Nebulized hypertonic saline
C. Therapeutic bronchoscopy
D. Mechanical insufflation-exsufflation (MIE)
E. Morphine

15. A 17-year-old female has recently developed signif-icant recurrent episodes of left upper extremity pain.

Her symptoms are worst when changing into and out of clothing. She also describes intermittent flushing of the skin and swelling of that same extremity. Prior to the onset of these symptoms, she suffered a distal radial fracture of the left upper extremity during cheerleading practice; this injury required surgical repair under general anesthesia. Her pain has led to numerous school days missed, and she no longer engages in any physical activity. She has required numerous hospitalizations for pain control. Multiple subspecialists have been involved in her care, including orthopedics, neurology, rheumatology, and psychology. As the pediatric hospitalist overseeing her most recent hospitalization, what is the best next step in management?

A. Schedule a family meeting involving all subspecialists
B. Reassure the patient and family that this patient does not have an organic diagnosis
C. Offer a short course of corticosteroids with close outpatient follow-up
D. Recommend electromyography
E. Discharge the patient and explain that her symptoms are psychosomatic

16. A full-term infant is born by cesarean section for maternal exhaustion after 24 hours of labor. The infant's oxygen saturation increases from 68% at 2 minutes of life to 94% by 10 minutes of life. Which of the following is accurate about this infant's cardiorespiratory changes after birth?

A. The infant had primary apnea causing initial hypoxia, which resolved with resuscitative efforts
B. Postnatal increases in oxygen caused pulmonary vasoconstriction so blood was shunted toward the infant's brain
C. After the infant's first breaths, pulmonary vascular resistance fell, which increased pulmonary blood flow
D. The initial oxygen saturation likely was an inaccurate value; monitoring infants via pulse oximetry is not useful until at least 60 minutes of life
E. Due to the mode of delivery, there was significantly impaired clearance of fetal lung fluid

17. A 14-year-old female with spastic quadriparetic cerebral palsy, epilepsy, and severe intestinal dysmotility with gastrojejunal tube and parenteral nutrition dependence is transferred from the pediatric intensive care unit (PICU) to the acute care unit. She has had increasingly frequent PICU admissions for central line–associated bacterial infection, ileus with recurrent pneumoperitoneum, and aspiration pneumonia. The patient's mother expresses that she feels guilty about her daughter's suffering and is anxious that she may die soon. You are concerned that these admissions may indicate a change in her functional status over time. Which of the following is the most accurate statement about advanced care planning?

A. When possible, children with a life-limiting medical condition should die in the hospital setting
B. Advanced care plans should only address healthcare decisions surrounding intubation and cardiopulmonary resuscitation
C. The physician's primary role in advanced care planning is to explain to parents which management plan is best for their child
D. It is unethical to ask children less than 18 years of age to contribute to the advanced care planning process
E. Parental anticipation of death may enhance the end-of-life decision-making process while the child is in a stable phase of care

18. A 12-year-old girl with cerebral palsy is hospitalized due to gastrostomy tube (G-tube) cellulitis that failed to respond to oral antibiotics in the outpatient setting. In the hospital, her peristomal cellulitis is improving with intravenous antibiotics. However, the nurse reports that her G-tube stoma has persistent leakage that worsens with feeds, and her parents note that her G-tube has been intermittently leaking for the past month. Despite optimization of nutrition, topical barrier cream, and appropriate dressing changes, the patient's peristomal skin is increasingly irritated by the leakage of gastric secretions. On your examination, the peristomal skin appears erythematous and eroded. What is your best next step?

A. Assess prealbumin
B. Exchange the G-tube to a larger diameter tube
C. Hyperinflate the interior retention balloon
D. Stop feeds and remove the G-tube temporarily
E. Resite the G-tube to another location

19. You admit a 16-year-old boy following reconstructive surgery after a self-inflicted gunshot wound. He denies suicidal thoughts and says that the injury was accidental. The family does not want an evaluation by the psychiatry service. Which of the following is true regarding suicide?

A. Suicide of a close family member increases a child's risk
B. Suicide attempts are more common in males
C. Frequently discussing suicide with a child can increase their risk

D. Enabling easy access to support services does not significantly decrease a child's risk
E. Patients who deny suicidal thoughts are at decreased risk

20. A large-for-gestational-age newborn presents with asymmetric arm movement. On examination, the newborn's left arm is extended along their side and internally rotated. There is full passive range of motion of the entire left arm. The palmar grasp reflex is intact, and there is no step-off or crepitus along the left clavicle. The infant is otherwise well appearing. What is the best next step in management?

A. Consult occupational therapy
B. Monitor for spontaneous recovery for 12 months
C. Obtain magnetic resonance imaging (MRI) of the cervical spine
D. Order electromyography (EMG)
E. Request urgent surgical consultation

21. A 7-year-old male with neurofibromatosis type 1, autism, epilepsy, renal artery stenosis, and optic glioma history is admitted for community-acquired pneumonia. Parents report that his diet is severely restricted to "a couple of foods he's used to." You note pinpoint bleeding around the hair follicles, kinked brittle hair, and flat, thin nails on physical examination. Which of the following additional findings is most commonly associated with this nutritional deficiency?

A. Temporal wasting
B. Diaper dermatitis
C. Hemarthrosis
D. Bitot spots
E. Skin depigmentation

22. A baby is born at 39 weeks' gestation after 17 hours of ruptured fetal membranes. The mother had a positive group B streptococcal (GBS) screening at 36 weeks' gestation. She received 2 doses of clindamycin during labor as she is allergic to penicillin and the culture was shown to be clindamycin sensitive. Two hours after delivery, there was a maternal temperature of 38.3°C. Screening laboratory tests on the infant reveal a white blood count (WBC) of 28,000/μL and a C-reactive protein (CRP) of 3.2 mg/dL. Which of the following is a risk factor for early-onset sepsis in this patient?

A. Prolonged rupture of membranes
B. GBS inadequately treated
C. Elevated WBC
D. Elevated CRP
E. Maternal fever

23. A 13-year-old boy is admitted with abdominal pain and nonbloody, nonbilious emesis. Over the past 8 months, he has missed 40 days of school due to recurrent episodes of intense abdominal pain, although he has not vomited until today. He describes the pain as sharp and stabbing, localized to the periumbilical area, and lasting up to several hours at a time. Associated symptoms include nausea and anorexia. He has had a thorough gastroenterology evaluation within the past month that did not identify a cause of his symptoms. Following fluid resuscitation and treatment with antiemetics, his pain resolves, and he is able to tolerate a regular diet. Which of the following represents the most appropriate discharge plan?

A. Prescribe an antiemetic for future use should the patient's symptoms recur
B. Provide a referral for outpatient cognitive behavioral therapy (CBT)
C. Encourage daily aerobic exercise and close outpatient follow-up with a psychologist
D. Ensure close outpatient follow-up with gastroenterology
E. Provide a note excusing the patient from school for the next several days

24. A 3-day-old infant born at term via planned repeat caesarian delivery has lost 11% of birth weight. The patient's mother breastfed her first child, and she intends to exclusively breastfeed this child as well. The infant is latching on well, and the mother reports that her breasts are engorged. The infant's urine output has been appropriate. Which of the following is the most accurate statement?

A. This degree of newborn weight loss is acceptable
B. Formula supplementation is indicated
C. The infant should be evaluated for a metabolic abnormality
D. The infant should have a swallowing evaluation
E. The weight measurements are likely inaccurate

25. A 17-month-old male with congenital hydrocephalus and ventriculoperitoneal shunt (VPS), infantile spasms, and cortical visual impairment presents with acute-onset sleepiness and three episodes of emesis. The patient has had no change in urine output, seizure, gaze palsy, irregular breathing pattern, or prior shunt failure. On examination, the patient's heart rate is 56 beats per minute, and blood pressure is 116/70 mm Hg. He has moist mucus membranes. Head computed tomography (CT) reveals no change in ventricle size when compared with imaging obtained 4 months prior. Electrocardiography demonstrates sinus bradycardia, and the patient has a capillary refill time of less than 2 seconds. The emergency room calls you, the admitting provider, for your recommendations. Which of the following is the most appropriate next step in management?

A. Administer 20 mL/kg normal saline
B. Discuss ventriculoperitoneal shunt tap with neurosurgery
C. Initiate cardiac pacing via transthoracic patches
D. Administer oral rehydration solution via nasogastric tube
E. Place an order for stool *Helicobacter pylori* antigen

26. A 2-year-old girl with a history of extreme prematurity at 24 weeks' gestational age and short-gut syndrome due to necrotizing enterocolitis is hospitalized for partial small bowel obstruction. The patient has been receiving intravenous fluids and nasogastric tube decompression for the past 2 days. The nurses note that her intravenous (IV) catheter was infiltrated and are unable to obtain IV access after multiple attempts using a vein finder and ultrasound. It has been 3 hours since IV access has been lost, and the patient's nasogastric tube has already drained 360 mL of pale greenish fluid. Her heart rate is 162 beats per minute, and blood pressure is 78/50 mm Hg. She is awake with warm and well-perfused extremities and capillary refill time less than 2 seconds. You start preparing to place a drill-assisted intraosseous needle. Which of the following potential complications of intraosseous access is the least common?

A. Compartment syndrome
B. Epiphyseal injury
C. Air embolism
D. Cellulitis
E. Osteomyelitis

27. You are performing an initial assessment on an ex–37-week baby girl born 7 hours ago. Which of the following infants have the lowest risk for significant neonatal hypoglycemia requiring treatment?

A. Exclusively breastfed infants
B. Infants of diabetic mothers
C. Large-for-gestational-age (LGA) infants
D. Late preterm (LPT) infants
E. Small-for-gestational-age (SGA) infants

28. A 9-year-old, 30-kg female with a history of thalamic infarct in the perinatal period, right hemiparetic cerebral palsy, and right hip subluxation was admitted after varus derotation osteotomy (VDRO) 4 days ago. The patient's pain is well controlled on oxycodone and diazepam. The patient was placed in a Petrie cast with

appropriate distal perfusion and pulses. She has voided, stooled, and demonstrated adequate oral intake. When considering discharge planning, which of the following is the most appropriate next step?

A. Coordinate ambulance transportation to an inpatient rehabilitation facility
B. Order a safety harness for car transportation
C. Discontinue oxycodone and diazepam
D. Consult physical therapy and occupational therapy to teach the family caregivers techniques for lifting and transfers
E. Request that orthopedic surgery bivalve the Petrie cast

29. A 3-week-old, full-term infant was treated for sepsis and dehydration at a community emergency department. A 45-mm drill–assisted intraosseous (IO) needle was used to administer two 20-mL/kg normal saline boluses, ampicillin, cefotaxime, and maintenance fluids via the right proximal tibia. The infant is transferred to your hospital 8 hours later. His nurse reports that his right calf is swollen, tense, and tender. Passive movement of the right ankle elicits outbursts of crying. The orthopedics team measures a posterior compartment pressure of 75 mm Hg and anterior compartment pressure of 30 mm Hg. What is the most likely cause of this complication?

A. Extravasation of fluid
B. Fracture of tibial metaphysis
C. Deep venous thrombosis
D. Popliteal artery thrombosis
E. Soft tissue necrosis

30. A newborn infant is noted to have progressive tachycardia and bogginess of the cranial subcutaneous tissues. Occipital frontal circumference (OFC) is remeasured and found to be increased from the measurement obtained at birth. The infant is immediately transferred to the neonatal intensive care unit (NICU) for continuous cardiopulmonary monitoring, serial hematocrits, and placement of venous access in anticipation of volume resuscitation. What is the most significant underlying risk factor for the infant's condition?

A. Female sex
B. Precipitous labor
C. Vacuum-assisted delivery
D. Meconium-stained amniotic fluid
E. Advanced maternal age

31. A 17-year-old male with a spinal cord injury from a gunshot wound to the spine, bladder dysfunction, and lower extremity paralysis is admitted for a urinary tract infection. You find a shiny, moist, shallow, open ulcer

with a red-pink wound bed along the sacrum on physical examination. The lesion is 3 cm along its greatest diameter, and there is no associated warmth, erythema, local tenderness, purulent discharge, or odor. Which of the following therapies is most indicated at this time?

A. Negative pressure wound therapy (wound vacuum)
B. Skin grafting
C. Restriction of dietary protein
D. Topical antiseptic
E. Debridement with normal saline cleanser

32. A 6-year-old girl with a history of extreme prematurity and short-gut syndrome due to necrotizing enterocolitis is transferred to your hospital for feeding intolerance. For the past week, she was treated at the community hospital with a specialty feeding formula and total parenteral nutrition (TPN), bags of which accompanied her on transfer. She was admitted just before change of shift and signed off to you for the overnight shift. At 21:00, you are called to the bedside by the nurse, who has spent the past hour trying to connect the TPN bag to her peripherally inserted central catheter (PICC) line. The patient's PICC is not a brand used by your hospital and has an unfamiliar connector. The room's lights are dim to allow the patient to sleep. Using a flashlight, you examine the tubing and agree that the connector shown to you by the nurse is not compatible with the PICC hub. What is your first step to ensure the safety of the patient?

A. Check the accuracy of the connections of the TPN and formula feeding bags
B. Consult the PICC team to exchange the PICC line catheter
C. Discontinue TPN for the night and order a new bag in the morning
D. Insert a peripheral intravenous (IV) catheter for peripheral infusion of TPN
E. Start intravenous fluids and order a new bag of TPN in the morning

33. A term infant is born to a mother who had negative group B streptococcal (GBS) screening during pregnancy at 36 weeks' gestation. The mother had a fever to 38.7°C during labor, and there was associated fetal tachycardia. No antibiotics were administered prior to delivery. The newborn's examination after delivery was normal, including vital signs, respiratory effort, and tone. Which of the following is most accurate regarding the newborn's risk of infection?

A. There is no risk of early-onset GBS disease due to negative maternal screening
B. There is no risk of late-onset GBS disease due to negative maternal screening

C. Due to intra-amniotic infection, the infant will develop early-onset sepsis
D. The infant is at risk of early-onset sepsis, including infection caused by GBS
E. If intrapartum antibiotics had been administered, the risk of neonatal sepsis would have been eliminated

34. You are asked to assess a 12-year-old with anorexia nervosa (AN) in the emergency department (ED) for possible admission. Her temperature is 37.2°C, heart rate is 53 beats per minute, blood pressure is 98/67 mm Hg, and respiratory rate is 18 breaths per minute. She appears pale and malnourished but has brisk capillary refill and normal mental status. She was diagnosed approximately 6 months ago and has been followed closely in the outpatient setting. She is adamantly refusing admission, but her mother is concerned about the slow pace of her weight gain over the past several weeks. The patient has refused to eat for the past 2 days. You review her medical record and note a weight gain of approximately half a pound a week over the past month. Her body mass index (BMI) is 15 kg/m² (50th percentile for her age is 19 kg/m²). Which of the following is an indication to hospitalize this patient?

A. Bradycardia
B. Body mass index
C. Failure of outpatient management
D. Acute food refusal
E. Poor weight gain

35. A newborn infant is noted to have upslanting palpebral fissures, epicanthal folds, bilateral single transverse palmar creases, and mild hypotonia. The infant has normal vital signs, has been feeding well orally, and has passed urine and stool. A chromosomal analysis is ordered, and the suspected diagnosis is discussed with the family. What other evaluation should be done during the first month of life?

A. Abdominal radiograph
B. Echocardiogram
C. Feeding evaluation by speech-language pathologist
D. Dilated fundoscopic exam
E. Cervical spine radiograph

36. A 4-month-old female with a suspected genetic disorder, diffuse hypotonia, and oromotor dysphagia with nasogastric tube dependence, is admitted with increased work of breathing. Her father reports that the patient has large-volume spit-ups and tends to cough frequently after nasogastric tube feeds, but she has gained weight appropriately. With the most recent feed, she appeared to choke after spitting up. She has had increased work

of breathing since that time. She showed aspiration on modified barium swallow and has not demonstrated improvement in oromotor coordination working with speech therapy as an outpatient. Which of the following is the best long-term recommendation for this patient?

A. Place a gastrostomy-jejunostomy tube
B. Place a nasojejunal tube
C. Place a peripherally inserted central catheter (PICC) for total parenteral nutrition (TPN)
D. Place a gastrostomy tube
E. Place a peripheral intravenous line for peripheral parenteral nutrition (PPN)

37. A 3-year-old boy with autism is hospitalized due to refractory functional constipation. A polyethylene glycol infusion is ordered by nasogastric tube (NGT). During insertion of the tube, the child becomes agitated, bucks, and flails his head. He has ongoing agitation after the procedure. He is crying and coughing and has an episode of nonbilious emesis with a streak of blood. There is a drop of blood present at the opening of the naris with the NGT in place. Position of the tube is confirmed by injection of air auscultated over the upper abdomen. The nurse asks you to assess the child, who remains agitated and coughing. What is the most common complication of NGT placement that can present with these clinical symptoms?

A. Epistaxis from nasal mucosal abrasion
B. Pulmonary insertion of the tube
C. Esophageal or gastric perforation
D. Pneumomediastinum
E. Nasal septum erosion

38. You are called to the bedside of a 7-year-old patient admitted with an asthma exacerbation. The respiratory therapist has been unable give him his last two respiratory treatments because the patient won't cooperate. The mother says he has always been difficult. She says her daughter stopped throwing tantrums around 3 years of age, but her son did not. He has frequent outbursts and "just won't listen." She wonders if he needs medication or should be evaluated by a psychiatrist. Which of the following is true regarding this diagnosis?

A. For diagnosis, episodes must occur once a month for 12 months
B. Medications are the most effective management option
C. Diagnosis cannot be made until a child is 5 years of age
D. Symptoms usually present before 8 years of age and rarely after adolescence

E. It is more prevalent in boys than in girls after puberty

39. You are called to the delivery of an infant whose mother received no prenatal care. The infant cries initially, but rapidly develops respiratory distress. On examination, you note a barrel chest and scaphoid abdomen; breath sounds are absent on the left side of the chest. Your immediate next step should be to

A. Arrange emergent transfer to a center with extracorporeal membrane oxygenation (ECMO) capabilities
B. Begin bag-valve-mask ventilation
C. Intubate and provide positive pressure ventilation
D. Place a naso- or orogastric tube to decompress the stomach
E. Perform needle decompression of the left chest

40. A 5-year-old male with Alagille syndrome and a history of liver transplantation was admitted overnight with increased work of breathing and post-tussive emesis. A respiratory pathogen panel ordered in the emergency room was positive for *Mycoplasma*, and the patient was started on azithromycin. He was given his home medications, including tacrolimus, and he also received ondansetron for persistent emesis. Overnight, the patient became unresponsive, and the code team was called. He required cardiopulmonary resuscitation for cardiac arrest, defibrillation, and medication administration, including epinephrine and magnesium sulfate. After reviewing the event, you realize that the patient's cardiac arrest was likely in part due to a medication interaction. Which of the following medications can also directly contribute to this adverse drug reaction?

A. Polyethylene glycol
B. Diphenhydramine
C. Acetaminophen
D. Ibuprofen
E. Amoxicillin

41. You are caring for a 4-year-old boy with severe global developmental delay and chronic hypercarbic respiratory failure with a tracheostomy tube and ventilator dependence, currently hospitalized for acute gastroenteritis. You are called to the bedside at 20:00 for tracheostomy tube dislodgement. The nurse was performing the weekly tracheostomy tube change alone and was unable to insert the tube with a small amount of lubricant. You enter the room with the nurse to find the patient agitated, turning his head side to side, and with suprasternal and subcostal retractions. His heart rate is 183 beats per minute, respirations 65 breaths per minute, and oxygen saturation 96% with blow-by oxygen.

Blood-tinged tracheal secretions are noted, but the tracheal stoma otherwise appears intact. He does not have a history of difficult tracheostomy tube exchanges. What is the most important next step in securing this patient's airway?

A. Apply more lubrication to the tracheostomy tube for reinsertion
B. Insert a smaller diameter tracheostomy tube.
C. Order a dose of intravenous lorazepam emergently
D. Reposition the head and reattempt tube insertion
E. Consult otolaryngology for surgical evaluation

42. A nurse pages you about a 2-day-old infant who is in the high-risk category for hyperbilirubinemia and would like to know if phototherapy should be initiated. Which of the following is true regarding the hour-specific Bhutani nomogram for total serum bilirubin?

A. It represents the natural history of neonatal hyperbilirubinemia
B. It can be applied to all newborns more than 36 weeks' gestation who have not received prior phototherapy
C. It can be applied to all healthy newborns, including those who have received prior phototherapy
D. It can be used to assess risk of developing hyperbilirubinemia in the future
E. It provides guidelines for the initiation of phototherapy

43. A 16-year-old female with a known seizure disorder is admitted following a prolonged seizure-like episode. Her mother describes a 10-minute period of abnormal movements, including arching of the back, head, and neck; bilateral arm stiffening; and pelvic thrusting. During this episode, her eyes were tightly shut. By the time emergency medical services arrived at her home, she was fully alert and responsive. Her seizures are well controlled on her current dose of levetiracetam. She endorses meticulous compliance in taking her daily medication. Her vital signs are within normal limits, and her neurologic examination findings are normal. Which test or study is most likely to reveal the underlying diagnosis?

A. Brain magnetic resonance imaging
B. Anti–epileptic drug level
C. Noncontrast head computed tomography
D. Cerebrospinal fluid studies
E. Video electroencephalography

44. You are called to attend a full-term delivery because of thick meconium staining in the amniotic fluid.

Under which of the following conditions should the newborn be intubated to suction the trachea?

A. All infants born through thick meconium should receive tracheal suctioning
B. A provider skilled at neonatal intubation is immediately available in the delivery room
C. The newborn is limp and apneic immediately after delivery
D. The newborn remains apneic after 60 seconds of tactile stimulation
E. The newborn requires positive pressure ventilation and there is evidence of airway obstruction

45. A 20-month-old female with global developmental delay, spasticity, tracheostomy, epilepsy, and recently diagnosed right vesicoureteral reflux is admitted with a urinary tract infection. The patient was also admitted 2 weeks ago for pyelonephritis. Following that admission, the patient developed antibiotic-associated diarrhea, and her parents stopped antibiotics the day after discharge because her fever had resolved. Which of the following is most likely to decrease this patient's risk of readmission?

A. Increased number of inpatient medical providers
B. Enrollment in public insurance
C. Documentation of a primary care physician follow-up plan at the time of discharge
D. Medical complexity with technology dependence
E. Family engagement through family-centered rounds

46. You are consulted by the emergency department (ED) physician for a 4-month-old infant with ventricular septal defect (VSD) and eczema who was referred to the ED for drainage of a first-time skin abscess. He is breastfed and receives furosemide. The mother has had recurrent skin abscesses on her forearms for the past few years. On your physical examination, the patient is nontoxic, with a temperature of 37.9°C, pulse 140 beats per minute, respiration rate 38 breaths per minute, and oxygen saturation of 96%. A fluctuant 1.5- by 2-cm skin abscess with a rim of erythema is seen on the left thigh. A healing diaper rash is present. White blood cell count is 11,000/μL without a neutrophil predominance. Which statement about incision and drainage (I&D) is correct for this patient?

A. Ultrasound should be performed to establish the diagnosis of abscess before I&D
B. After I&D, the patient should be discharged from the ED without antibiotics
C. After I&D, the patient should be discharged with a course of empiric antibiotics

D. One dose of antibiotic should be administered before I&D because of the patient's congenital heart disease
E. After I&D, the patient should be admitted for intravenous antibiotics because of age

47. You are called to the postanesthesia unit to assess a 4-year-old otherwise-healthy patient for agitation. He had multiple teeth extracted under sedation and has been persistently agitated for the past 15 minutes. He received halothane in the operating room. He is crying inconsolably and has pulled out his peripheral intravenous catheter. Which of the following laboratory tests are indicated?

A. Arterial blood gas, point-of-care blood glucose
B. Arterial blood gas, lactate
C. Blood culture, point-of-care blood glucose
D. Serum electrolytes, point-of-care blood glucose
E. Blood culture, lactate

48. A large-for-gestational-age infant is delivered by elective caesarean section at 37 weeks' gestation to a mother with poorly controlled gestational diabetes. The infant emerges vigorous and pink. He cries with minimal stimulation, but rapidly develops tachypnea, grunting, and subcostal and intercostal retractions. His breath sounds are clear and equal bilaterally. The infant is started on continuous positive airway pressure (CPAP), and he stabilizes. A chest radiograph shows a flattened diaphragm and fluid in the interlobar fissures. What most likely explains this presentation?

A. Aspiration of meconium-stained amniotic fluid
B. Bacterial pneumonia
C. Inadequate clearance of fetal lung fluid
D. Pulmonary surfactant deficiency
E. Transposition of the aorta and pulmonary artery

49. A 17-year-old male with muscular dystrophy, intellectual disability, progressive cardiomyopathy, recurrent aspiration, and gastrostomy tube dependence presents to the hospital with aspiration pneumonia. The patient has had frequent admissions over the last year, and the family feels that he is suffering. On echocardiogram, there is evidence of severe biventricular dysfunction compared to prior studies. After a multidisciplinary discussion with the family, the medical team initiates treatment with antibiotics to stabilize the patient, prepares a system to blow cool air on the patient's face for comfort, and administers morphine to manage dyspnea but plans to allow a natural death. After receiving moderate-dose morphine, the patient continues to appear uncomfortable and dyspneic.

Which of the following should you administer at this time?

A. Continuous enteral feeds via the gastrostomy tube
B. Additional morphine
C. Normal saline 20 mL/kg over 20 minutes
D. Vecuronium
E. Potassium chloride 150 mg/kg intravenous

50. While covering a community hospital, you are called emergently to the delivery room to resuscitate a full-term newborn. Thick meconium was noted at delivery, and the baby emerged cyanotic and floppy. Despite warming, drying, and providing positive pressure ventilation for the baby, his heart rate is 68 beats per minute at 1 minute of life. Chest compressions are begun, and the patient is successfully intubated. He remains limp, and his extremities are mottled and poorly perfused, with thready pulses and delayed capillary refill to 5 seconds. You prepare to place an umbilical venous catheter (UVC). The nurse suggests epinephrine administration as the next step. Which of the following is correct regarding UVC use in this situation?

A. The umbilical cord does not need to be tied because of the emergent nature of the situation
B. The UVC should be inserted to a depth of 3–5 cm below the skin or until blood return is seen
C. UVC location must be confirmed with a radiograph prior to use
D. Intraosseous needle (IO) insertion into the proximal tibia is faster and more reliable than UVC insertion for newborn resuscitation
E. Endotracheal epinephrine is more effective than intravenous

51. A 2-day-old, full-term baby has failed the newborn hearing screen in the right ear twice. In addition to referring to audiology for a repeat outpatient examination, which of the following types of studies would you recommend?

A. Renal imaging
B. Bag urine specimen
C. Post-feed saliva sample
D. Brain imaging
E. Serum infectious studies

52. A 14-year-old football player is admitted from the emergency department (ED) somnolent and disoriented. His speech is slurred, and he is unable to remember his address or the day of the week. He had been playing football in 90° F weather for the past 4 hours. He appears severely dehydrated and has a core

body temperature of 105°F. His urine drug screen is negative. A creatine phosphokinase (CPK) is 35,000 U/L (normal range is 10–120 U/L). What is the most likely cause of this patient's presentation?

A. Heat stroke
B. Heat exhaustion
C. Rhabdomyolysis
D. Drug intoxication
E. Head injury

53. You are notified that a 2-hour-old baby born at term is grunting. Which of the following best describes this finding?

A. Silent compensatory symptom that increases upper airway diameter and reduces resistance
B. Low-pitched sound heard over the extrathoracic airways that indicates nasopharyngeal obstruction
C. High-pitched sound that indicates obstruction at the larynx, glottis, or subglottic area
D. High-pitched sound that indicates tracheobronchial obstruction
E. Expiratory sound caused by partial closure of the glottis to keep alveoli patent

54. A 9-year-old female with gastroparesis, intestinal dysmotility, and gastrostomy-jejunostomy tube dependence is admitted. Currently, she is receiving feeds 16 hours daily (alternating 4 hours on, 2 hours off). Which of the following medications can be most effectively administered via the patient's jejunostomy tube?

A. Diazepam
B. Phenytoin
C. Ciprofloxacin
D. Ferrous sulfate
E. Lactobacillus

55. You are called to the bedside of a 6-month-old boy with Treacher Collins syndrome who was admitted for respiratory distress from bronchiolitis. As you enter the room, the respiratory therapist and nurse are already bag-mask ventilating the patient for persistent low oxygen saturations, increasing respiratory distress, and lethargy. The patient is unresponsive, and you notice that the respiratory therapist has placed an oral airway. There is a weak brachial pulse present on palpation, and oxygen saturation is at 82%, but you do not see adequate chest rise with bagging efforts. A pediatric code blue is called. Intubation is attempted twice unsuccessfully. You hear that it will take the surgical team and anesthesia 30 minutes to arrive because they are still in the operating room for an emergent case. What is the best next step?

A. Wait for the surgical team to evaluate the airway
B. Switch to nasal airway for difficult mask ventilation
C. Prepare for another intubation with a smaller endotracheal tube
D. Prepare for intubation with a supraglottic airway
E. Ask the nurse to administer albuterol

56. A 14-year-old female is admitted to the pediatric hospital medicine service for further workup of sudden-onset bilateral leg weakness and difficulty ambulating. She reports feeling as though she is going to fall and has significant pain in both legs when walking. Associated symptoms include headache, fatigue, and poor appetite. She does not appear to be worried about her symptoms and reports no recent life stressors. At baseline, she does endorse a high level of generalized anxiety in her ability to perform well in athletic, social, and academic activities. Her neurological examination remains inconsistent on serial assessments during her hospital stay, including a wide unsteady gait. The physical therapist notes she can walk appropriately when distracted. A magnetic resonance imaging (MRI) study of the spine is normal. What is the best next step in management?

A. Discharge home with physical therapy follow-up
B. Inpatient psychology consultation
C. Discharge home with primary care follow-up
D. Continue inpatient physical therapy services
E. Discharge home with outpatient psychology referral

57. A term neonate is born by cesarean section because of a maternal vaginal lesion suspicious for herpes simplex virus (HSV) infection that was noted on presentation to labor and delivery. The mother has not had a known history of prior HSV infection. The newborn's examination 30 minutes after birth is normal, with normal vital signs, normal tone, and no skin lesions. What is the best next step in management of the newborn?

A. Start intravenous (IV) acyclovir as soon as possible
B. Transfer the infant to the neonatal intensive care unit for continuous cardiopulmonary monitoring
C. Continue routine newborn care because the neonate was born by cesarean section
D. Request that the obstetrician send maternal HSV serologies and HSV polymerase chain reaction (PCR) and culture from the lesion
E. Immediately send HSV surface cultures, blood PCR, and cerebral spinal fluid (CSF) PCR from the neonate

58. A 14-year-old obese male with spina bifida, severe hypospadias, lower extremity paralysis, mild intellectual disability, and a history of recurrent pyelonephritis presents with urinary tract infection. The patient takes

oxybutynin as prescribed and self-catheterizes his urethra at home. He has some leaking between catheterization, but he wears a diaper and has no perineal skin
breakdown. He does not take antibiotic prophylaxis
and stopped consistently drinking cranberry juice
roughly 1 month before presentation. Which of the following puts this patient at the most significant risk of
ascending urinary tract infection?

A. Clean intermittent catheterization
B. Use of oxybutynin
C. Urinary leaking
D. Lack of antibiotic prophylaxis
E. Cessation of cranberry juice

59. An infant is admitted for failure to thrive, and multiple attempts for intravenous (IV) access have been
made without success. The baby has persistent vomiting
and oral intolerance, but she is alert and hemodynamically stable. Her parents agree to another IV placement
attempt. You are reviewing potential sites to insert your
IV and note the veins of the lower arms, hands, and feet
have already been attempted. What is the best next anatomic site to attempt another IV?

A. Superficial scalp
B. Basilic vein
C. Saphenous vein
D. Femoral vein
E. External jugular vein

60. A previously healthy 17-year-old male is admitted
following a witnessed event of self-injurious behavior at
home. His brother observed him cut his left forearm with
a kitchen knife, saying he was following the commands of
an internal voice. An extensive workup, including a complete blood count with differential, complete metabolic
panel, salicylate level, acetaminophen level, blood alcohol
level, urinalysis, thyroid-stimulating hormone level, and
vitamin B_{12} level are unremarkable. A urine drug screen is
positive for cannabinoids. His father has bipolar disorder,
and his paternal grandfather died by suicide as an adolescent. The child psychiatry team recommends starting an
atypical antipsychotic. Prior to initiation of this psycho-
tropic medication, what additional test should be ordered?

A. Fasting lipid panel
B. Serum glucose level
C. Repeat urine drug screen
D. Electrocardiogram
E. Echocardiogram

61. An infant is born at a gestational age of 36 weeks and
2 days and a birth weight of 2700 g. The night before her

anticipated discharge, she undergoes a car seat tolerance screening (CSTS), during which she has an apneic
episode lasting 30 seconds that resolves with minimal
stimulation. Which is the correct interpretation of this
result?

A. She failed the CSTS and cannot be cleared for
discharge
B. She failed the CSTS but can be discharged in a
car bed
C. She passed the CSTS and can be discharged
D. She was born near term, so a CSTS was not
indicated, and the brief apnea can be disregarded
E. She was not low birth weight (LBW), so a CSTS was
not indicated, and the brief apnea can be disregarded

62. A 2-year-old male with propionic acidemia and a
history of developmental regression following a metabolic stroke is admitted from an acute rehabilitation facility with 1 day of intractable, nonbilious, nonbloody
emesis. He is normally fed via a gastrostomy tube
due to dysphagia and receives six bolus feeds per day.
Laboratory tests have been collected and are pending.
What is the best next step in management?

A. Continue his home feeding regimen and start
dextrose-containing fluids intravenously to make up
for his gastrointestinal losses
B. Transition from bolus to continuous feeds
with the same total volume and start dextrose-
containing fluids intravenously to make up for his
gastrointestinal losses
C. Continue bolus feeds at smaller volumes and
more frequent intervals and start dextrose-
containing fluids intravenously to make up for his
gastrointestinal losses
D. Continue his home feeding regimen at half volume
and start dextrose-containing fluids intravenously at
maintenance rate
E. Stop feeds and start dextrose-containing fluids
intravenously at 1.5 times maintenance rate

63. A 10-year-old boy with cerebral palsy, intractable
epilepsy with a vagal nerve stimulator, and significant
delay with gastrostomy tube dependence is admitted
for pneumonia. He has been on antibiotics for the past
2 days with minimal improvement. This evening he
has had worsening agitation and increasing oxygen requirement. His vital signs are heart rate of 130 beats per
minute, respirations of 32 breaths per minute, blood
pressure of 134/78 mm Hg, and oxygen saturation
of 89% on 10 L/min 100% oxygen via high-flow nasal
cannula. An urgent chest radiograph is obtained and is
shown in Figure 2.2. What is the best next step?

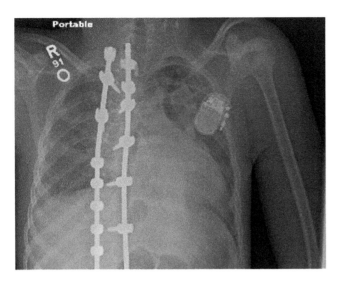

Figure 2.2

A. Place patient in lateral decubitus position, left side down
B. Confirm radiograph findings with an ultrasound
C. Place a needle in midclavicular second intercostal space
D. Prepare to perform intubation
E. Consult surgery for chest tube placement

64. A 14-year-old male with depression, oppositional defiant disorder, and posttraumatic stress disorder is admitted to the hospital for further workup of worsening paranoid behaviors noted by his group home caseworker. He is refusing to eat or drink. A nurse attempts to place an intravenous (IV) line, but the boy aggressively starts pacing across his hospital room and shouts that he will hurt anyone that touches him again. A behavioral response team is paged immediately. What is the best next de-escalation step while awaiting specialized assistance?

A. Physically restrain the boy using bodily force
B. Administer intramuscular lorazepam
C. Leave the patient alone in the room
D. Remove any dangerous objects from the room
E. Continue to engage verbally with the patient, explaining the medical need for IV placement

65. You are called to evaluate an 8-hour-old newborn in the special care nursery. The mother has a history of opioid abuse and took buprenorphine throughout her pregnancy. Both meconium and maternal urine drug screens are positive for opioids. The infant is jittery and has increased tone, but the jitters can be suppressed by holding the infant. Vital signs and the remainder of the physical examination are otherwise unremarkable. Which of the following is the best next step?

A. Treatment with morphine if the infant cannot feed, cannot sleep, or cannot be easily consoled
B. Treatment with paregoric and titrate the dose until the jitteriness resolves
C. Order an electroencephalogram as the jitters and increased tone may represent seizure activity
D. Nonpharmacological treatment with swaddling, on-demand feeding, and minimizing environmental stimulation
E. Finnegan score assessment and treatment with morphine if the score is elevated

66. A 14-year-old with a history of cerebral palsy, obstructive sleep apnea, and constipation is admitted for poor weight gain following an acute respiratory illness. His parents are divorced and his care is divided between two different medical centers. Both parents work night shifts and have missed his last two clinic appointments. The patient's current weight is 30 kg (0.1 percentile for age). His parents report that he had no difficulties with oral feeding before this illness. On examination, he is alert and nonverbal, with remarkable muscle wasting and joint contractures. What is the best next step?

A. Call Child Protective Services for possible child neglect
B. Check albumin and prealbumin to assess nutritional status
C. Obtain more history and a bedside swallow study
D. Consult a surgeon for a gastrostomy tube (G-tube) placement
E. Discharge home with gastroenterologist follow-up

67. A 20-day-old female infant presents to the emergency room for a temperature of 101.2°F, irritability, and poor feeding for 1 day. Previous attempts to catheterize the patient for urine collection have been unsuccessful. Which of the following is a contraindication to urethral catheterization in infants?

A. Imperforate hymen
B. Vaginitis
C. Pelvic fracture
D. Sepsis
E. Spinal cord injury

68. An 18-year-old female with oppositional defiant disorder, type 2 diabetes mellitus, and hypertension is admitted to the pediatric hospital medicine service for acute management of hyperglycemia. She was brought in to the emergency department by police after refusing to return home following a verbal altercation with her father at a gas station. On day 3 of hospitalization, she becomes visibly upset when told she is not being discharged. She attempts to elope from the pediatric

inpatient unit, becoming physically aggressive with staff as they attempt to redirect her. She requires a hospital security escort back to her room. She continues to shout and curse, visibly upset about having to remain in the hospital. De-escalation techniques to achieve a calm and cooperative state do not prove useful, and she refuses to take her scheduled oral medications. What is the best next step in management?

A. Place the patient in soft restraints for the remainder of her hospitalization
B. Administer intramuscular (IM) haloperidol and reassess her agitation in 15 minutes
C. Continue verbal de-escalation efforts
D. Place the patient in hard restraints and reevaluate her agitation in 1 hour
E. Administer IM lorazepam and titrate the dose to achieve sedation

69. You are called to evaluate a set of twins born full term with weights appropriate for gestational age (AGA). Twin A has equinovarus deformities of both feet, and twin B has torticollis. They are otherwise well appearing with unremarkable physical examinations. Twin A's feet and twin B's head can be brought back to the neutral position with gentle pressure. What is the most likely cause of these abnormalities?

A. A germline mutation
B. An inherited genetic trait
C. Birth trauma
D. Physical forces during fetal development
E. Toxic exposure in utero

70. You admit a 14-year-old with systemic lupus erythematosus (SLE) following an intentional acetaminophen overdose. Her lupus is well controlled with hydroxychloroquine and prednisone. She has recently become withdrawn and has struggled to complete her schoolwork. Her mother suffers from depression. What is the most important risk factor for depression in this child?

A. History of maternal depression
B. Female gender
C. Chronic illness
D. Age
E. Steroid medication

71. During an examination of a 7-month-old ex–24-week female with chronic lung disease, epilepsy, and obstructive hydrocephalus secondary to bilateral grade IV intraventricular hemorrhage with a ventriculoperitoneal shunt, you note increased tone in the bilateral upper and lower extremities along multiple joints. There is

increased resistance to motion on joint range of motion with increased velocity. Which of the following is recommended for this patient?

A. Lorazepam
B. Botulinum toxin injection
C. Baclofen
D. Deep brain stimulation
E. Levodopa (administered with carbidopa)

72. A 2-day-old infant in the newborn nursery is being evaluated for a petechial rash and is found to have periventricular calcifications on neuroimaging. What other finding would be expected?

A. Failure to pass the hearing screen
B. Cataracts
C. Macrocephaly
D. Extramedullary hematopoiesis
E. Bone deformities

73. A 17-year-old obese female with intellectual disability and lower limb spasticity undergoes a left hip osteotomy. Two days after the surgery, while casted, she develops a decubitus ulcer of the right heel. The wound consultant diagnoses a stage 2 pressure ulcer. The patient is on an anticoagulant and is currently non–weight bearing. Which one of the following is the least true of pressure ulcers?

A. Early assessment of risk factors reduces the risk of the development of pressure ulcers
B. Prescribing vitamin C and zinc can expedite wound healing
C. Instituting a turning schedule significantly reduces certain pressure ulcers
D. Reducing friction and shearing are helpful
E. Adequate nutrition is recommended

74. A 1-year-old male with well-controlled epilepsy is presenting for procedural sedation for brain magnetic resonance imaging. Routine sedation was started with propofol, but the patient started developing bronchospasm. The team was unable to effectively ventilate the patient due to bronchospasm, and the patient went into cardiac arrest. What is a known risk factor of cardiac arrest during procedural sedation?

A. Age younger than 1 year
B. American Society of Anesthesiologists (ASA) Physical Status I
C. Epilepsy
D. Propofol infusion
E. Pediatric sedation outside the operating room

75. A 15-year-old severely autistic boy is admitted for acute management of constipation requiring bowel cleanout with polyethylene glycol–electrolyte solution administered via a nasogastric (NG) tube. On day 2 of hospitalization, the patient develops abnormal facial movements. Painful, repetitive, involuntary twisting motions of his lips, tongue, and jaw are noted. His examination and vital signs are otherwise unremarkable. His mother is at bedside and notes that in the emergency department her son was given a medication to help calm him down. Which medication was most likely administered in the emergency department?

A. Lorazepam
B. Diphenhydramine
C. Haloperidol
D. Olanzapine
E. Risperidone

76. A full-term, large-for-gestational-age (LGA) newborn is born by vacuum-assisted vaginal delivery. On examination, there is an asymmetric Moro reflex with decreased movement of the right arm, and the infant cries with passive movement of the right shoulder. The infant has normal movement and reflexes of the right hand. An x-ray shows a mildly displaced midshaft fracture of the right clavicle. Which is the best next step in management?

A. Consult orthopedic surgery for possible operative repair
B. Recommend passive stretching and range of motion exercises
C. Immobilize the affected arm by pinning the right sleeve to the shirt front
D. Obtain magnetic resonance imaging (MRI) to assess the integrity of the brachial plexus
E. Report the injury to Child Protective Services (CPS)

77. A 15-year-old with muscular dystrophy and ventilator dependence is admitted following scoliosis surgery. During repositioning, the patient's tracheostomy tube accidentally becomes dislodged, and his oxygen saturation falls to 80%. The respiratory therapist replaces the tracheostomy tube and briefly performs bag-mask ventilation. The patient then develops increased work of breathing, anxiety, and worsening hypoxia. He is found to be febrile and tachycardic. What is the best next step?

A. Start intravenous antibiotics
B. Consult surgery for emergent chest tube placement
C. Give a normal saline bolus
D. Obtain a stat chest radiograph
E. Give lorazepam to relieve anxiety

78. A 3-week-old former 39-week infant was admitted to a community hospital this afternoon for bronchiolitis. You are called to the bedside because the baby is poorly responsive, head bobbing, and grunting. Deep intercostal and subcostal retractions are also seen. Respiratory sounds are coarsely crackly with poor air excursion and incomplete exhalation. You prepare to initiate bag-mask ventilation. Which statement below is correct?

A. The mask should fit from the bridge of the nose to just below the chin
B. Adequate ventilation is assessed primarily with a CO_2 detector
C. Continuous flow of oxygen can be provided passively through the reservoir portion of a self-inflating bag
D. In situations of poor lung compliance, use of a pressure pop-off valve is recommended to avoid pressure-related pneumothorax
E. Bag-mask ventilation is contraindicated in a spontaneously breathing child

79. A 7-year-old is transferred to the floor from the pediatric intensive care unit (PICU) after 29 days of hospitalization for bacterial myositis and sepsis. He has undergone multiple surgical procedures and was intubated and mechanically ventilated for the first 2 weeks of admission. He was previously healthy with normal development, but now he rarely speaks, sleeps 14–15 hours a day, does not recognize the alphabet, and is unable to count. Physical therapy is working with him as he has not gotten out of bed for a month. Which of the following is an appropriate medication for this patient?

A. Diazepam
B. Scopolamine
C. Methadone
D. Atropine
E. Olanzapine

80. You are preparing an educational session on the topic of breastfeeding for the nurses on the labor and delivery unit. Which of the following women should be counseled against breastfeeding?

A. A mother with a positive tuberculin skin test but no symptoms
B. A mother with herpetic lesions on her back
C. A mother with human immunodeficiency virus (HIV) and an undetectable viral load
D. A mother with a history of brucellosis
E. A mother with a history of substance abuse

81. The mother of a patient with hypoxic-ischemic encephalopathy signs a modified advanced care directive for her daughter. She wishes for her daughter to receive comfort

measures, no chest compressions, and no electrical shock or drugs to restart her heart. The mother would like to be contacted if there is a need for endotracheal intubation, which the family only wants in the case of a reversible medical condition. During your shift, the patient vomits and then develops increased work of breathing. You order a chest radiograph and start bilevel positive airway pressure (BiPAP), but the patient's respiratory status continues to deteriorate. The patient's mother is unreachable by phone. As the primary physician, what should be your next step?

A. Continue trying reach the mother to determine next steps
B. Start broad-spectrum antibiotics to treat aspiration pneumonia
C. Emergently intubate and ventilate the patient
D. Provide additional oxygen and pain medications
E. Contact the office of risk management

82. A 7-month-old female presents to the emergency department after a nonfatal drowning incident in a neighbor's pool. She is breathing spontaneously, but she is lethargic and her oxygen saturation is 85% on 10 liters per minute oxygen by face mask. You prepare to obtain arterial blood gas measurements. Which of the following statements regarding arterial puncture is true?

A. Overlying infection is a contraindication to the procedure
B. There is a high risk of ischemic complications
C. Sterile technique is necessary
D. Lack of pulsatile blood flow indicates the specimen is venous rather than arterial
E. The needle should enter the skin at a 90° angle

83. A 17-year-old female with anorexia nervosa is hospitalized for medical stabilization. Which of the following findings would you expect to see in this patient?

A. Hypernatremia
B. Supraventricular tachycardia
C. Metabolic alkalosis
D. Delayed gastric emptying
E. Thrombocytosis

84. An infant is born at 36 weeks' gestation with a birth weight appropriate for gestational age. Which of these is most likely to be normal and does not require additional monitoring?

A. Bilirubin level
B. Glucose level
C. Body temperature
D. Hematocrit level
E. Feeding ability

85. You are planning to discuss an advance care directive with the parents of a 17-year-old with antiphospholipid antibody syndrome, glomerular membranopathy, hypertension, and hemiplegia. The patient has normal cognition. Which of the following statements is true regarding this conversation?

A. It is best to avoid engaging the patient in this discussion until her prognosis is certain
B. Cultural differences should not impact your approach
C. You should discuss unnecessary therapies that prolong life
D. It is unnecessary to acknowledge the attitudes of patients, families, and clinicians
E. You should discuss financial burden and cost of providing care up front

86. A 15-year-old male is admitted for evaluation of new-onset ataxia. He is undergoing magnetic resonance imaging (MRI) of his brain today. He reports that he has claustrophobia but thinks he can be still for the duration of the study. Which of the following depths of procedural sedation is indicated for this patient?

A. None
B. Minimal sedation
C. Moderate sedation
D. Deep sedation
E. General anesthesia

87. A 17-year-old female is admitted for a recent 20-pound weight loss in the setting of regular bingeing and purging behaviors. This is her third admission this year for the same condition. She is undergoing nutritional rehabilitation and has been seeing a psychologist regularly between hospitalizations. Which of the following medications is recommended for this patient?

A. Bupropion
B. Olanzapine
C. Nortriptyline
D. Fluoxetine
E. Topiramate

88. While examining a newborn, you notice a pit in the skin in the gluteal cleft overlying the coccyx. You cannot see the bottom of the pit. There is no excessive hair, vascular malformation, or pseudo appendage in the area. The gluteal cleft is not deviated. The infant has no other congenital anomalies, and prenatal screening and ultrasounds were normal. Which of the following is the best next step?

A. Consult neurosurgery
B. Discharge the infant
C. Order lumbosacral magnetic resonance imaging (MRI)

D. Order a sacral ultrasound

E. Schedule neurology follow-up

89. A 2-year-old, nonverbal child with cerebral palsy, intractable epilepsy, dysautonomia, and obstructive sleep apnea is admitted with concern for an aspiration event. On examination you note significant drooling, pooling of salivary secretions in the posterior oropharynx, and increased work of breathing that improves with 0.5 liters per minute of supplemental oxygen via nasal cannula. You continue his home medications of rufinamide, clobazam, clonazepam, valproic acid, propranolol, and lorazepam. He underwent botulinum toxin injection of the salivary glands 3 weeks ago and was started on glycopyrrolate with minimal improvement in his secretions. His parents note that his drooling has worsened over the past year despite extensive work with an oral motor skills specialist. Which one of the following steps is the most effective intervention at this point?

A. Consult head and neck surgery for parotid gland ligation

B. Reduce daily free water intake to decrease secretions

C. Increase glycopyrrolate dose

D. Consider repeat botulinum toxin injection

E. Consult speech therapist for oral motor exercises

90. You are urgently called to evaluate a 2-hour-old newborn who "choked and turned blue" when her mother attempted to breastfeed her for the first time. When you arrive in the room, the infant is vigorous, pink, and crying loudly. The physical examination is unremarkable, with clear symmetrical breath sounds and no signs of a cleft palate. Which of the following is the best next step?

A. Check pre- and postductal pulse oximetry

B. Order a bedside swallowing evaluation

C. Order a head and neck computed tomography (CT) scan

D. Observe the next feeding session

E. Pass a suction catheter through both nares

91. You are caring for a previously healthy 17-year-old who was a restrained passenger in a motor vehicle accident. She suffered a mild concussion and fractures of the left tibia and right femur. She is currently on scheduled acetaminophen and ibuprofen. She is having difficulty sleeping in the hospital, and her exhaustion is making it difficult for her to work with physical therapy (PT). Which one of the following is the least preferred step?

A. Start amitriptyline at bedtime

B. Assess pain before and after PT and add oxycodone as needed

C. Ask her to keep a sleep log

D. Start melatonin at bedtime

E. Consult psychology

92. Shortly after birth, a family asks to speak with you regarding circumcision of their healthy newborn. Which of the following statements is true?

A. Evidence-based health benefits to circumcision include decreased risk of neonatal urinary tract infections, transmission of human papilloma virus (HPV), and rates of penile cancer

B. The American Academy of Pediatrics (AAP) recommends routine circumcision

C. It is appropriate to perform a routine circumcision on a patient with a webbed penis, but circumcision is contraindicated when hypospadias is present

D. Sugar water and appropriate swaddling technique provide similar analgesic effects with less risk than penile nerve blocks

E. There are higher risks when circumcision is performed in the neonatal period

93. A 2-month-old female with a history of necrotizing enterocolitis (NEC) requiring extensive bowel resection is admitted for postoperative fluid and nutritional support. The patient had 60 cm of small bowel resected, and her ileocecal valve is intact. She is currently receiving nasogastric feeds in addition to total parenteral nutrition (TPN). Which of the following factors confers the greatest odds to achieve full enteral autonomy?

A. Residual bowel length greater than 50 cm

B. Preservation of the ileocecal valve

C. Presence of primarily jejunal bowel remnant

D. Postoperative time to initiation of enteral feeds

E. Presence of intact oral-motor skills

94. On your initial examination of a full-term baby on day of life 1, you note a normal 3.1-cm phallus with a well-developed rugated scrotum but cannot palpate the testes. Which of the following is the best next step?

A. Abdominal ultrasound

B. Serum electrolytes

C. Urology consultation for immediate surgical correction

D. Watchful waiting for 6 months

E. Watchful waiting for 12 months

95. A 10-year-old female with newly diagnosed systemic lupus erythematosus (SLE) is admitted for management of a disease flare. Her home medications include hydroxychloroquine and nonsteroidal anti-inflammatory drugs. She is started on pulse-dose methylprednisolone. On examination the following morning, her mother comments that the patient has been more confused and disoriented for the last few days, but today is having hallucinations and delusions as well. Her vital signs and neurologic examination are normal. Which of the following is the most likely cause of this patient's symptoms?

A. Steroid-induced psychosis
B. Neuropsychiatric lupus
C. Stroke
D. Primary psychiatric disorder
E. Acute intoxication

96. You are preparing to discharge a 3-day-old infant born at 39 weeks' gestation to a primiparous mother via unscheduled cesarean section. Her mother has not yet noticed significant breast engorgement or mature milk leaking from her breasts, and she asks you why her milk has not "come in yet." Which of the following is the most appropriate response to this question?

A. It is too early to expect signs of lactogenesis II at this point
B. Progesterone levels are likely too low to allow for normal milk production
C. Prolactin levels are likely too high to allow for normal milk production
D. Frequent breastfeeding in the first 2 days of life has caused delayed lactogenesis
E. Primiparous mothers are more likely to have a longer time to the onset of lactogenesis II

97. A 17-year-old boy who is fed via a percutaneous endoscopic gastrostomy (PEG) tube presents to the emergency department due to persistent nonbloody, nonbilious emesis for the past 3 days. His PEG tube flushes easily and has been infusing feeds without resistance. The patient's pulse is 133 beats per minute, blood pressure 120/72 mm Hg, and oxygen saturation 97% while breathing room air. He has lost 10 kilograms over the past 3 months. His abdomen is nontender and soft with mild upper abdominal distention. An abdominal plain film is unremarkable. A complete blood count, basic metabolic panel, liver enzymes, and lipase are normal. What is your best next step?

A. Computed tomography (CT) of the abdomen with oral and intravenous contrast
B. Pediatric surgery consult
C. PEG tube contrast study
D. Trial of clear fluids by PEG tube
E. Stool studies

98. An infant is born at 39 weeks' gestation with a birth weight of 3200 grams. Maternal hepatitis B surface antigen (HBsAg) is unknown but was drawn on

arrival and has a laboratory turnaround time of 24–36 hours. Which of the following do you recommend?

A. Await the mother's results prior to giving the hepatitis B vaccine
B. Give the hepatitis B vaccine within the first 24 hours
C. Give both the hepatitis B vaccine and hepatitis B immune globulin (HBIG) within the first 12 hours of life
D. Give the hepatitis B vaccine within 12 hours of life and HBIG within 7 days if the mother's results return positive
E. Give HBIG within 12 hours of life and the hepatitis B vaccine within 7 days if the mother's results return positive

99. A 9-year-old female with chronic encephalopathy and recurrent aspiration is experiencing episodes of tachycardia and hypoglycemia in the postoperative period following a fundoplication. The episodes occur approximately 1 hour after her scheduled bolus feeds, which are given enterally through a gastrostomy tube. Of the following, which is the intervention most likely to improve the patient's symptoms?

A. Increase the rate of the bolus feeds
B. Vent the gastrostomy tube immediately following completion of the bolus feeds
C. Add a complex carbohydrate to the patient's formula
D. Initiate loperamide prior to feeds
E. Bowel rest for 1 week followed by resumption of current regimen

100. You are called to the delivery of an infant born at 39 weeks' gestation by cesarean section for arrest of descent. The baby emerges limp and apneic. You immediately place the infant on the warmer, dry, stimulate, and suction the mouth and nares. At 60 seconds of life, the infant is spontaneously breathing with a heart rate of 70 beats per minute. What is your next step?

A. Continue to dry, warm, and stimulate for an additional 30 seconds
B. Begin positive pressure ventilation (PPV) with a fraction of inspired oxygen (FiO$_2$) of 30%
C. Begin PPV with FiO$_2$ 21%
D. Begin chest compressions at a ratio of 15:2
E. Begin chest compressions at a ratio of 3:1

101. You are consulted in the emergency department (ED) to see a 12-year-old with abdominal pain. Her grandmother reports that she has been having abdominal pain daily for the past 3 weeks and has been unable to attend school. She has seen a pediatric gastroenterologist and has undergone a thorough outpatient evaluation that included imaging and stool and blood studies that

were normal. You note eight prior ED visits for this same complaint. Your physical examination is reassuring. You are considering a diagnosis of somatic symptom disorder (SSD). Which of the following is true regarding SSD?

A. The diagnosis requires a triggering event or stressor
B. Cognitive behavioral therapy (CBT) is the most effective treatment
C. Patients typically present to mental healthcare settings
D. Bullying is rarely associated with pediatric SSD
E. Thorough diagnostic testing is recommended to rule out organic causes

102. You are asked to review a new protocol for management of newborn hypoglycemia, which includes 40% dextrose gel as an option for treatment. Based on the available evidence, which of the following is true regarding the safety and efficacy of this treatment option?

A. Dextrose gel is more effective than feeding alone for treatment of neonatal hypoglycemia in the first 48 hours after birth
B. Newborns who receive treatment with dextrose gel should be transferred to the neonatal intensive care unit (NICU) for monitoring because of the risk of rebound hypoglycemia
C. A glucose level should be checked immediately after dextrose gel is administered
D. Newborns should not be fed for at least 30 minutes after receiving dextrose gel
E. Dextrose gel should be mixed with breast milk or formula and fed by syringe to the newborn

103. After a peripherally inserted central catheter (PICC) placement on a 6-year-old boy, you are notified by the nurse to confirm placement so she can use the catheter for medication administration. After reviewing the chest radiograph in Figure 2.3, what is the best next step?

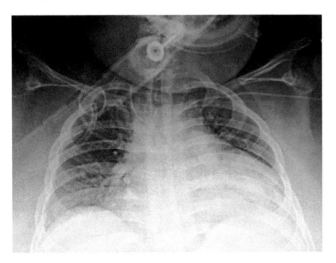

Figure 2.3

A. Immediate use of the catheter
B. Repeat the chest radiograph
C. Obtain a neck ultrasound
D. Consult the intensive care unit team
E. Consult the PICC team for repositioning

104. On admission to the nursery, a family asks you why the obstetrician waited until 1 minute of life to clamp the umbilical cord. You discuss that delayed cord clamping in a term infant for 30–60 seconds decreases the infant's risk of which of the following?

A. Necrotizing enterocolitis
B. Polycythemia
C. Hyperbilirubinemia requiring phototherapy
D. Hypothermia
E. Iron deficiency anemia in the first year of life

105. A previously healthy 13-year-old girl is brought to the emergency department (ED) with acute onset of an abnormal gait. She was recently enrolled in a new school, and her mother believes she is "faking it" because she is scared to go to school. A thorough physical examination is reassuring, although with ambulation the patient frequently falls onto an outstretched hand. You are considering a diagnosis of functional neurological symptom disorder. Which of the following is true regarding this condition?

A. Examination findings should be compatible with the patient's symptoms
B. Adolescent boys are at increased risk
C. Patients are typically distressed by their symptoms
D. The prognosis is generally poor
E. Symptoms most commonly involve motor function

106. You are examining a full-term baby on their second day of life and notice tremors, hypertonicity, a high-pitched cry, exaggerated sucking, and some colostrum regurgitation on the blanket. Based on these findings, you should ask the mother if she has a history of which of the following?

A. An autoimmune disorder
B. A viral infection during pregnancy
C. Antidepressant use during pregnancy
D. Marijuana use during pregnancy
E. A sexually transmitted disease

107. A 5-year-old patient with a history of severe traumatic brain injury resulting in intractable epilepsy and limited neurocognitive function is admitted for replacement of a dislodged gastrostomy tube. The nurse calls you to evaluate a sudden change in clinical status. On assessment, he is febrile, tachycardic, hypertensive, and diaphoretic

with dystonic posturing. He is started on broad-spectrum antibiotics and intravenous fluids. Two days later, he continues to have similar events intermittently despite continued antibiotics and a negative infectious workup. His father reports that he has events like this at home as well. Which of the following medications can be used as an abortive and preventive medication for these events?

A. Clonidine
B. Morphine
C. Gabapentin
D. Baclofen
E. Lorazepam

108. You are caring for a 2-day-old infant with hyperbilirubinemia. The infant has not been breastfeeding well, has passed one stool since birth, and is down 9% from birth weight. The bilirubin level is 15.5 mg/dL at 48 hours of life, so you initiate phototherapy. On recheck 12 hours later, the bilirubin level has decreased to 14 mg/dL. Which of the following explains the drop in bilirubin?

A. Bilirubin is being conjugated in the liver and excreted in the urine
B. Bilirubin is being converted to lumirubin and excreted in the urine
C. Bilirubin absorption by intestinal mucosa is increasing, facilitating excretion in the stool
D. Bilirubin is becoming unbound from albumin, allowing uptake in the liver
E. Bilirubin is being deconjugated by the kidneys and excreted in the urine

109. A neonate is being evaluated in the emergency department (ED) for sepsis. A lumbar puncture is attempted and is unsuccessful after multiple attempts. The parents are becoming increasingly upset and ask if there is any way to increase the success rate of the procedure. What is the best next step in management of this patient?

A. Attempt lumbar puncture with another provider
B. Attempt lumbar puncture in the upright position
C. Attempt lumbar puncture with bedside ultrasound
D. Admit the patient for fluoroscopy-guided lumbar puncture
E. Start intravenous fluids to hydrate the infant

110. You are preparing to discharge a 2-day-old infant. He was born at term without complications and has been breastfeeding exclusively. He has passed multiple stools, has voided three times in the past 24 hours, and his weight has decreased 3% since birth. A screening transcutaneous bilirubin is in the low-risk zone. The mother asks your advice on feeding patterns after discharge. Which is the most appropriate response?

A. Continue breastfeeding when the infant displays feeding cues, at least 8–12 times in a 24-hour period
B. Continue breastfeeding no more frequently than every 4 hours
C. Increase breastfeeding to every 2 hours because of the decreased urine output
D. If formula supplementation is desired, offer at least 2–3 ounces (60–90 mL) after each feeding from the breast
E. It is helpful to begin using a breast pump early on in addition to breastfeeding to increase milk supply

111. A 15-year-old male is brought to the emergency department (ED) by his parents out of concern for their safety because he threatened his mother with a butcher knife. They report that over the last several months he has become increasingly aggressive. He recently broke his sister's laptop with a hammer, has repeatedly hit the family pet, and has twice set fires in his closet. They have had to call the police to their home multiple times. There is no family history of psychiatric disorders, and he has been otherwise healthy with normal development. He recently started struggling with his schoolwork. What is the most likely diagnosis?

A. Bipolar disorder
B. Oppositional defiant disorder
C. Conduct disorder
D. Intermittent explosive disorder
E. Pyromania

112. A 3-year-old male with Pierre Robin sequence is admitted for dehydration due to acute gastroenteritis. During his hospital stay, he is noted to have loud snoring associated with episodes of apnea. His mother states that she often notes similar episodes at home. During one episode, his oxygen saturation is found to dip transiently to 80%. The team is discussing the possibility of sleep apnea in this patient and the risks and benefits of positive pressure ventilation devices at home. Which of the following statements about home positive pressure ventilation is true?

A. Continuous positive airway pressure (CPAP) is safe for children at risk for aspiration
B. It is preferable to initiate CPAP prior to performing a sleep study
C. Chronic use of CPAP can lead to abnormal facial development

D. Bilevel positive airway pressure (BiPAP) would likely be more effective than CPAP for this patient
E. Small children often initially require restraints in order to keep from removing the CPAP mask

113. A 2-week-old female presents to the emergency department for runny nose and a rash. She was born to a mother who received no prenatal care. Her vital signs are within normal limits. Her physical examination is notable for rhinorrhea, hepatomegaly, and a maculopapular rash on the back, buttocks, palms, and soles. Which of the following is a recommended part of this child's workup?

A. Respiratory pathogen panel
B. Computed tomography (CT) of the chest
C. Lumbar puncture
D. Abdominal ultrasound
E. Fungal blood culture

ANSWERS

1. ANSWER: D

Neonates have lower blood glucose levels in the first few hours of life, which then normalize in 24–48 hours. This is termed transitional hypoglycemia of the newborn and is thought to be part of normal adaptation to extrauterine life. Much research has been done to balance potential long-term neurologic sequelae from lack of glucose to the brain with overtreating, which leads to separation of the mother and baby, interferes with the establishment of oral feedings, and carries the inherent risks of intravenous access. Newborns who require screening for hypoglycemia include any newborn with symptoms such as tremors at rest, lethargy, exaggerated Moro reflex, tachypnea, or hypothermia, as well as asymptomatic newborns with risk factors such as prematurity, small or large for gestational age, and maternal gestational diabetes.

The American Academy of Pediatrics 2011 practice guidelines recommend that asymptomatic infants with risk factors for hypoglycemia should be fed within 1 hour of birth, with a plasma glucose checked 30 minutes after the initial feed. Based on the guidelines (summarized in Table 2.1), this infant should be refed and have a repeat glucose level 1 hour later. If the repeat level was again less than 25 mg/dL, then intravenous (IV) glucose should be initiated at a rate of 5 to 8 mg/kg per minute and titrated up as needed to maintain euglycemia.

Table 2.1 MANAGEMENT OF ASYMPTOMATIC INFANTS WITH RISK FACTORS FOR HYPOGLYCEMIA[a]

	0-4 HOURS OF LIFE	4-24 HOURS OF LIFE
Screening glucose level (mg/dL)[b]	<25 Refeed and recheck in 1 hour	<35 Refeed and recheck in 1 hour
Recheck glucose level (mg/dL)	<25: IV glucose / 25–40: Refeed and recheck in 1 hour; if persistent, consider IV glucose	<35: IV glucose / 35–45: Refeed and recheck in 1 hour; if persistent, consider IV glucose

[a] Adapted from Reference 1.

[b] If screening value greater than or equal to the cutoff listed, continue feeds every 2–3 hours with prefeed glucose checks.

[ABP 3.B.1. Hypoglycemia]

REFERENCE

1. Committee on Fetus and Newborn, Adamkin DH. Postnatal glucose homeostasis in late-preterm and term infants. *Pediatrics.* 2011;*127*(3):575–579.

2. ANSWER: A

This child's presentation is concerning for small intestinal bacterial overgrowth (SIBO). Her lack of an ileocecal valve, prior abdominal surgery and risk of stricture, and increased risk of poor motility all predispose her to SIBO. D-Lactic acidosis is a rare neurologic syndrome that can present in patients with SIBO associated with short-bowel syndrome after a carbohydrate-rich feed. The bacterial fermentation of unabsorbed carbohydrates can cause altered mental status, ranging from confusion to coma, slurred speech, seizures, or ataxia. Nephrolithiasis may be associated with some medications or dehydration that premature infants may experience; however, there is no association with SIBO. While a disrupted intestinal barrier may predispose to bacterial translocation, meningitis is not associated with SIBO. Anemia due to poor nutrition or anemia of chronic disease may be seen in infants with a history of prematurity or necrotizing enterocolitis (NEC). However, typically patients on TPN are appropriately supplemented to prevent this. Thrombocytopenia may be seen in the setting of sepsis or as a side effect of some medications; however, it is not associated directly with SIBO.

[ABP 4.B. Feeding and nutrition]

3. ANSWER: C

Normal newborn temperatures are defined as axillary temperatures of 36.5°C to 37.4°C. Late preterm infants are at increased risk of temperature instability. They have increased heat losses due to small size and a larger ratio of surface area to weight as compared to term infants. In addition, late preterm infants cannot generate heat from adipose tissue as effectively as their term counterparts because brown fat maturation increases with gestational age. Late preterm infants also have less white adipose tissue, which functions as insulation. For these reasons, the neonatal resuscitation program guidelines recommend taking steps to keep the late preterm newborn warm, including drying with warm towels, ensuring that the radiant warmer is preheated prior to the birth, initiating skin-to-skin contact when possible, and placing a hat on the newborn's head. For infants born prior to 32 weeks, the use of a polyethylene bag/wrap and a thermal mattress is recommended.

[ABP 3.B.5. Late preterm infant]

REFERENCE

1. Engle WA, Tomashek KM, Wallman C; Committee on Fetus and Newborn, American Academy of Pediatrics. "Late-preterm" infants: a population at risk. *Pediatrics.* 2007;*120*(6):1390–1401.

4. ANSWER: D

Central lines in pediatric patients must be carefully chosen based on the purpose, duration of use, size of the patient, risks to the patient, and overall family needs. Given parenteral nutrition commonly calls for therapy with high osmolar content and high vesicant properties (e.g., calcium solution), and the patient will most likely need to be accessed daily for many weeks to months, the best central line option for her is a single-lumen tunneled catheter. Tunneled central access devices like a Broviac or Hickman can be secured with a cuff, decreasing infectious risk and securing the line for greater than 6 weeks. This is preferable to a PICC, which is not as secure and has a higher infection risk. A single-lumen catheter is preferred to a double lumen given the patient's relatively small size and need for only one infusion therapy. An implanted port is not the preferred choice given that a port is typically reserved for intermittent therapies like monthly chemotherapy instead of therapies that require daily intravenous access.

[ABP 5.K. Peripheral intravenous placement]

REFERENCE

1. Ullman AJ, Bernstein SJ, Brown E, et al. The Michigan Appropriateness Guide for Intravenous Catheters in Pediatrics: miniMAGIC. *Pediatrics*. 2020;*145*(suppl 3):S269–S284.

5. ANSWER: A

Breastfeeding has been associated with decreased length of stay as well as decreased need for pharmacological treatment for neonatal opioid withdrawal syndrome. While methadone and buprenorphine are excreted into human milk at low concentrations, this may actually decrease clinical signs of opioid withdrawal. As such, the Academy of Breastfeeding Medicine encourages breastfeeding for women who are engaged in substance abuse treatment and consent to discussing their progress with their treatment counselor, have not relapsed in more than 90 days prior to delivery, and do not have a medical contraindication to breastfeeding (e.g., HIV). Rates of breastfeeding initiation and duration among mothers with OUD are low, and infants may have difficulty latching due to withdrawal symptoms, so additional lactation support is needed for these mother-infant dyads.

REFERENCE

1. Patrick SW, Barfield WD, Poindexter BB; Committee on Fetus and Newborn, Committee on SUBSTANCE USE and Prevention. Neonatal opioid withdrawal syndrome. *Pediatrics*. 2020;*146*(5):e2020029074.

6. ANSWER: B

This patient's respiratory Gram stain shows gram-negative rods, which increases suspicion for *Pseudomonas aeruginosa* infection, as rates of *Pseudomonas* colonization are high among patients with tracheostomy. Because ceftriaxone does not adequately cover *Pseudomonas*, cefepime would be a more appropriate empiric antimicrobial. Children with tracheostomy dependence are at increased risk of tracheitis because of higher bacterial colonization and mucosal injury rates. This patient has had multiple hospitalizations and is at higher risk of antimicrobial-resistant organisms, including methicillin-resistant *Staphylococcus aureus* (MRSA). As such, it is reasonable to continue clindamycin to cover MRSA empirically while awaiting respiratory culture results. Regional MRSA susceptibility patterns may also be of benefit in selecting an empiric antibiotic regimen.

Atypical bacterial organisms, such as *Mycoplasma* species and *Mycobacterium tuberculosis*, are unlikely to be the causative organisms, so empiric azithromycin and isoniazid are not warranted in this case. Ampicillin does not provide adequate coverage for MRSA or *Pseudomonas*, and it does not cover common organisms such as *Haemophilus influenzae*, *Moraxella catarrhalis*, or anaerobic microorganisms. This patient's presentation warrants empiric antimicrobial treatment because of clinical symptoms of tracheitis and 2+ PMNs on Gram stain.

[ABP 4.C. Device and technology management, including complications]

REFERENCE

1. Brook I. Bacterial colonization, tracheobronchitis, and pneumonia following tracheostomy and long-term intubation in pediatric patients. *Chest*. 1979;*76*(4):420–424.

7. ANSWER: D

Developmentally normative aggressive behaviors are commonly seen at age 2–3 years. Physical aggression is most common at this age, while verbal aggression presents in older children and increases into adolescence. Aggressive behaviors are associated with physical and mental health problems in adulthood, including violent crime, domestic violence, suicide, and drug abuse. While there are syndromes associated with high levels of aggression such as cri-du-chat and fragile X syndrome, trisomy 21 is associated with low levels of aggression. Cognitive behavioral therapy is the mainstay of treatment for reducing aggression due to mental illness.

[ABP 2.B. Acute aggression and psychosis]

8. ANSWER: D

This full-term infant presents with hyperbilirubinemia. Being exclusively breastfed, having significant weight loss, and having an older sibling who required phototherapy are all risk factors for hyperbilirubinemia, but they are not risk factors for neurotoxicity. A TSB of 9 mg/dL at 30 hours of life in an infant born between 35 and 37$^{6}/_{7}$ weeks' gestation with hyperbilirubinemia risk factors indicates a high risk of hyperbilirubinemia, but the lack of neurotoxicity risk factors means that this infant is only at medium risk for neurotoxicity (based on gestational age). Although older guidelines provide the option to start phototherapy for TSB levels 2–3 mg/dL below the levels shown in the nomogram, more recent recommendations from Choosing Wisely suggest that the risk of kernicterus below published values is low, so phototherapy would not be indicated in this case. The fact that the TSB did not fall much during phototherapy is somewhat concerning, but the matching maternal and infant blood types and the negative DAT are reassuring that there is likely no significant ongoing hemolysis. Even if phototherapy had been indicated, barring low birth weight, suspected sepsis, and ongoing hemolysis, there is no indication to hold up discharge in order to check a rebound TSB. Supplementation may be helpful for infants with hyperbilirubinemia and concerns for dehydration, but this may be done with expressed breastmilk. There is no indication to counsel the mother to stop breastfeeding.

[ABP 3.B.2. Neonatal hyperbilirubinemia]

REFERENCES

1. American Academy of Pediatrics Subcommittee on Hyperbilirubinemia. Management of hyperbilirubinemia in the newborn infant 35 or more weeks of gestation. *Pediatrics.* 2004;*114*(1):297–316.
2. Mackara N. Choosing Wisely: Pediatric Hospital Medicine—SHM, AAP, APA. January 11, 2021. Accessed March 18, 2021. https://www.choosingwisely.org/societies/pediatric-hospital-medic ine-shm-aap-apa/.

9. ANSWER: A

In patients with ineffective swallow mechanics, excessive secretion of thin saliva, or sialorrhea, can cause harm. These medically complex patients with drooling are at increased risk of skin breakdown, aspiration of saliva, dehydration, and salivary pooling, which may interfere with noninvasive ventilation. Management of sialorrhea may include speech therapy focused on lip seal and swallow for those able to participate, suctioning, anticholinergic medication such as glycopyrrolate or scopolamine, salivary gland botulinum toxin injection, radiotherapy, and surgical intervention.

This patient was started on an anticholinergic medication. Common side effects of anticholinergic medications include parched mouth, increased intraocular pressure, constipation, urinary retention, orthostatic hypotension, decreased perspiration with increased body temperature, change in vision due to pupillary dilation and impaired accommodation, confusion, and sedation. A common mnemonic is "blind as a bat, mad as a hatter, red as a beet, hot as a hare, dry as a bone, the bowel and bladder lose their tone." Myelosuppression, bronchoconstriction, tendonitis, and hepatotoxicity are not commonly associated with the use of anticholinergic medications.

[ABP 4.D. Medication management]

REFERENCES

1. McGeachan AJ, Mcdermott CJ. Management of oral secretions in neurological disease. *Pract Neurol.* 2017;*17*(2):96–103.
2. Hull J, Aniapravan R, Chan E, et al. British Thoracic Society guideline for respiratory management of children with neuromuscular weakness. *Thorax.* 2012;*67*(suppl 1):i1–i40.

10. ANSWER: E

In 2012, the American Academy of Pediatrics updated the circumcision policy statement to recommend that the health benefits of newborn male circumcision outweigh the risks, and that the procedure's benefits justify access to this procedure for families who choose it. Specific benefits identified included prevention of UTIs. There is fair evidence from multiple studies that the UTI incidence among boys under age 2 years is reduced in circumcised boys compared with uncircumcised boys. The benefits of male circumcision are therefore likely to be greater in boys at higher risk of UTI, such as male infants with underlying anatomic defects such as reflux or hydronephrosis in this case. It is estimated that 7 to 14 of 1000 uncircumcised male infants will develop a UTI during the first year of life, compared to 1 to 2 infants among 1000 circumcised male infants. The estimated risk of UTIs in boys is about 1%, and the reduction of UTIs with circumcision is 10-fold in boys with urinary tract abnormalities compared with healthy circumcised neonates.

While bleeding is the most common risk of circumcision, neonates with urinary tract abnormalities are not at higher risk of bleeding than other infants. A circumcision does not need to be delayed or conducted by a urologist unless there are urethral abnormalities like hypospadias. A renal ultrasound should be completed for additional workup of the urinary tract abnormality, but it is not a prerequisite to complete a circumcision.

[ABP 5.O. Circumcision]

REFERENCE

1. Ellison JS, Dy GW, Fu BC, Holt SK, Gore JL, Merguerian PA. Neonatal circumcision and urinary tract infections in infants with hydronephrosis. *Pediatrics.* 2018;*142*(1):e20173703.

11. ANSWER: C

All newborns exposed to HIV are at risk for perinatal transmission and should be prescribed postnatal antiretroviral prophylaxis. The specific regimen is determined by the mother's viral load and ART history. Infants born to mothers with high viral loads or who were not treated with combination ART during pregnancy may require a three-drug regimen for 6 weeks. Conversely, term infants born to mothers who received ART and had documented viral suppression during pregnancy are at lower risk and may require only zidovudine (ZDV) for 4 weeks.

For infants exposed to HIV, HIV PCR testing should be performed, but this testing should not be done from cord blood due to a high risk of false-positive results. The mode of delivery is determined by the mother's viral load, but does not inform the infant's ART regimen. If the mother's viral load is greater than 1000 copies per milliliter, the infant should be delivered via planned cesarean section prior to rupture of membranes. If viral load is less than 1000 copies per milliliter, cesarean section solely for the prevention of transmission is not recommended. In the United States, maternal HIV infection is a contraindication to breastfeeding as there is a risk of transmission via breastmilk regardless of the viral load, though this risk is significantly decreased with maternal ART. Maternal hepatitis C serologies do not determine the infant's ART regimen.

[ABP 3.B.4. Neonatal infections, including exposure]

REFERENCE

1. Chadwick EG, Ezeanolue EE; Committee on Pediatric AIDS. Evaluation and management of the infant exposed to HIV in the United States. *Pediatrics*. 2020;*146*(5):e2020029058.

12. ANSWER: D

Conduct disorder is associated with a number of comorbidities, including ODD, learning disabilities, depression, and attention-deficit/hyperactivity disorder. Oppositional defiant disorder is diagnosed in children under 8 years of age and is a common antecedent to CD. Conduct order is defined as a repetitive and persistent pattern of behavior in which the basic rights of others or major age-appropriate social rules are violated. Onset before 10 years of age is known as childhood-onset type and carries a worse prognosis. A diagnosis of conduct disorder would put this child at high risk for antisocial personality disorder as an adult. To make a diagnosis of CD, there must be three or more incidents within the last 12 months or at least one in the last 6 months.

[ABP 2.B. Acute aggression and psychosis]

13. ANSWER: C

Neonatal Resuscitation Program guidelines suggest that all births should be attended by at least one person whose only responsibility is for management of the newborn. This person should be skilled in the initial steps of newborn care and positive pressure ventilation. If a risk factor such as meconium-stained amniotic fluid is present, then one additional dedicated qualified person should attend the delivery. There are many other risk factors that increase the likelihood that a newborn will need resuscitation, such as prematurity, maternal preeclampsia or eclampsia, intrauterine growth restriction, emergency cesarean section, breech or other abnormal fetal presentation, or chorioamnionitis. For all deliveries, a team that includes people with full resuscitation skills, including endotracheal intubation, emergency vascular access, and medication administration, should be immediately available in case steps beyond initial resuscitation are needed.

[ABP 3.A. Delivery room care, including resuscitation and stabilization]

REFERENCE

1. Weiner GM, Zaichkin J. *Textbook of Neonatal Resuscitation (NRP)*. 7th ed. American Academy of Pediatrics and American Heart Association; 2016.

14. ANSWER: D

Cough supports airway clearance and expels secretions, which may otherwise worsen airway obstruction and inflammation. Patients with poor lung compliance, hypoventilation from intercostal or diaphragmatic weakness, bulbar muscle weakness, bronchial obstruction, chest wall deformity, and reduced lung parenchyma may have an ineffective cough. This patient has evidence of weak cough on physical examination, and parents report that his ability to clear secretions is impaired. Therefore, this patient would benefit from MIE for airway clearance, also known as "cough assist." MIE can be administered noninvasively via a face mask or mouthpiece or invasively via tracheostomy in children above 3 months of age.

Guaifenesin may reduce bronchial sputum surface tension and stimulate the cholinergic pathway, but its clinical efficacy has not been supported in randomized controlled trials. Nebulized hypertonic saline may increase ciliary motility and mucus liquefaction. The medication may also cause mucosal irritation and induce cough, but this may be of limited benefit in this patient with continuous coughing and ineffective cough mechanics. Therapeutic bronchoscopy is an invasive procedure and is not indicated in this patient. Morphine may be considered for palliative relief of "air hunger" during end-of-life care and would not be indicated for this patient.

[ABP 4.C. Device and technology management, including complications]

REFERENCE

1. Volsko TA. Airway clearance therapy: finding the evidence. *Respir Care*. 2013;58(10):1669–1678.

15. ANSWER: A

Complex regional pain syndrome (CRPS) is a chronic neurologic condition resulting from a traumatic insult. Being female, having sustained an upper extremity injury, and having suffered high-energy trauma all place an individual at increased risk for developing this disorder. It commonly presents with allodynia, hyperalgesia, skin temperature changes, and edema. When making the diagnosis of a somatic symptom disorder such as CRPS, five basic tenets should be followed: (1) explain what the patient has based on symptom presentation; (2) tell the patient what they do *not* have based on diagnoses of exclusion; (3) show belief in the patient's symptoms and disability; (4) explain how common somatic symptoms are; and (5) talk about effective treatments. A family meeting provides an ideal setting to meet these five tenets of sharing a somatic symptom disorder diagnosis. Reassuring the family that there is not an organic disease process only partially addresses aspects of making the diagnosis that should be discussed with the patient and family. Stating the patient's symptoms are all psychosomatic would be counterproductive. Electromyography has shown distinct types of myoclonus in patients with CRPS, but this test has very limited sensitivity and is unlikely to be helpful in this case. Data on the benefit of corticosteroids in patients with CRPS is equivocal. The best next step in management for a somatic symptom disorder, prior to initiating a treatment plan, is the appropriate delivery of a diagnosis.

[ABP 2.D. Psychosomatic disorders]

16. ANSWER: C

The Neonatal Resuscitation Program has guidelines that list target oxygen saturations by minute of life. Normal fetal oxygen saturation is approximately 60%, and this rises to over 90% by 10 minutes of life. This infant's oxygen saturations are within the normal ranges for age. The normal physiologic changes that occur after birth include pulmonary vasodilation caused by increased blood oxygen levels after the first breaths, which results in a fall in pulmonary vascular resistance. The resulting increase in pulmonary blood flow increases oxygen delivery throughout the newborn's body.

While pulse oximetry may not function if the infant has a low heart rate or poor perfusion, it is a useful tool to guide oxygen administration during a resuscitation. The mechanisms by which fetal lung fluid is cleared are complex, but they include sodium transport across alveolar epithelium (and subsequent fluid shifts) and elevated intrapulmonary pressure with the first breaths that drives alveolar fluid into the interstitium. A cesarean section without preceding labor is a risk factor for impaired clearance of fetal lung fluid as the physiologic mechanisms for resorption may not have begun. However, the physical squeezing of the infant's thorax during passage through the birth canal is thought to play a very minor role, so the mode of delivery after 24 hours of labor should not cause significant impairment in fluid clearance.

[ABP 3.A. Delivery room care, including resuscitation and stabilization]

REFERENCES

1. Weiner GM, Zaichkin J. *Textbook of Neonatal Resuscitation (NRP)*. 7th ed. American Academy of Pediatrics and American Heart Association. 2016.
2. Swanson JR, Sinkin RA. Transition from fetus to newborn. *Pediatr Clin North Am*. 2015;62(2):329–343.

17. ANSWER: E

Physicians may worry that discussing advanced care plans with parents may shift the focus of care away from clinical management. However, research suggests that parents appreciate open discussion and shared decision-making. When possible, these conversations can start and continue while the child is in a stable care phase. Avoidance of advanced care planning may lead to parental distrust and resentment. Shared decision-making should involve the child when possible, depending on their cognitive state and developmental stage. When possible, the physician should not make unilateral decisions.

Advanced care plans reflect the patient's and family's goals, values, and beliefs. The plan may include information on oxygen administration, airway clearance, time-limited bag valve mask ventilation, ideal location of death, and artificially administered nutrition. Physicians can guide parents by discussing what can be done during a crisis, rather than focusing solely on care limitations. For many families, the preferred location of death is the home. The home setting benefits may include privacy, less perceived judgment, and more opportunities to address spiritual or cultural needs.

[ABP 4.F. Palliative and end-of-life care]

REFERENCES

1. Duc JK, Herbert AR, Heussler HS. Paediatric palliative care and intellectual disability—a unique context. *J Appl Res Intellect Disabil*. 2017;30(6):1111–1124.
2. Fraser J, Harris N, Berringer AJ, Prescott H, Finlay F. Advanced care planning in children with life-limiting conditions—the Wishes Document. *Arch Dis Child*. 2010;95(2):79–82.

18. ANSWER: D

Peristomal leakage is a common G-tube complication. Risk factors that can contribute to leakage include infection, gastric hypersecretion, excessive cleaning with hydrogen peroxide, buried bumper syndrome (when the internal bumper of the tube erodes into the gastric wall), torsion on the tube, and lack of bolster (Figure 2.4) to stabilize the tube. Initial treatments, including optimizing nutrition and medical status, barrier creams, and skin protectants, were already completed in this patient. The best answer is to allow the tract to partially close, removing the G-tube for a few days, and placing a new tube along the same tract. A larger diameter tube could cause the tract to enlarge and exacerbate the leakage. Hyperinflating the interior balloon would temporarily stabilize the tube but could break the interior balloon. Surgically replacing the G-tube would be the next step if all other measures failed to improve the patient's symptoms.

[ABP 5.E. Gastric tube replacement/change]

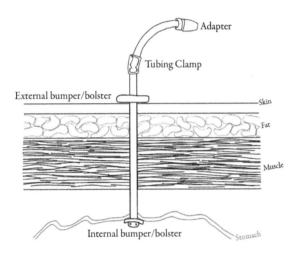

Figure 2.4 Clinical pathway to manage failed tracheostomy tube change. Figure reprinted with permission from Reference 1.

REFERENCE

1. Schrag SP, Sharma R, Jaik NP, et al. Complications related to percutaneous endoscopic gastrostomy (PEG) tubes. A comprehensive clinical review. *J Gastrointestin Liver Dis.* 2007;*16*(4):407–418.

19. ANSWER: A

A full assessment should be undertaken for patients who present with high risk factors for suicidality. Suicide of a close family member puts a child at increased risk for suicide. Suicide attempts are more common in girls than in boys. It is untrue that talking to children about suicide will increase their risk. Easy access to support services can reduce a child's risk. Denial of suicidal thoughts or behavior does not indicate a decreased risk of committing suicide.

[ABP 2.A. Self-harm/suicidality]

20. ANSWER: A

This newborn's clinical presentation is consistent with a brachial plexus injury. Neonatal brachial plexus injuries occur in 0.5 to 3 out of 1000 live births. Clinical presentations can range from Erb palsy with the affected arm weak, extended at the elbow, and internally rotated, to Horner syndrome if the sympathetic nerve roots are involved, to respiratory distress due to hemidiaphragmatic paralysis. Erb palsy should be distinguished from the much less common Klumpke palsy, which is an isolated hand paralysis caused by damage to only the lower nerve roots of C8 and T1. The degree and severity of palsy depend on which nerve roots are involved and how badly they have been damaged. Despite the historical teaching that "all neonatal brachial plexus palsy recovers," studies have found persistent deficits in 20%–30% of cases. Neonatal brachial plexus injury is generally a clinical diagnosis. MRI and EMG are technically difficult in newborns, and they do not reliably predict recovery or the need for surgical repair. The mainstay of initial treatment is occupational therapy referral to maintain range of motion and begin therapeutic exercise. Otherwise-well newborns with brachial plexus injuries should be observed for recovery for up to 1 month. Those who have not regained normal function by 1 month should then be referred for surgical evaluation at a subspecialty center.

[ABP 3.B.7. Birth trauma]

REFERENCE

1. Smith BW, Daunter AK, Yang LJ, Wilson TJ. An update on the management of neonatal brachial plexus palsy-replacing old paradigms: a review. *JAMA Pediatr.* 2018;*172*(6):585–591.

21. ANSWER: C

Children with medical complexity are at higher risk for micronutrient deficiency. This patient with autism and a restricted diet has hypovitaminosis C with consequent impairment of collagen synthesis. Manifestations of nutritional deficiencies are summarized in Table 2.2. In addition to looking for these symptoms, a nutrition-focused physical examination may include assessing fat stores, particularly in the face, arms, chest, and buttocks. Clinicians may assess muscle wasting due to protein-calorie malnutrition in the temple, clavicle, thigh, and calf.

Table 2.2 PRESENTING SIGNS AND SYMPTOMS OF MICRONUTRIENT DEFICIENCIES

MICRONUTRIENT	SYMPTOMS OF DEFICIENCY
Vitamin A	Corkscrew hair, follicular hyperkeratosis, and Bitot spots (buildup of keratin in the conjunctiva)
Vitamin C	Poor wound healing; corkscrew hair; gingival swelling; ecchymosis; hyperkeratosis; koilonychia (flat, thin nails often with concavity); hemarthrosis; bony lesions or brittle bones; ocular hemorrhages; perifollicular hemorrhages (particularly in the lower extremities)
Zinc	Alopecia and dermatitis, particularly affecting the perineum, chin, cheeks, and acral surfaces
Copper	Kinked hair, skin depigmentation, myelopathy presenting as sensory ataxia
Iron	Pallor, onychomadesis (periodic shedding of the nails), and koilonychia

[ABP 4.B. Feeding and nutrition]

REFERENCE

1. Foster BA, Lane JE, Massey E, Noelck M, Green S, Austin JP. The impact of malnutrition on hospitalized children with cerebral palsy. *Hosp Pediatr.* 2020;*10*(12):1087–1095.

22. ANSWER: B

Early-onset sepsis can have significant morbidity and mortality if not properly detected. The American Academy of Pediatrics guidelines currently describe three reasonable approaches for identifying infants at risk of early-onset sepsis (EOS): (1) categorical risk algorithms, (2) multivariate risk assessments (evidence-based sepsis calculators), and (3) enhanced observation protocols. With increasing data showing that evidence-based sepsis calculators lead to significant reductions in antibiotic use without a concomitant increase in EOS, there is a push to adopt this strategy universally. One of the main risk factors for EOS is GBS colonization without adequate treatment, which is defined as one dose of a penicillin or cephalosporin given at least 4 hours prior to delivery. Even if an isolate is known to be susceptible to clindamycin or vancomycin, they are not considered adequate treatment due to differences in pharmacokinetic profiles. When administered during labor, the penicillins and cephalosporins cross the placenta and are excreted by the fetal kidneys into the amniotic fluid more rapidly and efficiently than clindamycin or vancomycin. Prolonged rupture of membranes for more than 18 hours

is also a risk factor for EOS. Intrapartum maternal fever is a risk factor, but this mother's fever occurred postpartum. Multiple studies have shown that WBC and CRP levels are poor indicators of EOS.

[ABP 3.B.4. Neonatal infections, including exposures]

REFERENCE

1. Puopolo KM, Benitz WE, Zaoutis TE; Committee on Fetus and Newborn; Committee on Infectious Diseases. Management of neonates born at ≥35 0/7 weeks' gestation with suspected or proven early-onset bacterial sepsis. *Pediatrics.* 2018;*142*(6):e20182894.

23. ANSWER: C

This patient's presentation is consistent with a diagnosis of abdominal migraines. Rome IV diagnostic criteria for abdominal migraine must include all of the following occurring at least twice within 6 consecutive months: (1) paroxysmal episodes of intense, acute periumbilical, midline, or diffuse abdominal pain lasting 1 hour or more; (2) episodes that are separated by weeks to months; (3) pain that is incapacitating and interferes with normal activities; (4) stereotypical pattern and symptoms in the individual patient; (5) pain that is associated with two or more of the following: anorexia, nausea, vomiting, headache, photophobia, or pallor; (6) symptoms that cannot be fully explained by another medical condition after a complete evaluation.

Recovery from any functional disorder involves three concurrent treatment modalities: (1) physical activity, (2) cognitive behavioral therapy, and (3) supportive medical oversight. Referrals to outpatient CBT and gastroenterology each address only one aspect of recovery and are therefore not the best answer choices. Prescribing an antiemetic or providing a note excusing the patient from school will only provide temporary relief of symptoms and does not connect the patient with ongoing follow-up and therapy required for successful recovery.

[ABP 2.D. Psychosomatic disorders]

REFERENCE

1. Simren M, Palsson OS, Whitehead WE. Update on Rome IV criteria for colorectal disorders: implications for clinical practice. *Curr Gastroenterol Rep.* 2017;*19*(4):15.

24. ANSWER: A

Newborns typically lose weight in their first days of life. Infants are born relatively fluid overloaded, and they may have minimal early fluid and calorie intake; they lose weight initially as they diurese, and then they begin gaining weight once their intake increases—typically at 3–5 days of life. Infants born by caesarian section often have higher birth weights and greater early weight loss, likely due to large volumes of intravenous fluids given to mothers during delivery, and exclusively breastfed infants have particularly low intake until their mothers' milk supply is well established.

In one large study, at 48 hours of age, 5% of vaginally delivered newborns and 10% of infants delivered by caesarian had lost more than 10% of their birth weight. This degree of weight loss is therefore not abnormal or pathological, and it is not an explicit indication to begin formula supplementation. The infant's normal urine output is a reassuring sign of adequate oral intake. If the infant is latching well and swallowing easily, there is no indication for a feeding evaluation. An infant who is otherwise well and not hypoglycemic does not require workup for metabolic abnormalities. There is no reason to suspect that the weight measurements are inaccurate.

[ABP 3.B.9. Newborn feeding (including breastfeeding and formula feeding)]

REFERENCES

1. Flaherman VJ, Schaefer EW, Kuzniewicz MW, Li SX, Walsh EM, Paul IM. Early weight loss nomograms for exclusively breastfed newborns. *Pediatrics.* 2015;*135*(1):e16–e23.
2. Noel-Weiss J, Woodend AK, Peterson WE, Gibb W, Groll DL. An observational study of associations among maternal fluids during parturition, neonatal output, and breastfed newborn weight loss. *Int Breastfeed J.* 2011;*6*:9.

25. ANSWER: B

With shunted hydrocephalus, emesis, fatigue, and two components of Cushing triad satisfied, including bradycardia and hypertension, this patient's presentation is highly suggestive of intracranial hypertension and VPS failure even though the head CT showed no ventriculomegaly. Head CT alone, with a 53%–92% sensitivity in detecting shunt failure, cannot definitively rule out shunt malfunction when other clinical signs of shunt failure are present. It is reasonable to interrogate the shunt at this time via shunt tap to assess for obstruction. In cases in which impending herniation is suspected, emergency measures to reduce intracranial pressure may include intubation and hyperventilation, hypertonic saline, mannitol, or surgical decompression. Mechanisms for shunt pathology include intracranial infection, shunt tip migration, shunt fracture, increased intra-abdominal pressure from constipation, abdominal pseudocyst, catheter allergy, and erosion through the intestinal wall.

With stable urine output and moist mucous membranes in a child with suspected intracranial hypertension,

administration of intravenous fluid or oral rehydration solution is not the most urgent or appropriate next step. Similarly, with stable peripheral perfusion, hypertension, and sinus bradycardia on electrocardiogram, this patient's sleepiness and reflex bradycardia are likely secondary to intracranial hypertension rather than poor cerebral perfusion from a primary cardiac etiology. Cardiac pacing is not indicated. This patient's emesis is unlikely related to gastritis from *Helicobacter pylori* infection.

[ABP 4.C. Device and technology management, including complications]

REFERENCES

1. Boyle TP, Nigrovic LE. Radiographic evaluation of pediatric cerebrospinal fluid shunt malfunction in the emergency setting. *Pediatr Emerg Care.* 2015;*31*(6):435–443.
2. Hanak BW, Bonow RH, Harris CA, Browd SR. Cerebrospinal fluid shunting complications in children. *Pediatr Neurosurg.* 2017;*52*(6):381–400.

26. ANSWER: B

Intraosseous access is an option when standard venous access is not easily obtained in the hospital setting. Complications after successful intraosseous infusions are rare, with an incidence of less than 1%. Bone injury, deformity, or growth arrest due to disruption of the growth plate is an extremely rare complication. The most common complication is extravasation of blood, fluids, and drugs into the soft tissue, which on occasion leads to compartment syndrome. Other possible complications include air embolism, fat embolism, soft tissue infection, and osteomyelitis. Of note, intraosseous needles should not be placed in a long bone with a fracture or in patients with fragile bones due to conditions such as osteogenesis imperfecta or osteoporosis.

[ABP 5.B. Intraosseous access placement]

REFERENCE

1. Luck RP, Haines C, Mull CC. Intraosseous access. *J Emerg Med.* 2010;*39*(4):468–475.

27. ANSWER: A

Glucose crosses the placenta freely, so fetal glucose homeostasis is maintained by a combination of both fetal and maternal metabolic mechanisms. After delivery, the newborn must transition to maintain euglycemia independently. During this transition, plasma glucose concentrations may fall as low as 30 mg/dL, but most newborns remain asymptomatic and tolerate this transient "physiologic hypoglycemia" well. Newborns rely primarily on ketogenesis and gluconeogenesis until adequate calorie intake is established. Exclusively breastfed infants commonly receive lower caloric intake for a longer period than infants who are formula fed from birth, but this does not commonly result in significant or symptomatic hypoglycemia.

Newborns who are predisposed to insufficient ketogenesis and/or gluconeogenesis are at highest risk for developing symptomatic hypoglycemia requiring treatment. LPT and SGA infants may not have sufficient fat stores to provide an adequate substrate for ketogenesis and gluconeogenesis. Infants of diabetic mothers—whether due to preexisting diabetes or gestational diabetes—are often born with elevated insulin levels due to recurrent or chronic hyperglycemia in utero. These elevated insulin levels suppress ketogenesis and gluconeogenesis, which can predispose these infants to hypoglycemia. Infants born LGA may also be at risk of hypoglycemia as a consequence of in utero hyperglycemia due to unrecognized maternal diabetes or prediabetes, and/or they may have inadequate fat stores relative to their large lean body mass.

[ABP 3.B.1. Neonatal hypoglycemia]

REFERENCE

1. Committee on Fetus and Newborn, Adamkin DH. Postnatal glucose homeostasis in late-preterm and term infants. *Pediatrics*. 2011;*127*(3):575–579.

28. ANSWER: D

Ancillary services, including physical therapy, can be vital in preparing patients and families for safe disposition. In conjunction with the physical medicine and rehabilitation team, physical therapists may educate families on safe transfers within precautions, provide wheelchair measurements and modifications, and recommend durable medical equipment.

This patient postoperatively requires acute rehabilitation therapy, but she cannot yet participate in intensive inpatient therapy. She may benefit from inpatient rehabilitation to improve her strength and mobility once her weight-bearing precautions are lifted. Patients younger than 4 years of age require vehicular restraints when traveling home from the hospital (Table 2.3); a restraint is not necessary for a patient of this age and size. Given the high risk of spasticity and pain, it would be inappropriate to discontinue oxycodone and diazepam at this time. Bivalving a cast involves splitting the cast along both sides to allow for expansion and soft tissue swelling. This patient does not have significant lower extremity swelling.

Table 2.3 AMERICAN ACADEMY OF PEDIATRICS TRANSPORTATION GUIDELINES FOR PEDIATRIC PATIENTS IN SPICA CASTS[a]

Infants weighing up to 9.0 kg (20 lb)	Rear-facing, modified convertible car safety seat with cut-away sides and bottom (i.e., Spelcast by SnugSeat Inc.)
Toddlers weighing up to 18.0 kg (40 lb)	Front-facing, modified convertible car safety seat with cut-away sides and bottom (i.e., Spelcast by SnugSeat Inc.)
Older children weighing up to 47.2 kg (105 lb)	Modified vest system that secures the child's side against the vehicle seat (i.e., EZ-ON vest)
When not possible to fit child on a vehicle seat	Use of ambulance for transport

[a] Adapted from Reference 1.

[ABP 4.E. Care coordination]

REFERENCE

1. Gockley A, Hennrikus W, Lavin ST, Rzucidlo S, Rieghard C. Transportation of children in spica casts in the USA. *J Pediatr Orthop B*. 2015;*24*(4):277–280.

29. ANSWER: A

Compartment syndrome is a rare complication of IO access, primarily thought to be due to extravasation of fluid into the muscular compartments. The potential causes for this extravasation include incomplete penetration of the cortex, penetration of the needle through the posterior aspect of the cortex, extravasation through a previous IO puncture site, and extravasation through the nutrient vessel. To prevent extravasation, precautionary measures include using a fresh, large-bore needle, avoiding multiple breaches of the cortex, and confirming free flow of the fluid. Plain radiographs can also be used to confirm correct positioning of the needle. Other recommendations include securing the cannula properly, close monitoring, frequent neurovascular examinations, and serial measurement of the circumference of the extremity at the level of the IO site. IO sites should not be used for more than 24 hours, and alternative venous access should be obtained shortly after initial stabilization. Answer B is not a reported complication of IO access. The other choices are potential complications of IO access in general, but they are not related to the complication of compartment syndrome with IO access.

[ABP 5.B. Intraosseous access placement]

REFERENCE

1. Atanda A Jr, Statter MB. Compartment syndrome of the leg after intraosseous infusion: guidelines for prevention, early detection, and treatment. *Am J Orthop (Belle Mead NJ)*. 2008;*37*(12):E198–E200.

30. ANSWER: C

The infant in the vignette has signs consistent with a subgaleal hemorrhage. Prompt recognition of this diagnosis is imperative given the potential for significant blood loss into the subgaleal space and subsequent hypovolemia, consumptive coagulopathy, and shock. Infants with concerns for subgaleal hemorrhage should be closely monitored in a NICU setting.

The most important risk factor for subgaleal hemorrhage is operative vaginal delivery, particularly vacuum extraction. The incidence in noninstrumented deliveries is approximately 4 per 10,000 and as high as 64 per 10,000 in vacuum-assisted deliveries. Other associated risk factors include coagulopathy, prematurity, macrosomia, precipitous labor, male sex, prolonged labor, and cephalopelvic disproportion.

[ABP 3.B.7. Birth trauma]

REFERENCE

1. Prazad PA, Rajpal MN, Mangurten HH, Puppala BL. Birth injuries. In: Richard J Martin, Avroy A Fanaroff, Michele C Walsh (Eds.), *Fanaroff and Martin's Neonatal-Perinatal Medicine*. 11th ed. Elsevier; 2020:458–488.

31. ANSWER: E

With superficial destruction of the epidermis, this wound can be classified as stage II. Stage I wounds are characterized by nonblanchable erythema with intact skin, stage III wounds are characterized by full-thickness tissue loss and possible exposure of subcutaneous fatty tissue, and stage IV is characterized by exposed tendon, fascia, ligament, cartilage, or muscle. With all wounds, patients require frequent repositioning, pressure reduction surfaces, and adequate nutritional intake of zinc, vitamin C, iron, vitamin A, and protein.

Wound care for stage II wounds involves debridement and wound cleansing using sterile water or normal saline. Some wounds require autolytic debridement. This process involves using the body's endogenous enzymes to rehydrate and soften any eschar or slough, typically using a moisture-retentive dressing covered by an occlusive dressing that absorbs the exudate produced. Surgical debridement may be required if autolytic debridement is unsuccessful. If these interventions fail, adjunct therapies may include negative pressure wound therapy or reconstructive surgery with skin grafting or skin flap. Topical or systemic antimicrobials may be clinically indicated if there is a concern for active wound infection or surrounding cellulitis, which is not the case with this patient.

[ABP 4.A. Symptom management]

REFERENCES

1. Freundlich K. Pressure injuries in medically complex children: a review. *Children (Basel)*. 2017;*4*(4):25.
2. Stansby G, Avital L, Jones K, Marsden G; Guideline Development Group. Prevention and management of pressure ulcers in primary and secondary care: summary of NICE guidance. *BMJ*. 2014;*348*:g2592.

32. ANSWER: A

"Medical misconnection," defined as an attempt to connect two incompatible systems, has led to life-threatening events, such as sepsis and emboli. A review from 2000 to 2006 of the United States Pharmacopeia Medication Errors Reporting Program found 24 incidents in which an enteral feeding formula or other medication intended for the feeding tube was administered via the wrong route. Of those 24 incidents, eight resulted in sentinel events, including permanent injury, life-threatening situation, and/or death. Many of these cases resulted from using an intravenous syringe to dispense, prepare, and administer enteral medication and inadvertently attaching the syringe to the IV system, resulting in a medication being administered via the wrong route. Risk factors for misconnection in this case include rotating shift work, inadequate lighting, moving patients from one hospital system to another, and multiple medications and solutions needing to be administered simultaneously. Some strategies to decrease the risk of medical misconnection include ensuring that all connections are made under proper lighting conditions, avoiding modifications or adaptations to feeding devices, allowing only users knowledgeable about the use of the device to set up the connection, and labeling connectors. The other answers in this question stem can be completed after accuracy of connections is confirmed first.

[ABP 4.C. Device and technology management, including complications, ABP 8.F. Patient safety regulations]

REFERENCE

1. Miller SJ. Enteral feeding misconnections: a consortium position statement. *Nutr Clin Pract*. 2008;*23*(6):664–665.

33. ANSWER: D

The strongest predictor of GBS early-onset disease is maternal GBS colonization. However, GBS infection can occur even when the mother has screened negative for GBS because maternal colonization can be intermittent and because of the possibility of false-negative screening tests. Late-onset GBS infection can also be caused by horizontal transmission from other caregivers. Therefore, negative GBS screening does not rule out the possibility of early- or late-onset GBS disease.

The vignette describes a scenario consistent with suspected intra-amniotic bacterial infection (a single maternal intrapartum temperature of 39.0°C or greater or a temperature of 38.0°C to 38.9°C plus maternal leukocytosis, purulent cervical drainage, or fetal tachycardia), and the American College of Obstetricians and Gynecologists recommends consideration of intrapartum antibiotic therapy in this situation. The use of intrapartum antibiotics decreases but does not eliminate the risk of early-onset sepsis. The presence of intra-amniotic infection increases the infant's risk for early-onset sepsis, but this does not mean that neonatal infection will definitely occur.

[ABP 3.B.4. Neonatal infections, including exposures]

REFERENCE

1. Puopolo KM, Lynfield R, Cummings JJ; American Academy of Pediatrics, Committee on Fetus and Newborn, Committee on Infectious Diseases. Management of infants at risk for group B streptococcal disease. *Pediatrics*. 2019;*144*(2):e20191881.

34. ANSWER: D

This patient's acute food refusal is an indication for hospitalization. While her heart rate is low, a patient with an eating disorder and a resting heart rate greater than 50 beats per minute while awake does not require admission for medical stabilization. Her BMI is also low but is not less than 75% of her estimated median BMI ([15 kg/m²]/ [19 kg/m²] = 79%). Although her mother is concerned for poor weight gain, her daughter is showing some progress; the information provided in the vignette does not support hospitalization for failed outpatient management, although a direct conversation with her outpatient provider would be helpful.

Care of children hospitalized for eating disorders requires a multidisciplinary approach. Treating their disorder often requires long-term care in residential facilities. Children may require admission for medical stabilization, although clear criteria should be applied to prevent interruption of outpatient treatment or a delay in transfer to an appropriate treatment center. Box 2.1 outlines indications for admission. While close monitoring for the many medical complications associated with eating disorders is necessary, appropriate multidisciplinary treatment of the psychological and behavioral issues underpinning these diseases is also critical.

[ABP 2.F. Eating disorders]

> *Box 2.1* INDICATIONS FOR HOSPITALIZATION OF ADOLESCENTS WITH EATING DISORDERS[a]
>
> Less than or equal to 75% of estimated median BMI (Patient BMI/50th Percentile BMI for Age and Sex)
>
> Dehydration
>
> Abnormal electrolytes (low potassium, sodium, or phosphorus)
>
> Abnormal electrocardiogram (ECG) (e.g., prolonged QTc)
>
> Physiologic instability:
> Heart rate <50 beats per minute while awake, <45 beats per minute while asleep
>
> Blood pressure <90/45 mm Hg
>
> Temperature <96°F (35.6°C)
>
> Orthostasis (heart rate increase [>20 beats per minute] or blood pressure decrease [>20 mm Hg systolic or >10 mm Hg diastolic])
>
> Arrested growth, development
>
> Failure of outpatient management
>
> Acute food refusal
>
> Uncontrollable binge eating and purging
>
> Acute medical complications of malnutrition (e.g., syncope)
>
> Comorbid psychiatric or medical condition that interrupts outpatient treatment (e.g., severe depression, type 1 diabetes mellitus)
>
> [a] Adapted from Reference 1.

REFERENCE

1. Hornberger LL, Lane MA, American Academy of Pediatrics Committee on Adolescence. Identification and management of eating disorders in children and adolescents. *Pediatrics*. 2021; *147*(1):e2020040279

35. ANSWER: B

Many patients with Down syndrome are now diagnosed prenatally, with reports of detection rates as high as 95% using the combined first-trimester screening (nuchal translucency + maternal serum levels of free β-human chorionic gonadotropin and pregnancy-associated plasma protein A). Cell-free fetal DNA testing in maternal blood is also becoming increasingly available and has excellent sensitivity and specificity. If the diagnosis was confirmed prenatally with chromosome studies, a copy of the results should be placed in the chart. If not prenatally diagnosed, cytogenetic analysis should be done postnatally.

Children with Down syndrome have approximately a 50% risk of congenital heart defects, so an echocardiogram is recommended even if a fetal echocardiogram was performed. While duodenal atresia or anorectal atresia/stenosis are associated with trisomy 21, radiologic evaluation is not indicated unless there are suggestive findings on history and physical examination. Feeding problems are common, and infants who have significant hypotonia or signs of poor feeding should be referred for radiographic swallowing assessments. Assessment of red reflex is important to assess for cataracts, and ophthalmologic evaluation should be done yearly, but a dilated examination is not needed in the newborn period if there are no abnormalities noted. Atlantoaxial instability is an important problem for physicians and parents to be aware of, but routine radiologic evaluation is not recommended.

[ABP 3.B.8. Congenital anomalies, ABP 3.B.9. Newborn feeding (including breastfeeding and formula feeding)]

REFERENCE

1. Bull MJ; Committee on Genetics. Health supervision for children with Down syndrome. *Pediatrics.* 2011;*128*(2):393–406.

36. ANSWER: A

Patients with severe reflux, risk of aspiration, gastroparesis, or gastric outlet obstruction often benefit from postpyloric feeds. This patient with a suspected genetic disorder and oromotor dysphagia would likely benefit from a more permanent enteral feeding tube rather than a nasojejunal tube. Although gastric feeds do not cause reflux, they may worsen reflux symptoms in children with frank or subclinical reflux. This patient with clinically apparent gastroesophageal reflux disease, dysphagia, and symptoms concerning for aspiration pneumonitis would likely not tolerate gastrostomy tube feeds.

Because this patient has gained weight with appropriate enteral nutrition and will likely require long-term nutritional support, parenteral nutrition is not ideal. Long-term use of parenteral nutrition may be associated with cholestasis with biliary sludging and steatosis, nephropathy, metabolic bone disease, increased risk of insulin resistance, and, if administered through a central line, central line–associated bloodstream infection or thrombosis.

[ABP 4.B. Feeding and nutrition]

REFERENCES

1. Fortunato JE, Darbari A, Mitchell SE, Thompson RE, Cuffari C. The limitations of gastro-jejunal (G-J) feeding tubes in children: a 9-year pediatric hospital database analysis. *Am J Gastroenterol.* 2005;*100*(1):186–189.
2. DeRaddo JS, Skummer P, Rivera M, Kobayashi K. Conversion to gastrojejunostomy tubes in developmentally disabled children intolerant to gastrostomy tube feeding. *J Pediatr Gastroenterol Nutr.* 2019;*69*(3):e75–e78.

37. ANSWER: B

The most common complication of NGT placement is incorrect insertion of the NGT into the lung. The most common sequela of this is pneumothorax, followed by pleural effusion and aspiration events. Pneumonia is also associated with pulmonary insertion of the tube. Other adverse events include perforation of the nasopharynx and anterior carotid artery or internal jugular vein puncture due to the distal tip crossing the parotid gland. Other described adverse events include vocal cord paralysis, laryngeal harm, and very rarely fatal massive hemorrhage. Pneumomediastinum is not a documented adverse event of NGT placement. Nasal mucosal abrasion is likely the source of this patient's epistaxis but is unlikely to cause persistent coughing. Nasal septum erosion occurs with long-term NGT placement.

Insertion length is conventionally determined by the nose-ear-midxiphoid-umbilicus (NEMU) distance. To confirm placement of the feeding tube, radiography is the most accurate method and is typically recommended when a tube is used for the first time. The auscultatory method to predict tube location is unreliable and should not be the sole method used to check placement. Placement can also be confirmed with pH testing of NGT aspirate; pH under 5.0 indicates gastric placement. Visual confirmation of fluid aspiration is unreliable in differentiating gastric, pleural, and tracheobronchial fluid.

[ABP 5.D. Nasogastric tube placement]

REFERENCE

1. Motta APG, Rigobello MCG, Silveira RCCP, Gimenes FRE. Nasogastric/nasoenteric tube-related adverse events: an integrative review. *Rev Lat Am Enfermagem.* 2021;*29*:e3400.

38. ANSWER: D

Oppositional defiant disorder (ODD) is characterized by defiant, disobedient behaviors toward authority figures. Diagnosis requires weekly episodes for 6 months in children over 5 years of age or episodes on most days for 6 months in children under 5 years of age. Symptoms typically present before 8 years of age and are rare in adolescence. Prior to puberty, ODD is more common in boys, but there is less gender disparity after puberty. Antisocial behaviors are more commonly associated with conduct disorder than with ODD. Cognitive behavioral therapy and parent training are the most effective management strategies. Medication should be reserved for cases in which these interventions alone are insufficient.

[ABP 2.E. Behavioral and developmental disorders]

39. ANSWER: C

This newborn likely has a congenital diaphragmatic hernia (CDH). A CDH is defined by a defect in the diaphragm that allows abdominal contents to protrude into the thoracic cavity and compress the ipsilateral lung. During fetal development, this causes pulmonary hypoplasia, which can also lead to pulmonary hypertension. A large diaphragmatic defect prevents the neonate from generating a negative intrathoracic pressure. In the delivery room, the immediate concern is to establish adequate ventilation. All newborns with symptomatic CDH require positive pressure ventilation. Bag-valve-mask ventilation is contraindicated because excess ventilation distending the stomach will worsen the pulmonary compression, so endotracheal intubation is required. Decompressing the stomach with a naso- or orogastric tube helps to minimize the thoracic volume taken up by the abdominal contents, but it is not an adequate replacement for intubation and positive pressure ventilation. While many newborns with CDH will require ECMO, initial management should focus on attempting to establish ventilation. Needle decompression is not indicated, as the thoracic volume is taken up with abdominal contents, not free air.

[ABP 3.B.3. Respiratory distress]

REFERENCE

1. Kirby E, Keijzer R. Congenital diaphragmatic hernia: current management strategies from antenatal diagnosis to long-term follow-up. *Pediatr Surg Int.* 2020;36(4):415–429.

40. ANSWER: B

The child developed drug-induced QTc prolongation due to tacrolimus, ondansetron, and azithromycin. Medications commonly associated with prolonged QTc include macrolides, fluoroquinolones, azoles, antipsychotics, antidepressants, and opioids. Diphenhydramine is also known to prolong the QTc interval. The other answer choices do not have this direct effect.

In adult patients, a QTc greater than 500 milliseconds is associated with a two-fold to three-fold increase in risk for torsade de pointes. Every additional 10-milliseconds increases the risk of developing torsade de pointes by approximately 5% to 7%. The mechanism by which magnesium sulfate treats torsade de pointes remains unclear. Although the patient may convert back to normal sinus rhythm following magnesium sulfate administration, magnesium does not significantly shorten the QTc interval. Hypokalemia should be corrected before magnesium is repleted.

[ABP 4.D. Medication management]

REFERENCE

1. Riad FS, Davis AM, Moranville MP, Beshai JF. Drug-induced QTc prolongation. *Am J Cardiol.* 2017;119(2):280–283.

41. ANSWER: D

Management of patients with stable ventilator support can occur outside of an intensive care unit when a chronic tracheostomy tube is in place. Tracheostomy tubes must be changed at routine intervals, depending on manufacturer and institutional guidelines (Figure 2.5). Standard recommendations are for routine changes to occur when the

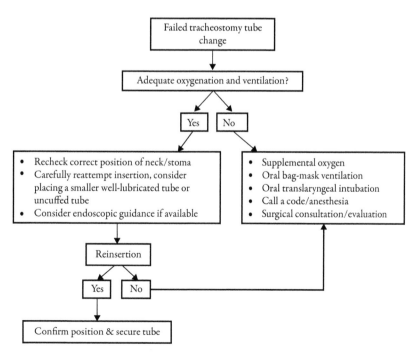

Figure 2.5. Clinical pathway to manage failed tracheostomy tube change. Figure reprinted with permission from Reference 1.

child is awake and least irritable. Positioning the patient's head and extending the neck are critically important. In the above case, the patient's agitated head turning makes re-insertion of a tracheostomy tube anatomically impossible. With a reassuring and firm hold, straightening a pediatric patient's head and elevation of the jaw can usually be accomplished without medication. At least two providers should participate in tube changes: one to maintain the tracheostomy tube and head position while the other removes the tracheostomy ties and prepares the new tube. Distortion of the tracheostomy tract can occur when the head is flexed and turned to the side, impeding insertion of a new tube.

One of the most feared complications of tracheostomy tube insertion is creation of a false passage into the anterior mediastinum, which would require emergent surgical intervention. Though false passages are most likely to occur at the first tube change after tracheostomy surgery, they can occur rarely if a tube is forcefully inserted and the caudal turn into the trachea performed too early. Because of the patient's chronic and well-established tract, false passage is unlikely in this case.

While supplemental oxygenation has been applied in this case with adequate response, the patient's airway needs to be secured urgently. Obtaining a new smaller tube is unnecessary and likely to lead to delay. Similarly, applying more than a small amount of lubrication is rarely necessary. Sedation with a benzodiazepine is reasonable and might improve procedural success but is not the most immediate next step.

[ABP 5.F. Tracheostomy tube change]

REFERENCE

1. White AC, Kher S, O'Connor HH. When to change a tracheostomy tube. *Respir Care*. 2010;55(8):1069–1075.

42. ANSWER: D

The Bhutani nomogram allows us to use a serum bilirubin level to evaluate the risk of a subsequent bilirubin level in that same infant being greater than the 95th percentile for age. It does not represent the natural history of neonatal hyperbilirubinemia. In addition, it does not provide guidance regarding when to initiate phototherapy. When using an evidence-based tool, it is important to keep in mind to which particular population it can be applied. The Bhutani nomogram is based on infants more than 36 weeks of age with birth weights above 2000 g or more than 35 weeks' gestation with birth weights more than 2500 g with no evidence of hemolytic disease and who have never received prior phototherapy. The nomogram may not accurately predict an infant's risk who falls outside these categories.

[ABP 3.B.2. Neonatal hyperbilirubinemia]

REFERENCE

1. American Academy of Pediatrics Subcommittee on Hyperbilirubinemia. Management of hyperbilirubinemia in the newborn infant 35 or more weeks of gestation. *Pediatrics*. 2004;114(1):297–316.

43. ANSWER: E

This seizure-like episode is most consistent with a psychogenic nonepileptic seizure (PNES). Pelvic thrusting, closed eyes resistant to opening, and lack of postictal confusion are typical of PNES. The majority of pediatric patients with somatic symptom–related disorders (including PNES) have comorbid organic medical diagnoses. In this case, video electroencephalography will help differentiate between epilepsy and PNES. Both brain magnetic resonance imaging and noncontrast head computed tomography can evaluate for a structural brain abnormality causing seizure, but such an abnormality is unlikely in this patient, and imaging is not diagnostic of PNES. Cerebrospinal fluid studies would be indicated if there was concern for meningitis. This is unlikely given the patient's normal vital signs and neurological examination. Low antiepileptic drug levels are also an unlikely cause of the seizure-like episode described given the patient reports appropriate compliance in taking her daily levetiracetam.

[ABP 2.D. Psychosomatic disorders]

44. ANSWER: E

Current guidelines indicate that direct laryngoscopy, intubation, and endotracheal suctioning "can be beneficial" for meconium-exposed newborns who require positive pressure ventilation and in whom there are signs of airway obstruction. However, it is important to note that this recommendation is based on expert consensus rather than rigorous evidence. Routine intubation and tracheal suctioning for infants born through meconium-stained amniotic fluid is no longer recommended. Vigorous, well-appearing, newborns with good respiratory effort should be allowed to remain with their mother. For nonvigorous newborns, the highest priority in the delivery room is to establish ventilation; stimulation and positive pressure ventilation (if indicated) should not be delayed for any reason, regardless of meconium-stained amniotic fluid or the skills of the providers participating in the resuscitation. Studies have shown no difference in outcomes between nonvigorous newborns born through meconium-stained fluid that undergo endotracheal suctioning and those who do not.

[ABP 3.A. Delivery room care, including resuscitation and stabilization]

REFERENCE

1. Aziz K, Lee CHC, Escobedo MB, et al. Part 5: neonatal resuscitation 2020 American Heart Association guidelines for cardiopulmonary resuscitation and emergency cardiovascular care. *Pediatrics.* 2021;*147*(suppl 1):e2020038505E.

45. ANSWER: E

Family engagement during hospitalization is associated with decreased readmission rates. Family-centered rounding is one means to increase family engagement. Families who participate in family-centered rounds feel less conflicted about treatment options, have higher patient and parent satisfaction rates, report increased comfort with transitioning to the home setting, and have increased compliance with the medical care plan.

Parents of children admitted to academic hospital centers report more problems with care coordination, in part because patients admitted to these centers are often cared for by a greater number of medical providers, increasing the risk of communication errors. Language barriers and culturally incompatible approaches to informed consent contribute to communication errors. Enrollment in public insurance and non-White race/ethnicity predict higher rates of pediatric readmission. Having a documented primary care physician follow-up plan at the time of discharge has not been proven to decrease the readmission rate significantly.

[ABP 4.E. Care coordination]

REFERENCES

1. Auger KA, Simon TD, Cooperberg D, et al. Summary of STARNet: Seamless Transitions and (Re)admissions Network. *Pediatrics.* 2015;*135*(1):164–175.
2. Sills MR, Hall M, Colvin JD, et al. Association of social determinants with children's hospitals' preventable readmissions performance. *JAMA Pediatr.* 2016;*170*(4):350–358.

46. ANSWER: C

Incision and drainage (I&D) is the mainstay of therapy for skin abscesses and may be sufficient treatment for uncomplicated cases. *Staphylococcus aureus* is the most common cause of purulent skin and soft tissue infections. The presentation of methicillin-resistant *S. aureus* (MRSA) is indistinguishable from that of methicillin-susceptible *S. aureus*. Diagnosis of skin abscess is made based on clinical findings of pain, fluctuance, and erythema. Though not required, bedside ultrasonography can be used to establish a clinically uncertain diagnosis of abscess or determine the dimensions and anatomy of the fluid pocket. While there is inconsistent evidence for systemic antibiotic treatment in conjunction with I&D, antibiotics are recommended for infants under 12 months of age, regardless of initial disease severity. Considerations for hospitalization after I&D generally include severe disease or clinical instability. Young age as low as 3 months has not been found to predict need for hospitalization, and because the patient in this case is clinically stable, hospitalization is not recommended.

Antibiotic prophylaxis for infective endocarditis is recommended by the American Heart Association (AHA) before certain procedures for patients with unrepaired cyanotic congenital heart disease (CHD), completely repaired CHD with prosthetic material or device for 6 months after procedure, or repaired CHD with residual defects at the site or adjacent to the site of a prosthetic patch or prosthetic device. Prophylaxis may be reasonable prior to I&D for these patients, but the patient in this vignette does not meet criteria.

[ABP 5.C. Incision and drainage]

REFERENCE

1. Stevens DL, Bisno AL, Chambers HF, et al. Practice guidelines for the diagnosis and management of skin and soft tissue infections: 2014 update by the Infectious Diseases Society of America. *Clin Infect Dis.* 2014;*59*(2):e10–e52.

47. ANSWER: A

Agitation in the postoperative recovery unit is common. Immediate consideration should be given to life-threatening conditions such as hypoxia, hypoglycemia, and hypercarbia. While postoperative sepsis is possible after an invasive procedure, it is unlikely that a patient would become symptomatic so soon after the procedure. Blood culture and serum lactate are therefore not immediate considerations. Serum electrolytes would be less helpful than an arterial blood gas for evaluating hypoxia and hypercarbia.

The most likely diagnosis in this case is emergence delirium, perhaps related to use of the inhalation anesthetic halothane. Emergence delirium is a generally benign, self-limited condition lasting 15–20 minutes. Observation without treatment is reasonable once hypoxia, hypoglycemia, and hypercarbia have been ruled out. However, pain control and sedatives may be needed. Recrudescence of symptoms is not typical. A prior episode of emergence delirium is not a risk factor for subsequent episodes.

[ABP 2.C. Delirium]

48. ANSWER: C

This infant most likely has transient tachypnea of the newborn (TTN), which is a self-limited condition involving inadequate clearance of fetal lung fluid that is present in less than 0.6% of term births. During fetal development, pneumocytes actively secrete chloride into the alveoli. This induces passive diffusion of sodium and water, which distend the alveoli and contribute to lung growth. Immediately prior to and during labor, increasing levels of fetal glucocorticoids and catecholamines reverse this process: pneumocytes are triggered to actively absorb sodium from the alveolar space, and fetal lung fluid is resorbed into the circulation. Scheduled caesarean delivery before any onset of labor is a major risk factor for TTN because the infant is born before any physiologic mechanism of fetal lung fluid reabsorption has begun. Infants who are large for gestational age and infants of diabetic mothers are also at increased risk, although those risks may be confounded by increased rates of elective caesarean deliveries in those populations.

Meconium aspiration syndrome (MAS) is a major cause of respiratory distress in newborns, but there is no history of meconium-stained amniotic fluid in this case, and the radiographic findings in this case are not consistent with the diffuse, patchy infiltrates typically seen in MAS. Bacterial pneumonia is unlikely in a newborn delivered by elective caesarean with no signs of maternal chorioamnionitis. Newborns with transposition of the great arteries or respiratory distress syndrome due to surfactant deficiency would be expected to have more persistent cyanosis and require more intensive ventilatory support.

[ABP 3.B.3. Respiratory distress]

REFERENCE

1. Alhassen Z, Vali P, Guglani L, Lakshminrusimha S, Ryan RM. Recent advances in pathophysiology and management of transient tachypnea of newborn. *J Perinatol.* 2021;*41*(1):6–16.

49. ANSWER: B

Providers are often hesitant to give large doses of narcotics at the end of life for fear that they may cause respiratory depression leading to death. However, when narcotics are dosed appropriately to treat dyspnea or pain, it is ethically and legally appropriate to accept that respiratory depression may hasten death in patients for whom life-sustaining treatment has been forgone. This patient received a modest dose of morphine and would likely benefit from the palliative effects of additional morphine.

It would be appropriate to withhold medically provided nutrition and fluids in this case if caregivers agree after discussion with the medical team. Given this patient's severe biventricular dysfunction, there is a risk of fluid overload, dyspnea, abdominal distension, nausea, and vomiting. Intravenous hydration may also prevent the natural decrease of secretion and urine production in dying patients and may cause more discomfort.

It is not ethically appropriate to administer medications with the sole purpose of hastening death in this case. Neuromuscular blocking agents and potassium chloride are examples of such medications. Neuromuscular blocking agents, such as vecuronium, may be particularly harmful because these medications limit the clinician's ability to assess for patient distress and pain.

[ABP 4.F. Palliative and end-of-life care]

REFERENCE

1. Burns JP, Mitchell C, Outwater KM, et al. End-of-life care in the pediatric intensive care unit after the forgoing of life-sustaining treatment. *Crit Care Med.* 2000;*28*(8):3060–3066.

50. ANSWER: B

The patient described in this vignette remains in shock despite an invasive airway and positive pressure ventilation. Intravenous epinephrine is the next step in resuscitation. During neonatal resuscitation, a low-lying UVC is the most rapid and reliable route for administration of epinephrine. Although the ideal location of the UVC tip is at the junction of the inferior vena cava and right atrium (RA/IVC), in this situation, radiographic confirmation will delay life-saving measures. A low-lying UVC route continues to be endorsed for emergency resuscitation of a newborn in the 2020 American Heart Association guidelines. When the patient is more stable, a low-lying UVC may be replaced or inserted to the higher RA/IVC position for longer use. The first essential step for UVC placement in any situation is to tie the umbilical cord base with a cord to reduce bleeding during and after cannulation.

While small case series and case reports have demonstrated success with the IO route for administration of medications and fluids in neonates, complications such as compartment syndrome and amputation have been reported, so a low-lying UVC is the safer option.

Pharmacokinetics, dose, and efficacy of epinephrine by the endotracheal route are poorly understood. Limited studies suggest that intravenous epinephrine is associated with more rapid time to peak plasma epinephrine concentration and shorter time to return of spontaneous circulation in perinatal asphyxiation.

[ABP 5.J. Umbilical artery catheter/umbilical vein catheter placement]

REFERENCE

1. Anderson J, Leonard D, Braner DA, Lai S, Tegtmeyer K. Videos in clinical medicine. Umbilical vascular catheterization. *N Engl J Med.* 2008;*359*(15):e18.

51. ANSWER: B

Congenital cytomegalovirus (cCMV) is the most common congenital viral infection worldwide and a leading cause of sensorineural hearing loss (SNHL). Although universal screening of newborns for cCMV is debated, the current recommendations are for targeted screening for those who fail the newborn hearing screen (unilaterally or bilaterally). Newborns should be tested within the first 3 weeks of life to differentiate between cCMV and postnatally acquired CMV. Therefore, it is reasonable to recommend cCMV testing in the newborn nursery prior to definitive diagnosis of SNHL with outpatient audiology.

Preferred testing for cCMV is polymerase chain reaction (PCR) analysis on a urine specimen, which does not require a sterile catheterized specimen. An alternative test is PCR on a saliva swab; however, this must be obtained at least 1 hour after breastfeeding to avoid false positives from CMV that has shed in maternal breastmilk.

Despite the known connection of ear and kidney development during embryogenesis, evidence does not support screening for renal anomalies in the setting of isolated SNHL. Brain imaging and serum studies are also not indicated for isolated SNHL.

[ABP 3.B.4. Neonatal infections, including exposure]

REFERENCE

1. Fowler KB, McCollister FP, Sabo DL, et al. A targeted approach for congenital cytomegalovirus screening within newborn hearing screening. *Pediatrics*. 2017;*139*(2):e20162128.

52. ANSWER: A

This patient has heat stroke, which is differentiated from simple heat exhaustion by the presence of delirium, obtundation, hallucinations, ataxia, slurred speech, and a core body temperature of 104°F (40°C) or greater. Increased environmental humidity and lack of fluid repletion adds to the risk of heat injury. While this patient does have rhabdomyolysis, it is a consequence of the primary cause of his presentation. The history and the presence of fever make heat stroke more likely than drug intoxication or head injury. The mainstay of treatment is aggressive hydration and cooling. Head imaging should be considered if his mental status does not improve with these interventions.

[ABP 2.C. Delirium]

53. ANSWER: E

Respiratory distress in a newborn is identified through a variety of physical findings that indicate increased work of breathing. Grunting is an expiratory sound caused by partial closure of the glottis during expiration in an attempt to maintain increased residual volume to prevent alveolar collapse. Nasal flaring is a compensatory symptom that increases upper airway diameter (choice A). Stertor is a sign of nasopharyngeal obstruction (choice B). A high-pitched sound from upper airway obstruction is stridor (choice C), and a high-pitched sound from tracheobronchial obstruction is wheezing (choice D).

[ABP 3.B.3. Respiratory distress]

54. ANSWER: E

Physicians must consider how postpyloric administration may affect medication absorption, delivery, and tolerance. These factors may depend on interactions between the medication and formula, the osmotic load of the liquid formulation of the medication, binding to the tubing, clogging of the tubing (especially in the case of crushed tablets), the acidity of the jejunum and distal intestine, and the intestinal absorption site for the medication. Diazepam solution binds extensively to tubing. Phenytoin may bind calcium and protein in a formula, and absorption may be significantly reduced if administered within 2 hours of feeds. Ciprofloxacin binds divalent cations in the formula and causes substantial absorption reduction when administered with meals. Ferrous sulfate requires gastric acid for activation and systemic absorption.

Lactobacillus remains in the intraluminal space and therefore can be administered via jejunostomy tube if necessary.

[ABP 4.D. Medication management]

REFERENCES

1. McIntyre CM, Monk HM. Medication absorption considerations in patients with postpyloric enteral feeding tubes. *Am J Health Syst Pharm*. 2014;*71*(7):549–556.
2. Wohlt PD, Zheng L, Gunderson S, Balzar SA, Johnson BD, Fish JT. Recommendations for the use of medications with continuous enteral nutrition. *Am J Health Syst Pharm*. 2009;*66*(16):1458–1467.

55. ANSWER: D

The best next step is placement of a supraglottic airway such as a laryngeal mask airway (LMA) given the difficult airway. Patients with Treacher Collins have micrognathia, which makes establishing an airway more difficult. Other patients who may have difficult airway anatomy include those with Pierre Robin sequence, Goldenhar syndrome, and anomalies of the external ear (microtia) and micrognathia. Other concerning signs for a difficult airway include the difficulty with mask ventilation and lack of chest rise despite an oral airway. LMAs are a useful tool for patients who are difficult to intubate and are associated with few complications. Contraindications for LMA include active vomiting of gastric contents or blood in the upper airway because the device cannot form an airtight seal around the larynx.

Nasal and oral airways are both effective in assisting with difficult mask ventilation, but switching from an oral to nasal airway would not be an effective escalation of airway management. Repeated conventional intubation could worsen laryngeal trauma, which can exacerbate the ongoing difficulty with mask ventilation. At this point in the case, the patient needs immediate ventilatory support, and waiting for a surgical airway will delay life-saving measures. Albuterol is not the correct answer in this situation because the difficult mask ventilation is caused by an anatomic reason and not bronchospasm.

[ABP 5.H. Endotracheal intubation and LMA placement]

REFERENCE

1. Benumof JL. Laryngeal mask airway and the ASA difficult airway algorithm. *Anesthesiology*. 1996;*84*(3):686–699.

56. ANSWER: B

This patient's presentation is consistent with functional neurological disorder, previously known as conversion disorder. Prognosis for this condition is better with early intervention. Involvement of the inpatient child psychologist early in the hospital course for any patient with suspected somatic symptoms is recommended. Continued inpatient hospitalization without psychology consultation would be suboptimal. A child psychologist's goals for inpatient admission would include completion of a thorough biopsychosocial workup, informing the family of the diagnosis and treatment plan, offering brief intervention sessions for symptom management and facilitation of outpatient care. These important services would be lacking with a simple discharge home with outpatient psychology, physical therapy, or pediatrician follow-up.

According to the *Diagnostic and Statistical Manual for Mental Disorders, Fifth Edition, (DSM-5)*, a conversion disorder must meet the following four criteria: (1) one or more symptoms of altered voluntary motor or sensory function; (2) clinical findings provide evidence of incompatibility between the symptom and recognized neurological or medical conditions; (3) the symptom or deficit is not better explained by another medical or mental disorder; and (4) the symptom or deficit causes clinically significant distress or impairment in social, occupational, or other important areas of functioning or warrants medical evaluation.

[ABP 2.D. Psychosomatic disorders]

57. ANSWER: D

The risk of neonatal HSV infection is much greater for newborns born to mothers with a first episode of HSV as compared to newborns born to mothers with recurrent HSV. The American Academy of Pediatrics has published guidance on the management of infants born to women with genital herpes lesions. The first step in management is to determine whether there was any maternal history of genital HSV prior to pregnancy. If yes (and thus the current episode is a recurrent infection), then the neonate should have HSV surface cultures and blood PCR sent at approximately 24 hours of age, but acyclovir does not need to be started as long as the infant remains asymptomatic. If there was no history of HSV prior to pregnancy, then HSV studies from the maternal lesion and typing if positive, paired with type-specific serology for HSV-1 and HSV-2, should be sent in order to confirm that the lesions represent a first-episode primary infection (evidence of virus in the genital tract in the setting of negative serologies) or a first-episode nonprimary infection (HSV-2 genital infection in the setting of preexisting HSV-1 antibody, or vice versa). In the case of first-episode infections, a full evaluation for neonatal HSV as listed in answer E should be done, and intravenous acyclovir should be started while awaiting results. As long as the infant is asymptomatic, this evaluation and treatment should be done at approximately 24 hours of age. Cesarean section reduces but does not eliminate the risk of neonatal HSV in infants born to mothers with active genital lesions; thus, the mode of delivery should not change management.

[ABP 3.B.4. Neonatal infections, including exposure]

REFERENCE

1. Kimberlin DW, Baley J; Committee on Infectious Diseases; Committee on Fetus and Newborn. Guidance on management of asymptomatic neonates born to women with active genital herpes lesions. *Pediatrics*. 2013;*131*(2):e635–e646.

58. ANSWER: A

Of the answer choices, clean intermittent catheterization puts this patient at the highest risk of urinary tract infection. There is insufficient evidence to universally recommend antibiotic prophylaxis and cranberry juice in this patient population. The use of oxybutynin may actually decrease the risk of urinary tract infection in patients with neurogenic bladder, but there is insufficient evidence to support this finding.

Patients with spina bifida are at increased risk of urinary tract infection for several reasons. There is direct inoculation of bacteria into the urinary bladder from catheterization and alteration of protective urinary flora from bacterial colonization in the perineum and urethra. Through catheterization, bacteria bypass secretory immunoglobulin A and a glycosaminoglycan (GAG) layer lining the urothelium. With urinary stasis, increased postvoid residual volume, and deficient mechanical cleansing from voiding, bacterial washout is decreased. The normal innate immune response, typically stimulated when bacterial components elicit pro-inflammatory signaling and leukocyte recruitment, is altered in the neurogenic bladder. Last, bladder ischemia from repeated distension may lead to tissue damage and decreased delivery of inflammatory cells and antibiotics.

[ABP 4.A. Symptom management]

REFERENCES

1. Frimberger D, Cheng E, Kropp BP. The current management of the neurogenic bladder in children with spina bifida. *Pediatr Clin North Am.* 2012;*59*(4):757–767.
2. Kaye IY, Payan M, Vemulakonda VM. Association between clean intermittent catheterization and urinary tract infection in infants and toddlers with spina bifida. *J Pediatr Urol.* 2016;*12*(5):284.e1–284.e6.

59. ANSWER: A

In neonates, superficial scalp veins (frontal, superficial temporal, posterior auricular, supraorbital, occipital, and posterior facial) are convenient access sites. The basilic and saphenous veins are typically reserved for peripherally inserted central catheter access. The femoral vein is generally saved for emergent situations and for shorter-term access given its close proximity to the groin and risk for infection. Care must be taken not to injure the femoral nerve or inadvertently cannulate the femoral artery. External jugular catheters are difficult to stabilize and can easily be dislodged by the patient.

[ABP 5.K. Peripheral intravenous placement]

REFERENCE

1. Stovroff M, Teague WG. Intravenous access in infants and children. *Pediatr Clin North Am.* 1998;*45*(6):1373–1393, viii.

60. ANSWER: D

Typical and atypical antipsychotic medications can cause prolongation of the QTc interval. A baseline electrocardiogram should always be obtained prior to the initiation of these medications to assess a baseline QTc interval. An echocardiogram would not provide any information regarding the patient's cardiac conduction system. Atypical antipsychotics are known to cause metabolic syndrome. While monitoring blood glucose and fasting lipid panels is recommended after prolonged use, obtaining baseline values prior to starting these medications is not necessary. A repeat urine drug screen would not impact the decision to initiate an atypical antipsychotic.

[ABP 2.B. Acute aggression and psychosis]

61. ANSWER: B

All infants born at less than 37 weeks' gestational age or with low birth weight (LBW, < 2500 g) should undergo a CSTS within 24–48 hours of hospital discharge. The infant is buckled securely into their own car seat, the car seat is positioned at the same angle it will sit at in a car, and the infant's pulse, respiration, and oxygen saturation are monitored continuously for 90–120 minutes. Criteria for failing the CSTS include any of the following: (1) apnea longer than 20 seconds, (2) bradycardia less than 80 beats per minute for more than 10 seconds, and (3) desaturation less than 90% for more than 10 seconds. This infant was born late preterm, so a CSTS was indicated, and she was apneic for 30 seconds, so she fails the CSTS.

Infants who fail the CSTS can still be discharged from the hospital in either of two ways: (1) The CSTS can be repeated 24 hours later, and the infant may pass on the second screen; (2) if the infant fails a second CSTS, or if the infant and the mother are otherwise ready for discharge before the repeat screening can occur, then the infant can be discharged home in a car bed that meets government safety standards.

[ABP 3.B.5. Late preterm infant]

REFERENCES

1. Bull MJ, Engle WA; Committee on Injury, Violence, and Poison Prevention and Committee on Fetus and Newborn; American Academy of Pediatrics. Safe transportation of preterm and low birth weight infants at hospital discharge. *Pediatrics.* 2009;*123*(5):1424–1429.
2. Magnarelli A, Shah Solanki N, Davis NL. Car seat tolerance screening for late-preterm infants. *Pediatrics.* 2020;*145*(1):e20191703

62. ANSWER: E

Children with organic acidemias can have persistent feeding intolerance. Although it is unconfirmed whether this patient is in a metabolic crisis at this time, prompt initiation of high-concentration dextrose and cessation of all protein intake is indicated to reverse or prevent a potential metabolic crisis (Table 2.4). If his laboratory work does not indicate an acute metabolic crisis, initiating feeds as tolerated, whether at smaller volumes or via continuous infusion, may be appropriate considerations.

Table 2.4 CONCEPTUAL FRAMEWORK FOR MANAGEMENT OF ORGANIC ACIDEMIAS[a]

CONCEPT	ACUTE MANAGEMENT	CHRONIC MANAGEMENT
Reverse or prevent catabolism	D_{10} with electrolytes	Avoid fasting
Decrease protein load	Hold protein ≤ 48 hours	Avoid nontolerated amino acids
Initiate "toxin" scavengers	Specific to disorder	Specific to disorder
Provide cofactors and supplements	For example, biotin, hydroxocobalamin	For example, biotin, hydroxocobalamin

[a] Adapted from Reference 1.

[ABP 4.A. Symptom management]

REFERENCE

1. Chapman KA. Practical management of organic acidemias. *Transl Sci Rare Dis*. 2019;4(3–4):121–131.

63. ANSWER: C

Based on the imaging as well as the patient's worsening agitation, respiratory distress, and hypoxemia, this patient has a moderate left-sided pneumothorax with clinical signs and symptoms concerning for a tension pneumothorax. A needle decompression is warranted for therapeutic removal of air. For needle decompression of a pneumothorax, the ideal position is supine with the head of the bed raised 30°. Insert the needle at the second intercostal space along the midclavicular line or the fourth intercostal space along the anterior axillary line. The needle should be inserted at a 90° angle. Waiting for a surgical chest tube will delay life-saving measures. Neither intubation nor decubitus positioning will definitively treat the underlying problem.

[ABP 5.I. Needle thoracentesis]

REFERENCE

1. Prestridge A. Thoracentesis. In: Goodman DM, Green TP, Unti SM, Powel EC, eds. *Current Procedures Pediatrics*. McGraw-Hill; 2011: Chap. 20.

64. ANSWER: D

If a patient's behavior becomes violent or his behavior poses risk of injury, activation of a specialized behavioral response team is the most appropriate next action step. While awaiting assistance, the following are important de-escalation and safety action steps to follow: (1) do not touch the patient; (2) remain calm and unhurried; (3) remove dangerous objects from the area and assist others not involved to leave the area immediately; (4) be nonpunitive and nonjudgmental; (5) reassure the patient they will be kept safe; and (6) set limits on inappropriate behaviors and avoid lengthy discussion related to conflicted issues. Leaving the patient alone in the room would increase the risk of potential self-harm and would not be an appropriate de-escalation step.

[ABP 2.E. Behavioral and developmental disorders]

65. ANSWER: D

This infant is showing signs of neonatal withdrawal, also known as neonatal abstinence syndrome (NAS). Treatment for NAS should be grounded in ongoing assessment of the severity of the infant's symptoms. The most common assessment tool used is a modified version of the Finnegan score, but mounting evidence suggests that the Eat-Sleep-Console (ESC) approach leads to shortened length of stay and decreased use of morphine. ESC is based on assessing the infants' ability to feed well, sleep for at least 1 hour at a time, and be consoled easily. Regardless of whether NAS severity is assessed using Finnegan scores or an ESC approach, nonpharmacological treatment should be attempted before beginning opioid replacement therapy. If opioid replacement is required, morphine is the preferred agent; paregoric has fallen out of use due to its high alcohol content and safety concerns. While tremors and increased tone can be signs of seizure activity in a newborn, the fact that a light touch suppresses the tremors makes seizures much less likely.

[ABP 3.B.6. Drug exposure/neonatal abstinence syndrome]

REFERENCES

1. Parlaman J, Deodhar P, Sanders V, Jerome J, McDaniel C. Improving care for infants with neonatal abstinence syndrome: a multicenter, community hospital-based study. *Hosp Pediatr*. 2019;9(8):608–614.
2. Patrick SW, Barfield WD, Poindexter BB; Committee on Fetus and Newborn, Committee on Substance Use and Prevention. Neonatal opioid withdrawal syndrome. *Pediatrics*. 2020;146(5):e2020029074.

66. ANSWER: C

A more complete history, including nutritional history, the family's resources at home, meal observation, and obtaining a bedside swallow evaluation will provide important insights to guide interventions. Care of medically complex children can be a challenge for working families. There is not enough information at this time to raise concerns for neglect. Assessment of nutrition is complicated in this group, and prealbumin is not helpful. He may benefit from a G-tube only after exhausting medical and nonsurgical management.

[ABP 4.B. Feeding and nutrition]

REFERENCES

1. Lark RK, Williams CL, Stadler D, et al. Serum prealbumin and albumin concentrations do not reflect nutritional state in children with cerebral palsy. *J Pediatr.* 2005;*147*(5):695–697.
2. Marchand V, Motil KJ; NASPGHAN Committee on Nutrition. Nutrition support for neurologically impaired children: a clinical report of the North American Society for Pediatric Gastroenterology, Hepatology, and Nutrition. *J Pediatr Gastroenterol Nutr.* 2006;*43*(1):123–135.

67. ANSWER: C

Pelvic fracture may result in urethral injury, which is a contraindication to urinary catheterization. Blood at the urethral meatus may be a sign of urethral trauma, and similarly catheterization should be avoided in these patients. Other contraindications include moderate or severe phimosis in a male. Vaginitis is not a contraindication to urethral catheterizations, but accidental catheterization of the vagina rather than the urethra is a common event because landmarks can be difficult on a young girl. None of the other answer choices are contraindications for urethral catheterization.

[ABP 5.M. Bladder catheterization]

REFERENCE

1. Plaza-Verduin MA, Lucas J. Suprapubic bladder aspiration. In: Ganti L, ed. *Atlas of Emergency Medicine Procedures.* Springer Verlag; 2016:717–720.

68. ANSWER: B

When faced with an agitated patient in the hospital setting, it is imperative to follow a stepwise approach to de-escalation and implementation of restrictive measures. Assessing the degree of agitation is an appropriate first step. The patient described in this vignette is moderately agitated as she continues to shout and curse, and unit staff no longer seem to be in control of the situation. Verbal de-escalation techniques to achieve a calm and cooperative state have already been trialed unsuccessfully. The best next step in management is administration of a medical restraint. IM haloperidol followed by reassessment of the degree of

agitation in 15 minutes is a much more appropriate option as compared to administration of IM lorazepam with a titration in dosing to achieve sedation. Sedation is never the desired endpoint in the management of agitation. Should medical restraint prove unsuccessful, manual restraints could be considered, with discontinuation as soon as the safety of the patient and staff are no longer threatened.

[ABP 2.B. Acute aggression and psychosis]

69. ANSWER: D

Congenital abnormalities can be divided into several broad categories:

- Malformations: defects caused by intrinsically abnormal fetal development (e.g., genetic syndromes such as trisomy 13 or trisomy 18)
- Disruptions: defects caused by destruction of or interference with tissues that were developing normally (e.g., limb defects caused by amniotic band syndrome)
- Deformations: abnormalities in the shape or positioning of tissue due to external forces affecting fetal development

With twins born full term with weights AGA, positional deformation caused by crowding in utero is the most likely cause of these congenital abnormalities. The fact that the deformities can be corrected with gentle pressure is further evidence that these are positional deformations and not inherent malformations. There is no obvious genetic syndrome—either inherited or a new mutation—or toxic exposure that links equinovarus deformity and torticollis, and these are not common injuries from birth trauma.

[ABP 3.B.8. Congenital anomalies]

70. ANSWER: A

The most important risk factor for developing depression is a parental history of mental illness. Other risk factors include medications such as glucocorticoids, isotretinoin, and some immunosuppressant and antiviral agents. Chronic illness also puts this child at increased risk. While depression is more common in adolescents and in females, this patient's family history puts her at greatest risk.

[ABP 2.A. Self-harm/suicidality]

71. ANSWER: C

Oral medications (baclofen, clonazepam, tizanidine, and dantrolene) are treatments of choice for generalized spasticity. There are three types of hypertonia: spasticity, dystonia, and rigidity. Spasticity is defined as velocity-dependent contraction of the muscle fibers, or "spastic catch," often more pronounced in one direction. Dystonia is the activation of an agonist-antagonist pair or two muscle groups with opposing actions. Rigidity is characterized by resistance to movement in all directions that is not velocity dependent. Rigidity is uncommon in the pediatric population. Because this patient has velocity-dependent resistance to movement and reason for upper motor neuron disease, the physical examination findings are most consistent with spasticity.

Lorazepam has a short half-life and may be associated with sedation and incoordination among other effects and is not commonly used for the long-term management of spasticity. Chemodenervation with botulinum toxin is considered the first-line treatment for focal spasticity rather than generalized spasticity. Deep brain stimulation is more widely used in children with dystonia after failure of medical therapy. Deep brain stimulation is not favored in infants given the high risk of lead displacement over time as the child's brain grows. Levodopa administered with carbidopa is most commonly used to treat Parkinson disease, not focal spasticity.

[ABP 4.A. Symptom management]

REFERENCES

1. Sanger TD, Delgado MR, Gaebler-Spira D, Hallett M, Mink JW; Task Force on Childhood Motor Disorders. Classification and definition of disorders causing hypertonia in childhood. *Pediatrics.* 2003;*111*(1):e89–e97.
2. Shamsoddini A, Amirsalari S, Hollisaz MT, Rahimnia A, Khatibi-Aghda A. Management of spasticity in children with cerebral palsy. *Iran J Pediatr.* 2014;*24*(4):345–351.

72. ANSWER: A

This patient likely has congenital cytomegalovirus (CMV), which is the most common nonhereditary cause of sensorineural hearing loss. Transmission can occur in utero (more likely if maternal primary exposure occurs during pregnancy) and postnatally through breast milk. Cataracts and extramedullary hematopoiesis are commonly associated with congenital rubella. Bone deformities can be seen with

congenital syphilis. Macrocephaly can be seen with congenital toxoplasmosis. See Table 2.5 below for comparison of various congenital infections.

[ABP 3.B.4. Neonatal infections, including exposure]

73. ANSWER: B

A pressure ulcer results from compromised nutrition to the local tissue. Hence avoiding pressure, ensuring adequate blood flow, and maintaining nutrition with adequate calories and protein are essential. Several types of occlusive dressings are applied to aid healing by providing moisture. Supplementation with vitamin C and zinc is reserved for wounds not healing after more than a week of appropriate interventions. Blood levels of vitamin C and zinc should be obtained prior to and during supplementation. Patients should be monitored for adverse effects, as zinc can reduce copper and iron absorption, and vitamin C predisposes patients to renal stones.

[ABP 4.A. Symptom management]

REFERENCE

1. Butler CT. Pediatric skin care: guidelines for assessment, prevention, and treatment. *Dermatol Nurs.* 2007;*19*(5):471–485.

74. ANSWER: A

Based on research from the Pediatric Sedation Research Consortium, age younger than 1 year and ASA physical status greater than II (Table 2.6) are two main factors that contribute to increased risk of cardiac arrest. Infants younger than 6 months are at higher risk for respiratory depression and apnea. It is generally recommended that an anesthesiologist or intensivist should sedate children under 3 months of age. Propofol infusion is generally well tolerated and has lower risk for adverse events when used without coadministration of other medications. Propofol is

Table 2.5 DISTINGUISHING FEATURES OF TORCH INFECTIONS

	EYE ISSUES	INTRACRANIAL CALCIFICATIONS	RASH	HEARING LOSS
Toxoplasmosis	+++ (chorioretinitis)	++ (intracerebral)	+ (maculopapular)	+
Syphilis	+ (interstitial keratitis)	−	+ (maculopapular)	+
Rubella	++ (cataracts)	−	++ (extramedullary hematopoiesis; blueberry muffin)	+++
CMV	+ (chorioretinitis)	++ (periventricular)	+ (petechiae; looks like blueberry muffin rash)	+++

TORCH, toxoplasma, other, rubella, CMV, herpes.

preferred for short procedures; adverse effects include hypotension, metabolic acidosis, and rhabdomyolysis. Medical conditions that put patients at higher risk for complications during sedation include significant craniofacial abnormalities or history of upper airway abnormalities. Caution should also be exercised with obese children with body mass index (BMI) greater than 95%. Studies have shown that there is no difference in adverse outcomes with pediatric procedural sedation performed outside the operating room versus inside, and there are no differences in either the adjusted or unadjusted rates of major complications among different pediatric specialists.

Well-controlled epilepsy is categorized as ASA II, and therefore there is low risk of adverse complications. The ASA classification should be determined for all patients to identify patients who require further anesthesia specialty care (Table 2.6). In general, children with ASA classification of I or II are appropriate for sedation by a trained sedation provider like a pediatric hospitalist.

Table 2.6 CURRENT ASA DEFINITIONS AND EXAMPLES[a]

ASA PHYSICAL STATUS CLASSIFICATION	DISEASE STATE	PEDIATRIC EXAMPLES
ASA I	A healthy patient	Healthy (with no acute or chronic disease), normal BMI for age
ASA II	A patient with mild systemic disease	Asymptomatic congenital cardiac disease, asthma without exacerbation, well-controlled epilepsy
ASA III	A patient with severe systemic disease	Asthma with exacerbation, poorly controlled epilepsy, insulin-dependent diabetes mellitus, morbid obesity
ASA IV	A patient with severe systemic disease that is a constant threat to life	Symptomatic congenital cardiac abnormality, congestive heart failure, shock, sepsis
ASA V	A moribund patient who is not expected to survive without the operation	Massive trauma, intracranial hemorrhage with mass effect, respiratory failure or arrest
ASA VI	A declared brain-dead patient whose organs are being removed for donor purposes	

[a] Adapted from Reference 1.

[ABP 5.N. Procedural sedation]

REFERENCES

1. Committee on Economics. ASA Physician Status Classification System. American Society of Anesthesiologists. October 15, 2014. Amended December 13, 2020. Accessed February 1, 2021. https://www.asahq.org/standards-and-guidelines/asa-physical-status-classification-system.
2. Daud YN, Carlson DW. Pediatric sedation. *Pediatr Clin North Am*. 2014;*61*(4):703–717.

75. ANSWER: C

This patient has developed an acute dystonic reaction, most likely a side effect of haloperidol. Haloperidol is a high-potency typical antipsychotic that can cause extrapyramidal symptoms (including dystonia and akathisia), neuroleptic malignant syndrome, and QTc prolongation. The risk of developing extrapyramidal symptoms with haloperidol is much higher than with administration of an atypical antipsychotic such as olanzapine or risperidone. The main side effects of lorazepam, a benzodiazepine, are sedation and respiratory depression. Benzodiazepines do not cause movement disorders but can lead to a paradoxical reaction. Antihistamines such as diphenhydramine can also cause paradoxical reactions in addition to anticholinergic symptoms (dry mouth, dizziness, constipation, urinary retention, delirium, cardiac conduction abnormalities, flushing, mydriasis, and dry skin).

[ABP 2.B. Acute aggression and psychosis]

76. ANSWER: C

Clavicle fractures are the most common skeletal injury sustained during delivery, occurring in 0.2%–4.4% of births. Risk factors include macrosomia, vacuum- or forceps-assisted delivery, and—most significantly—shoulder dystocia. Clavicle fractures should be considered in infants with an asymmetric Moro reflex, pain on passive movement of one arm, and any visible or palpable signs of fracture, such as bruising, swelling, crepitus, or a deformity over the clavicle. An x-ray of the infant's chest and both upper extremities can confirm the diagnosis and rule out concomitant injuries, such as shoulder separation or humerus fractures. The majority of clavicle fractures require no treatment but can be splinted for comfort by dressing the child in a long-sleeve shirt and pinning the sleeve across the chest with the elbow flexed at 90°. Orthopedics consultation is only indicated in cases of severely comminuted or multiple fractures. MRI to assess the brachial plexus is not necessary unless there are other signs of nerve injury, such as decreased movement in the lower arm or hand. In-hospital child physical abuse is extremely rare, so a CPS report is not warranted unless there are other reasons for concern. Physical therapy and range-of-motion exercises do not promote healing.

[ABP 3.B.7. Birth trauma]

REFERENCE

1. Hsu TY, Hung FC, Lu YJ, et al. Neonatal clavicular fracture: clinical analysis of incidence, predisposing factors, diagnosis, and outcome. *Am J Perinatol.* 2002;*19*(1):17–21.

77. ANSWER: D

Tracheostomy tube dislodgement is a medical emergency. This patient is deteriorating despite tracheostomy tube replacement. This patient is at risk for pneumothorax given that he received bag-mask ventilation after tube replacement. A chest radiograph can confirm tube dislodgement, a false tract, an air leak in the soft tissue of the neck, as well as a pneumothorax. While starting antibiotics, giving intravenous fluids, and treating anxiety may all be reasonable interventions, improving this patient's ventilation should take priority. While a chest tube may be indicated, a chest radiograph should first confirm the diagnosis of pneumothorax.

[ABP 4.C. Device and technology management, including complications]

REFERENCE

1. Bontempo LJ, Manning SL. Tracheostomy emergencies. *Emerg Med Clin North Am.* 2019;*37*(1):109–119.

78. ANSWER: C

The patient described in this vignette displays acute hypoxic and ventilatory respiratory failure due to bronchiolitis. Positive pressure ventilation is indicated. The vast majority of self-inflating bags include a reservoir interface that can provide continuous passive oxygen flow to a patient. An appropriate size face mask should be applied effectively using an "E-C clamp" configuration of fingers and thumb. The mask should fit from the bridge of the nose to the cleft of the chin. While CO_2 detectors may be used during resuscitation, adequate ventilation is assessed primarily by looking for chest rise. Pressure-limiting pop-off valves on self-inflating bags are usually manufactured to release at 35–45 cm H_2O to prevent excessive airway pressures. However, in diseases with poor lung compliance, closing the pop-off valve may be necessary to achieve adequate airway-distending pressure.

If the child is spontaneously breathing but ineffectively, positive pressure breaths should be synchronized. Failure to synchronize may prevent effective ventilation and stimulate coughing, gastric inflation, emesis, and laryngospasm. Consequently, the person performing bag-mask ventilation should monitor chest rise and patient effort continuously. The 2020 American Heart Association (AHA) Pediatric Advanced Life Support update recommends rescue breaths of 20–30 breaths per minute and pulse checks every 2 minutes in situations of respiratory arrest.

[ABP 5.G. Bag mask ventilation]

REFERENCE

1. American Heart Association. Managing respiratory distress and failure. In: *Pediatric Advanced Life Support Provider Manual eBook.* American Heart Association; 2020: part 8.

79. ANSWER: E

Delirium is treated primarily by identifying and treating the underlying cause and minimizing risk factors. Atypical antipsychotics such as olanzapine, quetiapine, and risperidone can be helpful in treating delirium, although their use is off label. Haloperidol has generally fallen out of favor due to its side-effect profile. Early ambulation, establishing a daily routine, clustering care, reducing noise and light pollution, minimizing caregiver turnover, using familiar objects (e.g., toys or blankets), and maintaining parental presence are all helpful in treating delirium. Medications should be reviewed to identify and minimize use of the most common deliriogenic medications: opioids, benzodiazepines, and anticholinergics. Of the answer choices, scopolamine and atropine are anticholinergics and should be avoided. Methadone, an opioid, and diazepam, a benzodiazepine, should both be avoided in patients with delirium. The use of melatonin and the sedative dexmedetomidine, an α_2-agonist, can help providers avoid the need for both benzodiazepines and opioids.

Symptoms of pediatric delirium include irritability, labile affect, agitation, sleep-wake disturbance, developmental regression, and reduced eye contact with primary caregivers. This child has shown significant regression with loss of milestones, and intervention to prevent persistence or worsening of these symptoms is required. Risk factors for the development of delirium include prolonged stay in an ICU environment, sleep disruptions, polypharmacy, use of restraints, hypoxia, surgeries, anesthesia, and prolonged periods of immobilization.

[ABP 2.C. Delirium]

80. ANSWER: C

Breastfeeding carries numerous benefits for both the mother and the newborn. Benefits to the newborn include decreased rates of gastrointestinal infections, respiratory infections (including otitis media), necrotizing enterocolitis, sudden infant death syndrome, allergies, celiac disease, inflammatory bowel disease, and obesity. For mothers, some evidence suggests decreased rates of rheumatoid arthritis, cardiovascular disease, and diabetes with increased cumulative lifetime breastfeeding.

There are few contraindications to breastfeeding. Absolute contraindications include active tuberculosis (TB), untreated brucellosis, and herpetic lesions on the breast. Latent TB infection, treated brucellosis, and herpetic lesions elsewhere on the body are not contraindications. In developing countries where malnutrition and waterborne infections cause high rates of infant mortality, the health benefits of breastfeeding may outweigh the risks of HIV transmission through breast milk, but in industrialized nations, any HIV infection is considered an absolute contraindication—no matter the mother's viral load. Substance abuse is considered a relative contraindication to breastfeeding; the risks conferred by the specific doses and types of substances must be weighed against the benefits of breastfeeding. Many prescription medications are similarly considered relative contraindications.

[ABP 3.B.9. Newborn feeding (including breastfeeding and formula feeding)]

REFERENCE

1. Section on Breastfeeding. Breastfeeding and the use of human milk. *Pediatrics.* 2012;*129*(3):e827–e841.

81. ANSWER: C

Advance directives with a modified clause can be challenging for providers. In such cases, when the parents are unreachable, a physician must take the next reasonable step as per the advance directive. Antibiotics and comfort measures are needed, but endotracheal intubation takes precedence due to the patient's worsening respiratory status despite BiPAP. Aspiration pneumonia, the most likely cause of this patient's respiratory distress, is a reversible condition, so intubation is allowed per the patient's advanced directive. There is no need to delay intubation in order to contact risk management or the patient's family.

[ABP 4.F. Palliative and end-of-life care]

REFERENCE

1. Hein K, Knochel K, Zaimovic V, et al. Identifying key elements for paediatric advance care planning with parents, healthcare providers and stakeholders: a qualitative study. *Palliat Med.* 2020;*34*(3):300–308.

82. ANSWER: A

Arterial puncture is a safe procedure that is useful to assess acid-base status as well as oxygenation and ventilation. The distal radial artery is the preferred site in children, though other sites, such as brachial and femoral arteries, can be considered if necessary. There are few contraindications to the procedure, but overlying infection is one of them. Ischemic complications are rare; however, patients undergoing arterial puncture of the radial artery should have the presence of collateral arterial perfusion of the hand assessed prior to the procedure. This can be performed with the modified Allen test: both the radial and ulnar arteries are compressed until the palm appears pale; the pressure is then released from the ulnar artery. Pink color should return to the palm within several seconds, indicating adequate collateral circulation. Sterile technique is necessary if blood cultures are being collected; otherwise, clean technique is sufficient. Blood flow may not be pulsatile in infants; bright red color generally indicates the specimen is of arterial origin. The needle should enter the skin at a 30° to 45° angle from horizontal.

[ABP 5.L. Arterial puncture]

83. ANSWER: D

Patients with eating disorders have several known complications; examples are included in the Table 2.7.

Table 2.7 EXAMPLES OF COMPLICATIONS OF EATING DISORDERS

Gastrointestinal complications	Delayed gastric emptying, dysmotility, superior mesenteric artery syndrome, constipation, hypercholesterolemia, pancreatitis, transaminitis
Fluid/electrolyte derangements	Dehydration, low phosphorus, low potassium, low sodium
Cardiac complications	Prolonged QTc, bradycardia
Endocrine dysfunction	Impaired glucose tolerance, sick euthyroid syndrome, amenorrhea
Hematologic complications	Leukopenia, anemia, thrombocytopenia

In addition to these complications, once patients are receiving adequate nutrition they are also at risk for refeeding syndrome. A drop in phosphorus is often the first sign of refeeding syndrome, which can progress to multiorgan dysfunction (e.g., edema, seizures, respiratory failure, rarely congestive heart failure).

[ABP 2.F. Eating disorders]

84. ANSWER: D

Infants born between $34^0/_7$ and $36^6/_7$ weeks' gestation are termed "late preterm." This population needs to be separated from term infants as they have increased rates of morbidity and mortality due to underlying physiologic and metabolic immaturity and decreased compensatory capabilities. Late preterm infants are more likely than term infants to have temperature instability, hypoglycemia, respiratory distress, apnea, hyperbilirubinemia, and feeding difficulties. Recommended guidelines have been suggested to safely monitor this population during the birth hospitalization.

Late preterm infants are not at increased risk for polycythemia, defined as a venous hematocrit level of more than 65%. Newborns at risk for polycythemia include those who are large for gestational age or small for gestational age, infants born to mothers with preeclampsia or diabetes, and those who undergo delayed cord clamping or are born at high altitude.

[ABP 3.B.5. Late preterm infant]

REFERENCE

1. Phillips RM, Goldstein M, Hougland K, et al. Multidisciplinary guidelines for the care of late preterm infants. *J Perinatol.* 2013;33(suppl 2):S5–S22.

85. ANSWER: C

Unrealistic expectations and an uncertain prognosis contribute to increased aggressive, unnecessary treatments at the end of life. It is imperative that such therapies be a central part of any discussion of end-of-life care. Involving patients early in these discussions is recommended. It is not necessary, and could in fact be detrimental, to hold off engaging a child in advance care planning until his or her prognosis is certain. Cultural differences can have a significant impact on end-of-life discussions. To make a proper decision about advance directives, physicians need to gain trust and build a relationship with the patient and family. Always acknowledge the emotions surrounding the discussion, for families and patients as well as the healthcare team. Ensure adequate time for these conversations and avoid distractions as much as possible. Although the cost of providing care and the financial burden on the family are significant concerns, they are not central to advance directive planning.

[ABP 4.F. Palliative and end-of-life care]

REFERENCE

1. Zinner SE. The use of pediatric advance directives: a tool for palliative care physicians. *Am J Hosp Palliat Care.* 2008;25(6):427–430.

86. ANSWER: B

This patient's history of claustrophobia in the context of being in an enclosed MRI machine for up to 1 hour warrants minimal sedation, also known as anxiolysis. With minimal sedation, the patient is still awake and able to interact, but is relaxed. Moderate sedation involves depressed consciousness, but the patient retains the ability to protect their airway and respond to commands or touch. With deep sedation, the patient may only respond to painful stimuli and may need airway support. With general anesthesia, the patient is completely unarousable and requires full airway and ventilatory support.

[ABP 5.N. Procedural sedation]

87. ANSWER: D

This patient has bulimia nervosa, a disease characterized by cycles of binge-eating behaviors and inappropriate compensatory behaviors, such as inducing vomiting or abusing diuretics, laxatives, or other medications, accompanied by a preoccupation with body image. There is ample data demonstrating that pharmacotherapy in combination with psychotherapy is most effective in reducing bingeing and purging behaviors, as well as achieving disease remission. Fluoxetine, a selective serotonin reuptake inhibitor (SSRI), is the first-line choice for both efficacy and side-effect tolerability. Second-line treatments include other SSRIs, such as sertraline. Third-line treatments include tricyclic antidepressants (e.g., nortriptyline) and topiramate. Bupropion has been associated with seizures in bulimic patients and is contraindicated. Olanzapine is not a treatment for bulimia nervosa.

[ABP 2.F. Eating disorders]

88. ANSWER: B

Midline skin pits over the sacral and coccygeal areas, commonly known as sacral dimples, have historically been considered possible cutaneous stigmata of occult spinal dysraphisms (OSDs) such as spina bifida or tethered cord syndrome. MRI is the definitive diagnostic tool for OSD, but ultrasound is also a highly sensitive and specific cost-effective alternative in newborns because the cartilaginous posterior spinal structures provide excellent acoustical windows. However, mounting evidence has questioned the utility of routine spinal imaging for sacral dimples. Several reviews have found that simple sacral dimples with no other abnormal history or physical examination findings have an extremely low positive predictive value for OSD. A simple sacral dimple is located on midline, within the gluteal cleft, no more than 2.5 cm above the anal verge, and not associated with hypertrichosis, hemangioma, or a caudal appendage (i.e., tail or pseudotail). A sacral dimple that meets all of these criteria indicates a 0–0.2% probability of OSD requiring future medical or surgical intervention, so imaging and subspecialty consultation or follow-up are not indicated. The apparent depth of the dimple and whether or not its end can be visualized do not affect that risk.

[ABP 3.B.8. Congenital anomalies]

REFERENCE

1. Ben-Sira L, Ponger P, Miller E, Beni-Adani L, Constantini S. Low-risk lumbar skin stigmata in infants: the role of ultrasound screening. *J Pediatr.* 2009;*155*(6):864–869.

89. ANSWER: C

Sialorrhea due to oromotor dysfunction is a common complication in children with cerebral palsy. Oral secretions can be anterior, causing visible drooling, or posterior, causing pooling in the posterior oropharynx. Behavioral and pharmacological interventions should be trialed before moving on to surgical interventions. The most commonly used medications for sialorrhea are the anticholinergic drugs glycopyrrolate and scopolamine. Doses should start low given the side-effect profile, then increased every 5 to 7 days until symptoms are controlled or the maximum dose is reached. Restricting free water intake in developmentally delayed children puts them at risk for severe dehydration. Botulinum toxin injections are often helpful and should be trialed before moving on to surgical interventions. However, they should only be repeated every 3–6 months; side effects include irritation at the injection site, hematoma, thickened secretions, and aspiration risk. Finally, while behavioral interventions with a speech therapist are critical first steps, they have not been effective for this child. Speech therapists can perform an oromotor assessment (focused on head control, positioning, mouth closure, and swallowing) and provide oral-motor exercises.

[ABP 4.D. Symptom management]

REFERENCE

1. Fairhurst CB, Cockerill H. Management of drooling in children. *Arch Dis Child Educ Pract Ed.* 2011;*96*(1):25–30.

90. ANSWER: E

This infant appeared well initially, developed respiratory distress and cyanosis during feeding, and was once again well appearing on subsequent examination while crying vigorously. This is a classic presentation of choanal atresia, which occurs in 1 out of 7000–8000 live births. That classic presentation is very rare because two-thirds of cases are unilateral, so those infants still have an open airway even when they cannot breathe through their mouth. Choanal atresia is definitively diagnosed by identifying no connection between the nasopharynx and the larynx on either CT or endoscopy; however, the diagnosis can be ruled out if a suction catheter can be passed more than 3.2 cm through each nostril. Since the newborn only became cyanotic during feeding and returned to baseline while crying immediately afterward, choanal atresia is much more likely than a cardiac defect, so pulse oximetry is not indicated. This incident was so severe and so early in life that it is unlikely to be due to a swallowing defect. The severity of the event and the ease and safety of passing nasal suction catheters also make it inappropriate to simply wait and observe for a recurrence.

[ABP 3.B.3. Respiratory distress]

REFERENCE

1. Myer CM 3rd, Cotton RT. Nasal obstruction in the pediatric patient. *Pediatrics.* 1983;*72*(6):766–777.

91. ANSWER: A

The adolescent in this vignette had no previous sleep problem, and it is common to have a disordered sleep cycle with prolonged hospitalization. She has circadian rhythm disturbances for which sleep hygiene and melatonin can be beneficial. Sleep logs aid parents and patients who may otherwise struggle with recall. This patient's sleep quality could certainly improve with optimization of pain control. A psychologist may help a patient cope with the stresses of her hospitalization. Other helpful interventions include maintaining daily routines, avoiding naps, "winding down" before bedtime, creating a quiet and dark setting for sleep, reducing media exposure, and rescheduling medications due at night.

[ABP 4.A. Symptom management]

REFERENCE

1. Stickland A, Clayton E, Sankey R, Hill CM. A qualitative study of sleep quality in children and their resident parents when in hospital. *Arch Dis Child.* 2016;*101*(6):546–551.

92. ANSWER: A

The AAP published an updated circumcision policy statement in 2012, which was then endorsed by the American College of Obstetricians and Gynecologists and the American Urological Association. Recommendations came from a multidisciplinary Task Force on Circumcision (TFOC), which first performed a systematic review of current literature. They concluded that there was sufficient evidence of health benefits that outweighed the risks of the procedure. These benefits included prevention of urinary tract infections; acquisition of human immunodeficiency virus; transmission of some sexually transmitted infections, including HPV; and penile cancer.

Although the TFOC concluded that benefits outweigh risks, they also stated that the benefits were not enough to formally recommend circumcision to all newborns but enough to make it accessible if a parent chooses. Circumcision in the neonatal period is associated with lower risks and greater benefits. Contraindications to routine circumcision include congenital abnormalities such as hypospadias, congenital chordee, or penoscrotal fusion (webbed penis). Penile nerve blocks are safe and the preferred analgesia for newborn circumcision. Sugar water and swaddling are only appropriate as analgesic adjuncts.

[ABP 3.B.8. Congenital anomalies]

REFERENCE

1. American Academy of Pediatrics Task Force on Circumcision. Circumcision policy statement. *Pediatrics.* 2012;*130*(3):585–586.

93. ANSWER: A

Short-bowel syndrome (SBS) is a malabsorptive disease process that occurs as a result of significant bowel resection or other defects limiting bowel absorption. Patients with SBS due to bowel resection often require fluid and nutritional support in the postoperative period to help them maintain appropriate growth and development. There are a number of different factors that can help predict a patient's odds of attaining full enteral autonomy. Residual bowel length is the factor that confers the greatest chance to achieve enteral autonomy. Patients with less than 20 cm of viable bowel are less likely to be able to be weaned from intravenous fluids and TPN. While the preservation of the ileocecal valve is another known positive predictive factor, its impact is less than residual bowel length. The presence of a primarily ileal bowel remnant is favored given the ileum's ability to adapt following resection.

[ABP 4.B. Feeding and nutrition]

94. ANSWER: B

The possibility of a disorder of sexual development (DSD) should be considered in any newborn with bilateral undescended testicles, severe hypospadias, or a unilateral undescended testicle with any degree of hypospadias and/or micropenis (phallus length of <1.9 cm). A newborn with a male phallus and bilateral undescended testicles could be a genetic female with congenital adrenal hyperplasia. These newborns are often unable to regulate their electrolytes, which can lead to hyponatremia, hyperkalemia, and shock. In addition to electrolyte monitoring, these patients should also have a karyotype and 17-hydroxyprogesterone level.

Abdominal imaging has shown to have poor diagnostic performance for locating undescended testicles with both false-positive and false-negative results. If this patient had a unilateral undescended testicle without any abnormality of the phallus, then watchful waiting with the pediatrician for 4–6 months would be appropriate. Spontaneous descent is unlikely to occur after 6 months.

[ABP 3.B.8. Congenital anomalies]

REFERENCES

1. Kolon TF, Herndon CD, Baker LA, et al. Evaluation and treatment of cryptorchidism: AUA guideline. *J Urol.* 2014;*192*(2):337–345.
2. Wu WJ, Gitlin JS. The male genital system. *Pediatr Rev.* 2020;*41*(3):101–111.

95. ANSWER: B

Patients with SLE are at risk for developing acute neuropsychiatric manifestations, including strokes, seizures, and rarely psychosis. Of the answer choices listed, lupus psychosis is the most likely diagnosis in the setting of active SLE. Initial treatment includes pulse steroids as well as steroid-sparing therapies such as cyclophosphamide or mycophenolate. It is important to rule out other potential etiologies for acute psychosis. While steroids may induce psychotic features, this is typically only seen in patients who are on prolonged courses of higher-dose steroids and would not be expected after one dose of methylprednisolone. A patient with a stroke is unlikely to have a normal neurologic examination. Acute intoxication is also less likely in a monitored hospital setting, but should be ruled out. A primary psychiatric disorder is rare in children.

[ABP 2.B. Acute aggression and psychosis]

96. ANSWER: E

Lactogenesis I, or secretory initiation, occurs during pregnancy and includes the development of the synthetic capacity of the mammary glands. Lactogenesis II, or secretory activation, starts after delivery and is the process by which mature milk is produced. The onset of lactogenesis II, or "milk coming in," usually occurs at approximately 2–3 days postpartum. After birth, the delivery of the placenta triggers a drop in progesterone levels, which is a major factor in initiation of lactogenesis II. Other important factors are increasing prolactin levels and oxytocin release that is triggered by the infant suckling at the breast. Risk factors for delayed lactogenesis II include primiparity; cesarean delivery; hormonal factors such as maternal diabetes, obesity, or hypothyroidism; early use of non–breast milk fluids such as formula; and low breastfeeding frequency.

[ABP 3.B.9. Newborn feeding (including breastfeeding and formula feeding)]

97. ANSWER: C

The best answer is PEG tube contrast study to assess for gastric outlet obstruction, which is a rare and commonly misdiagnosed complication of gastrostomy tube placement. Migration and malposition of the gastrostomy tube can lead to gastric outlet obstruction, which is clinically characterized by nausea, postprandial nonbilious vomiting, epigastric pain, early satiety, abdominal distention, and insidious weight loss due to mechanical obstruction in the distal stomach, pylorus, or duodenum. Simple adjustment of the gastrostomy tube after visualization by a PEG tube contrast study can resolve the problem without unnecessary imaging, medical tests, and aggressive interventions. A trial of clear fluids would not identify the underlying problem and could worsen the patient's vomiting.

[ABP 5.E. Gastric tube replacement/change]

REFERENCE

1. Shah J, Shahidullah A. Gastric outlet obstruction due to malposition of gastrostomy tube: a rare and commonly misdiagnosed condition. *Case Rep Gastroenterol*. 2020;*14*(2):409–414.

98. ANSWER: D

Hepatitis B virus is highly infectious, and chronic infection may lead to cirrhosis and liver cancer. To eliminate perinatal transmission of hepatitis B virus, routine testing of maternal HBsAg and universal newborn management protocols have been implemented. Infants born to mothers with a negative HBsAg who are more than 2 kilograms should receive their first hepatitis B vaccine dose within the first 24 hours of life. Infants born to mothers with a positive HBsAg should be given both the hepatitis B vaccine and HBIG within the first 12 hours of life. If a mother's HBsAg is unknown, it is recommended to give the hepatitis B vaccine within the first 12 hours of life as this intervention is recommended regardless of the mother's status without any additional risk to the newborn. If the mother's status is able to be tested, then the HBIG can be held for a maximum of 7 days until the results return.

[ABP 3.B.4. Neonatal infections, including exposure]

REFERENCES

1. Committee on Infectious Diseases; Committee on Fetus and Newborn. Elimination of perinatal hepatitis B: providing the first vaccine dose within 24 hours of birth. *Pediatrics*. 2017;*140*(3): e20171870.
2. Schillie S, Vellozzi C, Reingold A, et al. Prevention of hepatitis B virus infection in the United States: recommendations of the Advisory Committee on Immunization Practices. *MMWR Recomm Rep*. 2018;*67*(1):1–31.

99. ANSWER: C

The patient's symptoms are consistent with dumping syndrome, a known complication following fundoplication. Dumping syndrome occurs when gastric contents are delivered more quickly to the small intestine due to the decrease in gastric volume after a fundoplication. The rapid delivery of undigested carbohydrates to the small intestine induces a hyperinsulinemic response that results in subsequent hypoglycemia. Addition of complex carbohydrates such as cornstarch to the formula can help prevent rapid glucose shifts and mitigate the risk of hypoglycemia in patients with dumping syndrome. Slowing the rate of feeds and transitioning to continuous feeds represent alternative strategies for managing dumping syndrome. Venting the gastrostomy tube may improve discomfort associated with feeds following fundoplication but would not address dumping. Similarly, there is no evidence to support antimotility agents such as loperamide or bowel rest for management of dumping syndrome.

[ABP 4.B. Feeding and nutrition]

100. ANSWER: C

Per evidence-based algorithms developed by the American Heart Association, neonatal resuscitation is required when a newborn is preterm or emerges with poor tone or apnea. Initial steps of resuscitation include warming, drying, stimulating, positioning the airway, and suctioning the mouth and nares as needed. If by 1 minute of life the newborn remains apneic/gasping or the heart rate is less than 100 beats/min, the most important and effective next step is providing PPV. In infants born at more than 35 weeks' gestation, it is reasonable to start with 21% FiO_2 and titrate up if needed. PPV for younger infants may start with an FiO_2 as high as 30%. If the heart rate does not improve to more than 100 beats/min after effective ventilation, then chest compressions should begin at a compression-to-ventilation ratio of 3:1.

[ABP 3.A. Delivery room care, including resuscitation and stabilization]

REFERENCE

1. Wyckoff MH, Aziz K, Escobedo MB, et al. Part 13: neonatal resuscitation: 2015 American Heart Association guidelines update for cardiopulmonary resuscitation and emergency cardiovascular care. *Circulation*. 2015;*132*(18 suppl 2):S543–S560.

101. ANSWER: B

Somatic symptom disorder should be suspected when a patient's somatic symptoms are associated with excessive thoughts, behaviors, or feelings about the symptoms and cause significant distress. The most common presenting symptoms are abdominal pain and headache. While somatization can be a developmentally appropriate coping mechanism, it should be considered a disorder when it impairs a patient's function, as it clearly does in this case. Cognitive behavioral therapy (CBT) is the most effective treatment for SSD and can provide active coping strategies related to the experience of illness. The diagnosis of SSD does not require identification of a trigger or stressor.

Patients with SSD tend to present to medical rather than mental healthcare settings. Bullying is a major risk factor for the development of SSD. Although a thorough evaluation is important, unnecessary, invasive evaluations risk reinforcing the patient's disability and increasing the family's anxiety.

[ABP 2.D. Psychosomatic disorders]

102. ANSWER: A

In a study comparing 40% dextrose gel massaged into the buccal mucosa to feeding alone, dextrose gel was found to be more effective in reversing neonatal hypoglycemia. The use of dextrose gel did not increase the risk of rebound (within 6 hours) or recurrent hypoglycemia or other adverse effects, and thus observation in NICU is not required after its use. The study intervention included administration of dextrose gel followed by feeding. Therefore, it is important to consider dextrose gel as an adjunct to feeding for treatment of hypoglycemia, rather than a singular intervention.

[ABP 3.B.1. Hypoglycemia]

REFERENCE

1. Harris DL, Weston PJ, Signal M, Chase JG, Harding JE. Dextrose gel for neonatal hypoglycaemia (the Sugar Babies Study): a randomised, double-blind, placebo-controlled trial. *Lancet*. 2013;*382*(9910):2077–2083.

103. ANSWER: E

The best position for the tip of a peripherally inserted central catheter (PICC) is in the distal third of the superior vena cava or at the cavoatrial junction. Tip position should be confirmed with fluoroscopy or postprocedure radiograph. This radiograph shows the PICC line turning superiorly into the superior vena cava and needs to be repositioned by the PICC team. Malposition is one of the most common postinsertion complications of placement of a PICC. Ultrasound of the neck can be helpful to confirm placement during the procedure but would be redundant in this scenario given the malposition is confirmed by radiograph. Other complications from vascular access devices are listed in the Table 2.8.

Table 2.8 COMPLICATIONS OF VASCULAR ACCESS DEVICES

ON INSERTION	POSTINSERTION
Air embolism	Accidental dislodgement
Arrhythmias	Arrhythmias
Arterial puncture	Catheter-associated bloodstream infections
Brachial plexus injury	Catheter migration/displacement
Cardiac tamponade	Device occlusion
Failure of placement	Extravascular infusion
Guidewire knotting/fracturing	Infection at exit site
Hematoma at insertion site	Line fracture with or without embolization
Hemorrhage	Right atrial perforation with or without cardiac tamponade
Hemothorax	Subcutaneous extravasation
Phrenic nerve injury	Venous perforation
Pneumothorax	Venous stenosis
Thoracic duct trauma with or without chylothorax	Venous thrombosis
Tricuspid valve damage	
Vascular damage (e.g., perforation/dissection)	

[ABP 5.K. Peripheral intravenous placement]

REFERENCE

1. Scott-Warren VL, Morley RB. Paediatric vascular access. *BJA Education*. 2015;*15*(4):199–206.

104. ANSWER: E

Delayed cord clamping (DCC) for 30–60 seconds in term and preterm infants who do not require immediate resuscitation has been recommended by the American College of Obstetricians and Gynecologists and endorsed by the American Academy of Pediatrics.

During the initial breaths of the newborn, placental transfusion increases due to the negative intrathoracic pressure from lung inflation. The additional blood that transfers to the newborn increases their hemoglobin level as well as their iron stores, which has been shown to reduce iron deficiency anemia in the first year of life. In preterm infants, DCC is associated with decreased rates of necrotizing enterocolitis, need for blood transfusion, and intraventricular hemorrhage. An initial barrier to implementing DCC was concern for hypothermia. Data show that thermoregulation is maintained with DCC, but there are no statistically significant data that it decreases hypothermia. DCC has not been shown to increase risk of polycythemia, but there is a slight increase in the number of infants who have hyperbilirubinemia who meet criteria for phototherapy.

[ABP 3.A. Delivery room care, including resuscitation and stabilization]

REFERENCE

1. American College of Obstetricians and Gynecologists' Committee on Obstetric Practice. Delayed umbilical cord clamping after birth: ACOG Committee opinion, number 814. *Obstet Gynecol.* 2020;*136*(6):e100–e106.

105. ANSWER: E

Functional neurological symptom disorder (also known as conversion disorder) should be considered when a patient's symptoms and functional deficits suggest a physical disorder that is not supported by a thorough examination. Conversion disorder is most common between the ages of 10 and 15 years and is more common in girls than in boys. Symptoms are most commonly related to motor function and can include paralysis, discoordination, and gait disturbances as well as loss of speech or any combination of these symptoms. Sensory symptoms may also be present. A complete and reassuring physical examination is required. Patients with conversion disorder are typically less bothered by their disability than expected (known as "la belle indifference"). While comorbid depression and anxiety or a history of sexual abuse indicate a less-favorable prognosis, over 85% of patients will achieve full recovery. Favorable outcomes are more likely with early diagnosis.

[ABP 2.D. Psychosomatic disorders]

106. ANSWER: C

Rarely, infants exposed in utero to selective serotonin receptor inhibitors (SSRIs) may experience neonatal adaptation syndrome. There are competing theories on whether this is a result of withdrawal from the medication or from overstimulation of the infant's serotonergic system. Symptoms include tremors; gastrointestinal disturbances (exaggerated sucking, poor feeding, regurgitation); sleep disturbance; high-pitched cry; hypertonicity; and tachypnea. Although some studies have shown that exposure to SSRIs increases the risk of persistent pulmonary hypertension of the newborn, the majority of neonatal adaptation syndrome cases are transient and mild. It is important for pediatric providers to recognize neonatal adaptation syndrome from SSRI exposure so they can provide appropriate monitoring, supportive care, and reassurance and avoid unnecessary diagnostic work-up.

[ABP 3.B.6. Drug exposure/neonatal abstinence syndrome (NAS)]

REFERENCES

1. Levinson-Castiel R, Merlob P, Linder N, Sirota L, Klinger G. Neonatal abstinence syndrome after in utero exposure to selective serotonin reuptake inhibitors in term infants. *Arch Pediatr Adolesc Med.* 2006;*160*(2):173–176.
2. Nörby U, Forsberg L, Wide K, Sjörs G, Winbladh B, Källén K. Neonatal morbidity after maternal use of antidepressant drugs during pregnancy. *Pediatrics.* 2016;*138*(5):e20160181.

107. ANSWER: A

This patient's symptoms are consistent with paroxysmal sympathetic hyperactivity, also known as dysautonomia. It can be seen in patients with a history of severe traumatic brain injury that disrupts autonomic regulation. Symptoms may overlap with a broad differential of life-threatening diagnoses such as sepsis. All of the answer choices listed may be used in the treatment of dysautonomia. Clonidine is used as an abortive and preventive medication. Morphine and lorazepam are typically used as abortive therapies, while gabapentin and baclofen are used as preventive therapies.

[ABP 4.A. Symptom management]

108. ANSWER: B

Bilirubin is transported to the liver primarily bound to albumin. Bilirubin metabolism is facilitated by the uridine diphosphoglucuronosyltransferase (UGT) enzyme, which conjugates bilirubin that is taken up by hepatocytes. Once conjugated, bilirubin is excreted in bile. Newborns have low activity of the UGT enzyme, which causes a buildup of unconjugated bilirubin. In addition, poor feeding contributes to increased enterohepatic circulation of bilirubin, allowing it to be reabsorbed through the intestinal mucosa back into circulation. During phototherapy, light changes the conformation of bilirubin into lumirubin, which can be excreted in both the urine and bile without being conjugated.

[ABP 3.B.2. Neonatal hyperbilirubinemia]

REFERENCE

1. Maisels MJ, McDonagh AF. Phototherapy for neonatal jaundice. *N Engl J Med.* 2008;*358*(9):920–928.

109. ANSWER: C

Lumbar puncture (LP) failure or the inability to obtain cerebrospinal fluid (CSF) is common—as high as 50%. The traditional landmark technique for performing an

LP involves palpation of the iliac crests and interspinous space, ensuring the needle enters the L3 to L4 or L4 to L5 interspace. Bedside ultrasound allows for identification of these major landmarks, including the subarachnoid space and conus medullaris. It can therefore provide evidence of sufficient CSF within the canal space, identify a hematoma from previous LP attempts, and recognize anatomic cord abnormalities before insertion of the needle. Several studies reported higher success rates with the use of ultrasound compared to the landmark technique. In a systematic review and meta-analysis study, the use of ultrasound improved LP success with an odds ratio (OR) of 2.22 (95% CI = 1.03 to 4.77) in favor of the ultrasound-assisted group and led to fewer traumatic LPs, shorter time to successful LP, fewer mean needle passes, and lower patient pain scores.

Although fluoroscopy-guided lumbar puncture is another option to increase success of a difficult LP, it increases hospital costs and unnecessary hospital days if the patient could be discharged based on CSF results in the ED. There is currently no standard or recommended optimal position for children undergoing lumbar punctures. Changing providers to complete the procedure would not guarantee an increased success rate and could increase parental distress. There is insufficient data to indicate that hydration of the infant increases the success of an LP.

[ABP 5.A. Lumbar puncture]

REFERENCE

1. Gottlieb M, Holladay D, Peksa GD. Ultrasound-assisted lumbar punctures: a systematic review and meta-analysis. *Acad Emerg Med.* 2019;26(1):85–96.

110. ANSWER: A

This infant is showing signs of successful breastfeeding, including adequate voiding and stooling patterns, minimal jaundice, and weight loss that is not excessive. Continued breastfeeding should be encouraged. Frequent feeding based on feeding cues is recommended, and breast emptying at least 8–12 times a day will facilitate more robust milk supply. Formula supplementation is not medically necessary given the normal parameters described in the vignette. If supplementation were required, volumes should be consistent with normal volumes of colostrum produced and the infant's stomach size. Typical volumes in the first few days of life for a healthy term breastfed infant are 5–15 mL per feeding at 24–48 hours of age and 15–30 mL at 48–72 hours of age. Timing of pumping breast milk for storage is always an option based on a family's needs. If direct feeding is going well, there is no need to recommend pumping at this time as breastfeeding sessions will effectively maintain and increase maternal supply as needed.

[ABP 3.B.9. Newborn feeding (including breastfeeding and formula feeding)]

REFERENCE

1. Kellams A, Harrel C, Omage S, Gregory C, Rosen-Carole C. ABM clinical protocol #3: supplementary feedings in the healthy term breastfed neonate, revised 2017. *Breastfeed Med.* 2017;12:188–198.

111. ANSWER: C

Conduct disorder (CD) involves repetitive, persistent behaviors violating the basic rights of others or major age-appropriate societal norms, typically manifesting as aggression toward people or animals and disregard for property. This should be differentiated from oppositional defiant disorder (ODD), which can be diagnosed in a child less than 8 years of age who demonstrates defiant, disobedient, and hostile behaviors toward authority figures. This child is too old to present with ODD, and his behavior is more consistent with CD. The mainstay of treatment for CD is cognitive behavioral therapy. An individual with intermittent explosive disorder demonstrates reactions that are out of proportion to the trigger and may include violence, temper tantrums, lack of impulse control, and property destruction. Pyromania is an irresistible urge to set fire. Although this patient has a history of setting fires, his overall presentation is more consistent with CD. Bipolar disorder in children presents with episodes of mania or hypomania beyond what would be expected for a child's developmental stage, as well as recurrent episodes of major depression. There is not enough information in this vignette to support this diagnosis.

[ABP 2.B. Acute aggression and psychosis]

112. ANSWER: C

Pierre Robin sequence is a craniofacial abnormality syndrome characterized primarily by micrognathia, either as a single condition or in association with other genetic disorders. Upper airway obstruction and obstructive sleep apnea (OSA) are common conditions associated with this disorder. Given this patient's nighttime snoring, apnea, and desaturations, it is reasonable to suspect OSA. Nasal mask or nasal pillows are the form of CPAP best tolerated in children because they allow unrestricted ability to speak and cough. One possible complication of chronic CPAP in children, particularly with nasal interfaces, is the development of midface hypoplasia due to the constant pressure on the maxillary bones. This can be prevented by providing as loose a fit as possible without resulting air leak, switching between face mask and nasal interfaces over time, and monitoring closely with regular follow-up.

In otherwise-healthy children, most OSA is due to adenotonsillar hypertrophy, and tonsillectomy and adenoidectomy (T&A) is the first-line treatment. However, in patients with craniofacial abnormalities, T&A is unlikely to be useful; positive pressure ventilation via CPAP is an effective nonsurgical treatment option. Patients at high risk of aspiration should generally not receive home CPAP as it can enhance the risk of aspiration and worsen gastric distension from the airflow. It is always preferable to perform a sleep study to properly diagnose OSA and tailor therapy prior to the initiation of home positive pressure ventilation. BiPAP is usually recommended for patients with hypoventilation, central apnea, or accumulation of carbon dioxide; there is no evidence of any of those issues in this patient. Small children often require a slow and thoughtful approach to introducing the mask, taking into account the child's age and developmental level. Positive reinforcement can be helpful. The use of restraints is not recommended.

[ABP 4.C. Device and technology management, including complications]

113. ANSWER: C

This patient has a physical examination concerning for congenital syphilis. While most neonates are asymptomatic at birth, signs and symptoms of early congenital syphilis typically appear within the first several weeks of life and include lymphadenopathy, hepatomegaly, rhinorrhea ("snuffles"), a maculopapular rash particularly on the palms and soles, and jaundice. Virtually any organ system may be involved; other findings include, among others, skeletal abnormalities, pneumonia, fever, and ophthalmologic manifestations. Congenital syphilis may be suspected based on a maternal history of a positive rapid plasma reagin (RPR) test during pregnancy, but this patient's mother did not receive prenatal care. According to the Centers for Disease Control and Prevention, workup for any infant with an examination consistent with congenital syphilis, regardless of maternal testing, should include at a minimum a serum nontreponemal test such as an RPR or Venereal Disease Research Laboratory (VDRL) test; complete blood count with differential; and cerebrospinal fluid VDRL, cell count, and protein. Other studies, such as liver function tests, chest radiograph, long-bone radiographs, head ultrasound, and ophthalmologic examination, may be indicated at a provider's discretion. Concurrent maternal testing for syphilis is generally also recommended to aid in the diagnosis. None of the other diagnostic testing options would aid in the diagnosis of congenital syphilis. Treatment consists of penicillin G intravenously for 10 days.

If a mother of a newborn is known to have a positive RPR and the infant has a normal examination:

1. Determine the results of a maternal treponemal test such as fluorescent treponema antibody absorption (FTA-ABS) as false-positive RPRs are common
2. In the case of a positive maternal treponemal test, investigate whether or not the mother has been adequately treated (with penicillin at least 4 weeks prior to delivery and without evidence of reinfection or relapse)
3. If the maternal treatment criteria *have not* been met, the newborn should be treated. If they *have* been met, the infant should have an RPR/VDRL test and be treated if titers are greater than fourfold the maternal titer.

[ABP 3.B.4. Neonatal infections, include exposure]

REFERENCE

1. Workowski KA, Bolan GA; Centers for Disease Control and Prevention. Sexually transmitted diseases treatment guidelines, 2015. *MMWR Recomm Rep.* 2015;*64*(RR-03):1–137.

3.

HEALTHCARE SYSTEMS: SUPPORTING AND ADVANCING CHILD HEALTH

QUESTIONS

1. You are working with a group of physicians across the United States to establish a clinical practice guideline (CPG) for evaluating and managing acute asthma exacerbations. You have created a multidisciplinary group without any conflicts of interest. The team has done a thorough systematic review of the literature and has agreed on a list of recommendations. Which of the following is considered a best practice for the creation of CPGs?

    A. Publish the guidelines on a private server
    B. Avoid making statements about the strength of recommendations
    C. Include all interested participants in the guideline development group (GDP)
    D. Establish best practices from evidence of consensus review and case reports
    E. Plan to update the guidelines regularly

2. The quality and safety committee at your hospital has noticed an increase in preventable adverse events over the last few months. After a series of root cause analyses, it was determined that several of these errors were related to communication gaps that occurred during resident handoff in the evening. Which of the following interventions related to the handoff process has been shown to decrease the rate of preventable adverse events?

    A. Implementing separate handoffs for interns and senior residents
    B. Moving the location of handoffs from workrooms to the ward nurses' stations
    C. Implementing a standardized handoff model for verbal handoffs
    D. Implementing a handwritten handoff tool
    E. Teaching residents to read the patient's history of present illness during their handoffs

3. You are evaluating the utility of a new diagnostic test for a novel disease. Due to the utmost importance of early detection, you want to find a cutoff value that detects all patients with the disease with as few false-positive cases as possible. Based on the receiver operating characteristic (ROC) curve seen in Figure 3.1, which of the following values should be used as the cutoff?

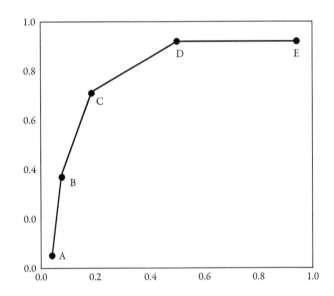

Figure 3.1 ROC curve for new diagnostic test

    A. A
    B. B
    C. C
    D. D
    E. E

4. A recent adverse event occurred on the pediatric ward of a hospital due to an incomplete medication reconciliation form. Review of the hospital's recent quality data shows that the form is completed within 24 hours of admission for only 60% of patients. A pediatric hospitalist is asked to lead a quality improvement initiative to improve timely completion of the medication reconciliation forms. The improvement team has developed a draft aim statement as follows: "Our quality improvement team will increase completion of medication reconciliation forms within 24 hours from 60% to more

than 85%." Which of the following should be added in order to optimize this aim statement?

A. "By creating an electronic prompt alert"
B. "Over the next 9 months"
C. "Through multiple tests of change"
D. "Without increasing medication errors"
E. "With assistance from the pharmacy staff"

5. A healthy, fully immunized 8-month-old male presents to the emergency department in December with a 2-day history of rhinorrhea and cough. He is afebrile with normal vital signs for age. He has fine crackles and mild wheezing in the lung bases on auscultation. The infant is alert, interactive, feeding well, breathing comfortably, and actively moving all extremities. Which of the following is the best next step?

A. Admit for observation on continuous pulse oximetry
B. Administer a bronchodilator
C. Discharge from the emergency department with return precautions
D. Obtain a chest radiograph
E. Obtain complete blood count

6. A Caucasian teenage daughter of a wealthy donor family receives peritoneal dialysis for end-stage renal failure. She has a history of depression with previous suicide attempts, drug abuse, and defiance of her parents. Another patient, a Hispanic teenage boy from south-central Los Angeles who often misses healthcare visits because of lack of access to transportation is hospitalized in the intensive care unit with severe heart failure associated with idiopathic cardiomyopathy. Both patients require transplant of their respective failing organs. The girl is offered a kidney transplant, but the boy is disqualified for a heart transplant due to his history of missing healthcare visits and lack of insurance coverage for posttransplant care. Which ethical principle is the predominant concern?

A. Beneficence
B. Nonmaleficence
C. Justice
D. Autonomy
E. Negligence

7. An infant is born at 36 weeks' gestational age weighing 3.1 kg to a mother who is hepatitis B surface antigen (HBsAg) negative. The mother states that he has been feeding and latching well and has urinated and stooled once. The parents ask you what you recommend regarding the hepatitis B (Hep B) vaccine. Which of the following is correct?

A. Hepatitis B vaccination and immunoglobulin should be given prior to discharge
B. Hepatitis B vaccination should be given within 24 hours of birth
C. The mother's HBsAg is negative, so the newborn can receive the first vaccine with the primary care provider
D. Since the infant is preterm, he should wait until he is 37 weeks corrected gestational age
E. The complete hepatitis B vaccination series is a two-dose series

8. A pediatric hospitalist is reviewing clinical characteristics in 40 patients with bronchiolitis who received treatment with high-flow nasal cannula (Table 3.1). Which patient characteristic is presented as an ordinal variable?

Table 3.1 PATIENT CHARACTERISTICS OF INPATIENTS WITH BRONCHIOLITIS RECEIVING HIGH-FLOW NASAL CANNULA

PATIENT CHARACTERISTIC	N = 40
Sex	
Male	25 (63%)
Female	15 (37%)
Age in months (median, interquartile range)	5 (2, 9)
Race	
White	26 (65%)
Black	8 (20%)
Asian	2 (5%)
Other	4 (10%)
Pediatric Early Warning Score (PEWS) (mean ± standard deviation)	3.2 ± 2.4
Pediatric Respiratory Score (PRS)	
Mild (<7)	10 (25%)
Moderate (7–9)	20 (50%)
Severe (10–12)	10 (25%)

A. Sex
B. Age
C. Race
D. PEWS
E. PRS

9. You receive a call from a newborn nursery nurse who suspects that a newborn has features of Down syndrome. The baby was born at 38 weeks via vaginal delivery and her weight is appropriate for gestational age. The nurse describes the baby as having low tone, upslanting palpebral fissures, a large tongue, a single palmar crease, and a positive sandal sign. The baby is 3 hours old, has demonstrated a good latch at the breast, and is breathing

comfortably in room air. You examine the baby and agree with the nurse that there are several features consistent with Down syndrome. Which of the following is the best approach to communicating with the family?

A. After sitting with the family, ideally with both parents present, express that you are sorry, but that you suspect their baby has trisomy 21, also known as Down syndrome
B. Since the baby is doing well, defer discussion of your suspicion of Down syndrome until after genetic testing is back
C. After congratulating the family on the birth of their baby, share that you have some news that may be unexpected
D. After discussing your suspicion for Down syndrome, explain to the family that you will need to coordinate transfer to the neonatal intensive care unit for further workup and management
E. Obtain a point-of-care glucose and echocardiogram prior to discussing your diagnostic suspicion

10. A 2-day-old female is born at term to a 28-year-old mother who tested positive for opioids on urine toxicology. The mother has been taking methadone for the past month for chronic pain. The newborn has been crying excessively for more than 10 minutes. She also demonstrates an exaggerated Moro reflex and has jitteriness throughout her body. What is the best next step in management for this newborn?

A. Score the patient on the Finnegan Neonatal Abstinence Scoring System (FNASS)
B. Start the patient on methadone
C. Tell the mother to stop breastfeeding
D. Attempt to breastfeed the baby for at least 10 minutes
E. Give the patient morphine

11. You are caring for a 2-year-old female with global developmental delay, chronic lung disease, epilepsy, and oromotor dysphagia requiring gastrostomy feeds who has been admitted for aspiration pneumonia and hypoxia. On day 3 of hospitalization, her hypoxia has resolved, and she is breathing comfortably. During the hospitalization, her enteral bolus feeding regimen was changed from four times a day to five times a day to minimize risk of aspiration at home by providing less volume of formula per feed. You plan on discharging the patient to complete a 10-day course of clindamycin to treat her aspiration pneumonia. Of the following, which intervention is most likely to decrease the patient's risk of readmission?

A. Teaching and then asking the patient's mother to verbalize the new feeding regimen and antibiotic duration at time of discharge

B. Faxing the patient's complete inpatient medical record to the patient's primary care provider (PCP)
C. Ordering a nasopharyngeal suction machine to be delivered to the patient's home
D. Encouraging the patient's mother to purchase a pulse oximeter to monitor the patient's oxygen saturations at home
E. Scheduling a follow-up appointment with the patient's PCP in 3 weeks

12. There has been a recent increase in nosocomial infections in a children's hospital. A pediatric hospitalist is leading the hospital effort to increase adherence to handwashing guidelines to decrease the rate of such infections. Of the following, which is the most appropriate process measure?

A. Surveys testing staff knowledge of hospital handwashing guidelines
B. Average amount of time spent between patient encounters
C. The number of nosocomial infections per month
D. The proportion of witnessed handwashing opportunities compliant with guidelines
E. The rate of nosocomial infections per 1000 patient-days

13. Your mentee was recently offered a leadership opportunity chairing a hospital committee. This is her first leadership experience, and you teach her a common leadership organizing principle called goals, roles, procedures/processes, and interpersonal relationships (GRPI). Which of the following statements about GRPI is correct?

A. Roles and responsibilities are best established on a rolling basis
B. Interpersonal relationships encourage groupthink
C. It is most productive to establish interpersonal relationships prior to goals, roles, or procedures/processes
D. Procedures/processes include openly dealing with conflict
E. GRPI principles do not apply to leading clinical teams

14. A 15-year-old female is admitted to the pediatric floor with community-acquired pneumonia. The pediatric hospitalist performs a confidential assessment of the patient with her parents outside of the room. The adolescent discloses to the hospitalist that she has been sexually active with one male partner in the last year. She has not used birth control, and her partner has "sometimes" used condoms during intercourse. She reports no vaginal discharge and states that her menses

are regular and her last menstrual period began approximately 3 weeks ago. In addition to a urine pregnancy test, which are the best next steps for the care of this patient?

A. Perform screening for human immunodeficiency virus (HIV), gonorrhea, and chlamydia, and counsel the patient on safe sex
B. Perform screening for gonorrhea and chlamydia, and counsel the patient on safe sex; perform HIV testing after obtaining consent from the adolescent
C. Counsel the patient to see her primary care doctor after hospital discharge for workup of sexually transmitted infections
D. Perform screening for human immunodeficiency virus (HIV), gonorrhea, and chlamydia, and counsel the patient on safe sex after getting consent from the patient's parents
E. Treat the patient empirically with single doses of oral azithromycin and intramuscular ceftriaxone

15. You have been asked to put together a curriculum to help interns learn how to manage cross-cover calls on the busy hospital medicine service at your institution. After reviewing the pediatric professional society recommendations for graduate medical education, you search the relevant online databases for examples of similar curricula at other institutions. What is the best next step?

A. Identify learning objectives for the curriculum
B. Select educational strategies to employ in the curriculum
C. Determine what barriers may exist for implementation
D. Perform a targeted needs assessment of residents on service
E. Outline evaluation metrics for learners and the curriculum

16. A 17-year-old female is admitted to the hospital for malodorous, bloody diarrhea in the setting of recurrent otitis media, for which she was recently treated with amoxicillin/clavulanic acid. On admission, her *Clostridium difficile* toxin test result is positive, and she is started on therapy. On reviewing her orders the following day, the pediatric hospitalist discovers that the patient has been receiving metformin 250 mg every 6 hours rather than the intended metronidazole. Of the following, which intervention might have made this error less likely to occur?

A. Admission medication reconciliation
B. Avoidance of "do not use" abbreviations

C. Coined names
D. Leading zeroes
E. Tall man lettering

17. A pediatric hospitalist is asked to examine the length of stay at her institution and summarize it compared to other hospitals. Based on the distribution in Figure 3.2, which of the following is the most appropriate summary statistic(s) for this data set?

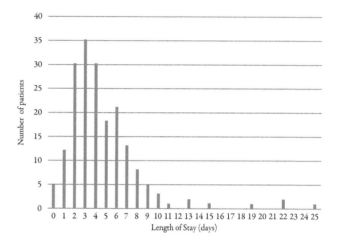

Figure 3.2

A. Mean and standard deviation
B. Mean and standard error
C. Median and interquartile range
D. Median and range
E. Mode

18. You are leading family-centered rounds (FCR) where the nurse, learners, and family are together for rounding and share in the control of the discussion. The senior resident mentions several patients on your census for the day for whom they think FCR should be avoided, suggesting table rounds for these patients instead. Which of the following statements about FCR is true?

A. Table rounds should be performed in lieu of FCR for patients admitted with suicidality
B. FCR should be avoided for patients admitted with concern for nonaccidental trauma
C. For non–English-speaking families, it is best to table round and then have one person update the family after rounds with an interpreter
D. FCR have been shown to lead to better resource utilization
E. A best practice of FCR is for the learner to present the patient formally to the team without the family present and then to follow up with the family to clarify questions

19. An 18-year-old male with a history of global developmental delay, restrictive lung disease requiring oxygen support, and severe dystonia is admitted for respiratory distress. He is typically admitted two or three times per year with similar symptoms. On the day of discharge, you are discussing the patient's follow-up plan with his mother. She tells you that the patient's pediatric pulmonologist has suggested transitioning to an adult medicine provider, but that she is hesitant to transition from providers who have known her son his entire life. What is the best advice to provide to the patient's mother about transitioning to adult medicine providers?

A. Advise that the patient should continue to be seen by pediatric providers
B. Provide the patient's mother with a list of adult pulmonologists in the area
C. Elicit the mother's concerns about transitions to adult care and offer to discuss the matter with the patient's pediatrician
D. Encourage the mother to discuss the matter with the patient's pediatrician at their next visit
E. Explain that you think it is in the best interest of the patient to be seen by adult providers

20. Several hospitalists have recently been concerned about delayed laboratory results for their patients leading to an inability to make a timely, informed decision about the patient's care. They would like to assemble a team to examine what factors may be causing the delayed laboratory tests. Which of the following tools would be most appropriate to identify multiple potential root causes that are impacting laboratory delay?

A. Scatter diagram
B. Pareto chart
C. Key driver diagram
D. Fishbone diagram
E. Process map

21. When creating a clinical practice guideline for your hospital, you encounter many different types of research articles with varying treatment and management recommendations. Which of the following types of research article provides the highest quality of evidence for the development of your clinical practice guideline?

A. Randomized controlled trial
B. Observational study
C. Case report
D. Cohort study
E. Case series

22. Several members of your hospitalist group are burned out, and you are motivated to implement changes to encourage well-being. Your division director is supportive of making improvements and asks you to use change management theory. Which of the following is part of Kotter's eight-step model for successful change efforts?

A. Create a sense of convenience
B. Form a bottom-up approach
C. Produce long-term wins
D. Create a new culture
E. Remain focused on one project

23. A 13-year-old boy is admitted with Hodgkin lymphoma. After one round of chemotherapy, the boy refuses further medical treatment. Instead, he plans to treat himself using alternative medicine in accordance with his religious and cultural beliefs. You find the boy to have low health literacy and an inadequate understanding of his disease or the consequences of treatment alternatives. The boy's parents insist on his right to administer his own alternative treatments and refuse additional chemotherapy. The oncology team considers chemotherapy to be standard of medical care and predicts 80%–95% likelihood of full remission if completed. What is your best next step?

A. Call Child Protective Services to enforce chemotherapy administration
B. Consult Spiritual Care to explore the family's religious traditions
C. Arrange a multidisciplinary family meeting
D. Discharge the patient from the hospital because he is not following medically recommended protocols
E. Consult psychiatry to determine if the patient has decision-making capacity

24. You have been asked to give grand rounds at your institution on the importance of evidence-based clinical guidelines in pediatrics. You plan to talk about four clinical guidelines used by your pediatric hospital medicine department as examples. In preparation for your talk, you outline the learning objectives for the session. Which of these learning objectives represents the highest cognitive level of learning?

A. Describe the importance of evidence-based clinical guidelines
B. Design an evidence-based clinical guideline for their clinical area
C. Assess whether a proposed clinical guideline meets the standards outlined in the talk
D. Implement one of four clinical guidelines examples when caring for a patient
E. Define evidence-based medicine

25. A hospitalist wants to trial a new intervention to reduce length of stay for bronchiolitis. The hospitalist develops a hypothesis: "In children under 2 years old with bronchiolitis, daily treatment with a nasal decongestant will change length of stay." The hospitalist's null hypothesis is that the length of stay in children either receiving or not receiving the treatment is the same. Which statistical value gives the maximum probability of committing a type 1 error (false positive; rejecting the null hypothesis when it is true)?

A. Alpha
B. Beta
C. Power
D. Effect size
E. Sample size

26. A pediatric hospitalist is asked to help decrease the time between asthma patients being clinically ready for discharge and vacating their room. Of the following, which represents a potential key driver?

A. Begin the discharge preparation 4 hours prior to meeting discharge criteria (i.e., after the first 4-hour cycle of albuterol)
B. Delays in prescription delivery from the pharmacy to the bedside
C. Improve the asthma discharge process
D. Increase the proportion of patients discharged within 90 minutes of receiving their second 4-hour albuterol from 30% to 75% within 6 months
E. Seven-day readmission rate among patients discharged for asthma exacerbation

27. A previously healthy, full-term, 5-day-old male was admitted to your service 1 day ago for hyperbilirubinemia and phototherapy. He was born at 39 weeks via a nontraumatic spontaneous vaginal delivery to a 30-year-old woman with a B+ blood type and negative group B *Streptococcus* screen. There were no complications prior to delivery or during the newborn nursery time period. The newborn's blood type is also B+. He has been exclusively breastfeeding and is at 9% weight loss from birth. Triple phototherapy was started for a bilirubin of 21 mg/dL at 85 hours of life. Overnight, the baby had a normal examination except for jaundice and was able to feed 8–10 times. He urinated six times and stooled twice. This morning his bilirubin is 14 mg/dL at 98 hours of life with a phototherapy threshold for low-risk patients of 20 mg/dL. What is the best next step in management?

A. Continue phototherapy
B. Stop phototherapy and discharge the patient with follow-up
C. Begin exchange transfusion
D. Stop phototherapy and repeat bilirubin in 8 hours in the hospital
E. Obtain complete blood count and reticulocyte count

28. You are a member of your hospital's diversity, equity, and inclusion committee working to address implicit biases in patient care. When considering change management, which of the following is a common error to organizational change that is important to avoid?

A. Creating a strong change team
B. Declaring victory too soon
C. Celebrating short-term wins
D. Anchoring changes in the culture
E. Allowing for personnel turnover

29. A 15-year-old girl is hospitalized due to acute lymphoblastic leukemia. She develops anemia after receiving the initial round of chemotherapy but refuses a blood transfusion despite your recommendation and against her parents' wishes. The patient is previously healthy except for a pregnancy termination at age 12 years. The patient has been living with her aunt for the past 3 years; she has not spoken to her parents during this time but they have not legally lost custodial rights. After embracing her aunt's faith last year, the patient was baptized to the Jehovah's Witness denomination and has been very active in the church. In your evaluation of the patient, you find her to be mature and to have a full understanding of her decision. The state has a mature minor law. After an ethics committee review, the hospital administrator discusses decision-making with you. What is the best course of action?

A. Consult social work
B. Follow the parents' wishes to transfuse
C. Obtain transfusion consent from the aunt
D. Acquiesce to the patient's wishes because she meets emancipated status based on her prior pregnancy
E. Acquiesce to the patient's wishes because she is a mature minor

30. A new test is being developed to detect a novel respiratory virus. Of the 100 patients tested, 60 had the virus. Only 50 of these patients tested positive, while 5 patients who did not have the virus also tested positive. What are the sensitivity and specificity of this test?

A. 0.88, 0.83
B. 0.83, 0.88
C. 0.91, 0.78
D. 0.78, 0.91
E. 0.78, 0.88

31. A pediatric hospitalist serving on a patient safety committee is asked to make a recommendation to decrease the number of central line–associated blood stream infections in the hospital. Of the following choices, which intervention, in isolation, is most likely to produce safe, sustainable improvement?

A. A lecture series to nurses and physicians on prevention of hospital-associated infections
B. A required daily form listing indications for a central line that suggests discontinuation if the patient does not meet those indications
C. An updated hospital policy consistent with evidence-based strategies to prevent hospital-associated infections
D. An automated order to discontinue all central lines after 7 days
E. Safe placement checklists on all central line supply kits

32. You are in the newborn nursery about to discharge a healthy 2-day-old baby who was born full term and has passed both the hearing and congenital heart defect screens. The parents inquire about home cardiorespiratory monitoring as they are worried about sudden infant death syndrome (SIDS). What is the best statement to tell them?

A. "Home cardiorespiratory monitors are safe and have been proven to reduce SIDS."
B. "Your baby is at low risk for SIDS and does not require rooming in for the first 6 months of life."
C. "In-hospital cardiorespiratory monitoring has been shown to detect infants at risk of SIDS."
D. "Apnea of greater than 30 seconds is more common in full-term infants."
E. "Home cardiorespiratory monitors have not been found to decrease the incidence of SIDS."

33. During a faculty development workshop, you discuss the importance of a learning environment that prioritizes psychological safety. When you mention this to a colleague, they admit that they are not familiar with that term. How would you best describe for them what it means to provide psychological safety in the clinical learning environment?

A. Minimizing the risk that learners will be exposed to microaggressions and overt discrimination from patients
B. Ensuring learners are appropriately trained in de-escalation techniques to apply if a patient suddenly becomes aggressive
C. Providing structured debrief sessions for learners after emotionally difficult cases or rotations
D. Allowing learners to express their opinions and concerns about a case without concern that their evaluations might be negatively impacted
E. Mindfully adhering to a traditional hidden curriculum in the clinical learning environment

34. Table 3.2 below provides the pre- and posttest scores for a residency class after receiving training on auscultation of murmurs. Which of the following is the most appropriate test to determine whether there is a statistically significant improvement?

A. Chi-square test
B. One-way analysis of variance (ANOVA) test
C. Paired t test
D. Rank sum test
E. Two-group t test

35. A resident you are working with asks you if there are any questions that you can ask a parent to gauge their health literacy. Which of the following is a validated question to assess health literacy?

A. "What is the highest level of education you have completed?"
B. "Do you prefer to read books or listen to audio books?"
C. "If a doctor told you to take a medicine BID, would you know what that meant?"

Table 3.2 RESIDENT SCORES ON MURMUR AUSCULTATION PRE- AND POSTTEST

RESIDENT	PRETEST	POSTTEST	RESIDENT	PRETEST	POSTTEST
1	57	74	6	59	67
2	57	80	7	35	53
3	32	51	8	18	47
4	60	73	9	32	52
5	58	60	10	71	73

D. "How often do you have someone help you read hospital materials?"

E. "How often do you find it difficult to interpret a graph or chart?"

36. A 3-year-old boy is admitted to the pediatric floor for hypoxemia in the setting of influenza pneumonia. On performing the history with a certified Spanish interpreter, the resident discovers that the child has not seen a primary care provider or other clinician since he was 12 months old. The family recently immigrated from Honduras, and the family speaks Spanish at home. The mother states that the child has approximately 15 words and does not speak in sentences. Aside from crackles in the right lower lobe on lung auscultation, the rest of the physical examination is normal. During the examination, the resident notes that the child makes repetitive flapping movements with his arms. Of the following, which is the most appropriate next step to care for this child?

A. Perform an electroencephalogram (EEG)
B. Obtain brain magnetic resonance imaging (MRI)
C. Screen for hearing, vision, and lead toxicity
D. Obtain serum immunoglobulins
E. Obtain serum mercury level

37. You are caring for a 5-month-old female who is admitted for pyelonephritis at a community hospital. Two hours after admission, the patient develops tachycardia, delayed capillary refill time, and lethargy. There is no improvement in symptoms despite ceftriaxone and 60 mL/kg normal saline fluid boluses. You are concerned that she is developing septic shock and plan to transfer her to the nearest pediatric intensive care unit. Which of the following strategies would be the most effective at preventing a handoff error during this transfer of care?

A. Call the receiving physician from the patient's bedside
B. Send detailed written documentation of your history and physical examination with the patient
C. Ask the receiver to "read back" the antibiotics and fluid volume the patient has received
D. Complete your handoff before asking the receiver if they have questions
E. Include an assessment of the patient's illness severity at the conclusion of your handoff

38. An adverse event recently occurred during a patient transfer from the medical floor to the pediatric intensive care unit (PICU) of a children's hospital. In the subsequent root cause analysis, the hospital quality improvement team discovered that the adverse event was related to poor handoff communication. After settling on an aim statement and measures, the team decided to design and test a handoff checklist to use for each floor-to-PICU transfer for 1 week. The checklists were collected at the end of the first week. Which of the following is the most appropriate next step in the team's Plan-Do-Study-Act (PDSA) cycle(s)?

A. Plan: the specifics of a subsequent PDSA cycle in which the checklist is implemented permanently
B. Do: continue to collect checklists from each floor to PICU transfer over the next week
C. Study: evaluate the checklists completed and interview participants in the transfers
D. Act: discuss with the quality improvement team in general terms what the next test of change should be
E. Spread: work to implement a similar checklist for emergency department-to-PICU transfers

39. A fully immunized 10-year-old female presents to the emergency room with a progressive productive cough for 1 week and 2 days of fevers. She has tachypnea to 32 breaths per minute, subcostal retractions, and an oxygen saturation of 88%. She is noted to have a consolidation in her left lower lobe on chest radiograph. She is admitted for oxygen support and started on antibiotics. She has no known allergies and is fully immunized. Which of the following antibiotic choices is correct for this child?

A. Clindamycin
B. Ceftriaxone
C. Ampicillin
D. Azithromycin
E. Vancomycin

40. Your institution currently screens caregivers for social determinants of health in the clinic setting. You would like to expand screening to the inpatient units of the hospital. What are examples of social determinants of health that might be included in the screening survey?

A. Access to healthcare services
B. Exposure to toxic substances
C. Surrounding parks and green spaces
D. Type of school setting
E. Housing and community design

41. A 4-month-old breastfeeding infant is hospitalized for failure to thrive. His parents recently immigrated to the United States and have not yet established medical care. On examination, the patient appears frail, thin, and irritable and has moderate jaundice. The social worker informs you that the father divulged his personal status as human immunodeficiency virus (HIV)

positive but asked to keep that information private from the mother. The mother asks why you are testing for HIV as she has no known exposures. How should you respond?

A. Do not share the father's HIV status and explain that unusual causes of failure to thrive need to be considered
B. Share the father's HIV status because he is not your patient and therefore does not have protected privacy rights
C. Share the father's HIV status because the mother is owed information to protect her from communicable disease
D. State that HIV testing is standard for infants with failure to thrive
E. Order HIV testing for mom

42. You are working with a resident on an educational session on hand hygiene and wish to study its effectiveness with the hopes of publishing your results. Which of the following represents the highest level of educational outcomes?

A. An observed handwashing audit 3 months later showing increased compliance with appropriate hand hygiene technique among those who had taken the session compared to an audit a month before the session
B. An immediate post-session survey with a 100% response rate showing that 55% of the learners felt more confident in their ability to effectively wash their hands
C. An immediate post-session survey with a 55% response rate showing that 100% of the learners felt more confident in their ability to effectively wash their hands
D. A survey administered 6 months later with 100% response rate showing that the learners scored significantly better than their presession assessment
E. A randomized controlled trial where learners who attended the session had a significantly greater increase in performance from a pre- to immediate post-session assessment than those who did not attend the session

43. A hospitalist is investigating the use of prophylactic anticoagulation in patients with medical complexity and prolonged hospitalization. Currently, about half of the attendings in her group routinely start anticoagulation. The researcher reviewed all patients on the complex care service over the past 5 years and recorded the incidence of deep venous thrombosis (DVT) in this population.

	DVT	NO DVT	TOTAL
Prophylaxis	10	90	100
No prophylaxis	30	70	100

What is the *relative risk* of developing DVT in the treated population compared to those who did not receive prophylaxis?

A. 0.20
B. 0.26
C. 0.33
D. 3.00
E. 3.86

44. You are participating in your institution's quality committee meeting. The committee is developing a plan to increase delivery of high-value care and reduce costs. Which of these has been shown to be effective in reducing costs for both the hospital and the patient?

A. Reducing nonclinical support staff
B. Reducing the number of operating rooms
C. Encouraging patient-physician conversations about cost
D. Encouraging variability in physician prescribing practices
E. Reducing clinic visit time from 15 minutes to 10 minutes

45. A pediatric resident receives a call from the emergency department (ED) about an admission. Thus far this evening, the team has admitted three infants with bronchiolitis, a child with pneumonia, a teenager with chronic abdominal pain, and a child with osteomyelitis. The ED doctor says, "Well, I've got another wheezer for you. Six-month-old girl, been sick for a couple days." The residents head in to see the patient and talk with her family. What cognitive bias does this handoff put the residents at risk for at this moment?

A. Omission bias
B. Visceral bias
C. Outcome bias
D. Availability bias
E. Aggregate bias

46. You are caring for a 6-month-old boy born at 24 weeks' gestation admitted to the hospital for failure to thrive. He is diagnosed with oromotor dysphagia due to prematurity and has a nasogastric tube placed for bolus feeds. He gains adequate weight in the hospital, and you plan to discharge him after educating the family on care and maintenance of the tube. Of the following, which

is the best next step to ensure a successful transition to the outpatient environment and ongoing success with weight gain?

- A. Refer the patient to your hospital's surgery clinic for gastrostomy tube placement
- B. Discuss the patient's discharge plan with the primary care provider (PCP) and inquire about services available in the provider's office
- C. Tell the family you will call them in 1 week to check on the patient's status
- D. Refer the patient to your hospital's occupational therapy clinic
- E. Refer the patient to a local nutritionist in the community

47. A pediatric hospitalist has developed a template to improve documentation of asthma severity and level of control. She has incorporated feedback from multiple providers on the template and has successfully used a paper version of it for five patients. A reasonable next step would be to

- A. Discuss the aims of the project with multiple stakeholders to ensure buy-in
- B. Find a volunteer to use the template three to five times over the next 2 weeks
- C. Place a request to incorporate the template into the electronic medical record
- D. Share the template with her division for others to use going forward
- E. Use the template herself consistently over the next 2 weeks

48. A 14-week-old male presents to the emergency department for an episode of "blue color" around his lips and face and a pause in his breathing while being held by his father. The parents report that this is the first time it has happened. The father, who is not a trained provider, started performing cardiopulmonary resuscitation (CPR) at about 30 seconds. The event completely resolved within 1 minute. Otherwise, he is vaccinated, healthy, and growing appropriately. In the emergency room, he is well appearing, alert, and awake without respiratory distress. His vitals are temperature 37°C, heart rate 120 beats per minute, respiratory rate 33 breaths per minute, and oxygen saturation 99%. He was born at 33 weeks' gestation and was in the neonatal intensive care unit for 3 weeks while feeding and gaining weight. What is the best next step in management?

- A. Educate caregivers and discharge with close follow-up
- B. Obtain laboratory testing, including complete blood count and blood culture

- C. Admit the patient for observation
- D. Prescribe medications for gastroesophageal reflux
- E. Discharge with home cardiorespiratory monitoring

49. You are caring for a hospitalized child with obesity and newly diagnosed type 2 diabetes. He is accompanied by his mother, who breaks down crying as you begin to council her on the importance of her child losing weight. She lets you know that she has been feeling overwhelmed since she and her husband were laid off from work in the past year. Their Supplemental Nutrition Assistance Program benefits are not enough to feed their family a nutritious diet. The family had to sell their car to help pay the bills, and she has to take at least two buses to get anywhere from her house. In discussing the difficulty of the case with your group, one colleague references "health in all policies." Of the following, which is the best definition of health in all policies?

- A. All policies should ensure the health of children
- B. Impact on health should be the primary consideration of all policies
- C. Improved health is a shared goal across all areas of government
- D. All decisions and actions in government policy determine health outcomes
- E. Health policy is part of all government policies

50. A 15-year-old girl with a history of pelvic Ewing sarcoma is hospitalized for pneumonia. Computed tomography (CT) of the chest, abdomen, and pelvis suggests recurrence of the tumor in her original site and new metastases in her lungs and vertebrae. The parents note that the patient had major depression and prevalent thoughts of suicide during her first course of cancer treatment and still shows signs of post-traumatic stress disorder and generalized anxiety. A multidisciplinary family meeting is held, in which the parents are informed that their daughter's predicted survival is 3 months. The parents demonstrate a full understanding of the prognosis and treatment options. They ask the clinical team not to reveal the likely recurrent sarcoma diagnosis and decide against further evaluation or cancer treatment. They want to sign a physician's order for life sustaining treatment (POLST) to limit life-sustaining measures with a goal of comfort care only and "do not resuscitate" (DNR) status. What is the best next step?

- A. Have a confidential meeting with the patient to inform her of her diagnosis
- B. Evaluate the patient for emotional and cognitive decision-making capacity to assist in emancipating her

C. Compel the family to move forward with surgical biopsy
D. Sign the POLST as requested and discharge the patient home with her parents under hospice care
E. Comfort the patient by telling her that her sarcoma is stable

51. A pediatric hospitalist is investigating the effect of total daily sodium consumption (Na, in g/d) on systolic blood pressure (SBP, in mm Hg) in overweight adolescents. While analyzing the results of an observational study she performed, she concludes that the best-fit linear regression line is

$$SBP = 5.73 \times Na + 108.7 \ (r^2 = 0.257)$$

The best interpretation of the reported r^2 value is

A. Of the variation in SBP, 25.7% is explained by knowing Na
B. For every g/d increase of sodium consumption, SBP is expected to increase by 0.257 on average
C. For every mm Hg increase of SBP, sodium consumption is expected to increase by 0.257 on average
D. There definitely is no statistically significant association between Na and SBP
E. There definitely is statistically significant association between Na and SBP

52. You are caring for a 2-year-old boy admitted to the hospital following a traumatic brain injury. Tracheostomy and gastrostomy tubes were placed during the hospitalization. You are working on educating the family on the patient's care in anticipation of discharge. However, the patient's mother and father are struggling with managing his tracheostomy and failed at replacing the patient's tracheostomy tube during a teaching session with the respiratory therapist (RT). The patient's parents verbalize that they feel "judged" by the care team and hospital staff for not being successful in tracheostomy education, and that they are under a lot of stress due to the financial burden of the patient's hospitalization and future care. Of the following, what is the best strategy to help improve the patient's discharge process?

A. Transfer the patient to a different physician team
B. Encourage the patient's parents to leave the hospital for several days to rest
C. Make a referral to Child Protective Services (CPS) out of concern for potential medical neglect
D. Coordinate a care conference with the parents, hospitalist, nursing staff, RT, and social worker to discuss the parents' concerns
E. Arrange for the parents to undergo tracheostomy education with a different RT

53. The quality improvement team of a children's hospital began a project to reduce the length of stay for patients admitted with asthma exacerbations. The team chose to measure the weekly average length of stay, in hours, demonstrated on the run chart in Figure 3.3. They are presenting the data to the leadership. Which of the following data points on the chart appropriately denotes the beginning of a trend in the data?

A. A
B. B
C. C
D. D
E. E

54. A previously healthy 15-year-old male is admitted to the hospital for fever and right femur tenderness and is diagnosed with osteomyelitis. He is started on 4 days of intravenous (IV) ceftriaxone and vancomycin and found to have methicillin-sensitive *Staphylococcus aureus* (MSSA) growing from his bone debridement. His initial C-reactive protein (CRP) was 10 mg/dL on

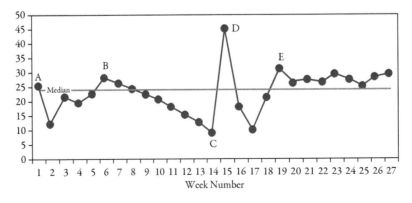

Figure 3.3 Run chart for asthma length of stay data

admission and has been 2 mg/dL for the past 2 days. He has been afebrile since the start of antibiotics and is now without tenderness or pain on his femur. He has no known drug allergies. What is the best next step?

A. Continue treatment on IV ceftriaxone and vancomycin
B. Transition to IV cefazolin
C. Stop vancomycin but continue ceftriaxone
D. Transition to oral cephalexin
E. Transition to oral clindamycin

55. You are taking care of a child whose mother is Spanish speaking only. You enter the room for family-centered rounds, and the resident caring for the child confirms that the mother requires Spanish interpretation. You remind the team that it is a professional responsibility and a Joint Commission standard to provide fluent translation services. Which of the following is a true statement about using interpreter services for caregivers with limited English proficiency?

A. Joint Commission requires that video remote interpretation services be available in the absence of a live interpreter
B. Although not formally required, it is best practice to document a patient's race/ethnicity, preferred language, and any communication needs
C. The pediatric patient or patient's sibling providing in person translation is preferable to video remote interpretation services
D. Prior to the encounter, the provider should prepare the interpreter for what will be discussed during the visit
E. During the encounter, the provider should address the interpreter directly and maintain eye contact with the interpreter

56. A 20-year-old young woman with a history of anorexia voluntarily presents for her fourth hospitalization after developing severe malnutrition with bradycardia and symptomatic orthostatic hypotension. She has agreed to have all details of medical assessment and treatment withheld from her, including vital signs, weight, laboratory values, calories offered or taken in, and names and doses of medications. As a high-achieving student at the local university, the patient is able to describe her disease accurately and understands the consequences of her choices. What is the ethical construct understood by the patient when she gives permission to withhold information from her?

A. Therapeutic privilege
B. Nonmaleficence

C. Lack of capacity
D. Respect for person
E. Human rights

57. While attending on the pediatric wards, you note the medical student on the team has been late to rounds the past 4 days, and his presentations are disorganized and incomplete, despite the fact that the senior resident gave him feedback yesterday. During his last presentation, he froze completely and turned bright red with embarrassment. What is the best next step regarding this struggling learner?

A. Carefully document his performance concerns for the clerkship director, using statements of fact rather than opinions
B. Ask the senior resident to talk with the student again to ensure he understands what the expectations are for rounds and presentations
C. Publicly praise the performance of the other medical student on the team to give the struggling student an example of a well-organized presentation
D. Sit down with the student after rounds to discuss expectations, explore any barriers he is experiencing, and work together to create a plan for performance improvement
E. To create psychological safety, avoid having the study student carry any patients the next day so that he can learn by observation without the stress of presentations

58. A new biomarker has been identified in cerebrospinal fluid (CSF) that may be able to identify bacterial meningitis. A researcher collected CSF from 100 selected patients, 50 of whom had bacterial meningitis and 50 of whom did not. They looked at the performance of the biomarker in these samples to identify meningitis. Which of the following test characteristics can be calculated and has the lowest value?

	HAS MENINGITIS	DOES NOT HAVE MENINGITIS
Biomarker positive	20	5
Biomarker negative	30	45

A. Negative predictive value
B. Positive predictive value
C. Prevalence
D. Sensitivity
E. Specificity

59. Your team is performing family-centered rounds with a patient, Tommy; his parents; and the nurse at the bedside. After rounds you wish to highlight effective communication skills, specifically the use of person-first language by the resident. Which of the following best exemplifies person-first language?

A. [Resident outside of the room to team] "Tommy is a 9-year-old boy with cystic fibrosis."
B. [Resident to patient] "Before we get started, Tommy, what do you want to make sure we talk about today?"
C. [Resident to patient] "Tommy, would you prefer we chatted with your parents in the room or in the hall?"
D. [Resident to nurse] "How did you think Tommy did last night?"
E. [Resident to Tommy's parents] "How does Tommy seem to be doing since we saw you last?"

60. A pediatrician at a rural clinic approximately 45 minutes away from your tertiary care center is evaluating a jaundiced 4-day-old male infant born at 37 weeks' gestation. The patient is otherwise asymptomatic, and his examination is nonfocal. He is breastfeeding every 2 hours for 10–15 minutes. The pediatrician has obtained a total serum bilirubin level of 19.1 mg/dL (indirect 18.6 mg/dL, direct 0.5 mg/dL). He calls to ask your advice on the patient's disposition. Of the following, what is the best advice to provide?

A. Transfer the patient to the nearest emergency department (ED) for further evaluation
B. Discharge the patient home with a biliblanket and follow-up in clinic the next day
C. Transfer the patient to the neonatal intensive care unit (NICU) at your hospital for admission
D. Transfer the patient to the general pediatrics floor at your hospital for admission
E. Ask the pediatrician to obtain a complete blood count (CBC) and Coombs test prior to determining disposition

61. A pediatric hospitalist is involved in a quality improvement project to increase the proportion of patients discharged with prescription medications delivered to the bedside. The quality improvement team has obtained baseline information and continues to track monthly data. Eight months ago, they implemented a new opt-out system for prescription delivery. The team is using a statistical process control chart to follow the progress of their outcome measure. Of the following,

which is the best interpretation of the data points marked in red on Figure 3.4?

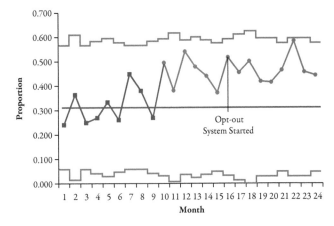

Figure 3.4 P-chart of Patients Discharged with Prescriptions Delivered to Bedside

A. Because all points are within the control limits, no change has occurred
B. The existence of common-cause variation demonstrates that an unexplained change has occurred
C. The existence of special-cause variation demonstrates that an unexplained change has occurred
D. The intervention successfully led to a shift in prescription delivery proportion
E. The intervention was associated with worsening of the outcome variable

62. A fully immunized 3-year-old female presents in January with rapid breathing in the setting of a month of polyuria, polydipsia, and weight loss. She is diagnosed with diabetic ketoacidosis and started on an insulin drip. She is transitioned to subcutaneous insulin, and her parents are educated about calories, carbohydrates, and administration. What vaccine(s) should be offered prior to discharge?

A. Pneumococcal 13-valent conjugate vaccine (PCV13)
B. Pneumococcal 23-valent polysaccharide vaccine (PPSV23)
C. Influenza vaccine
D. PCV13 and influenza vaccine
E. PPSV23 and influenza vaccine

63. On entering the room of an 8-month-old infant admitted with bronchiolitis, you find the mother praying over the child with an unbroken egg. The mother stops and explains that in her culture, it is believed that the egg can absorb negative forces and heal the child. The mother has been compliant with all of your recommendations. The premise that healthcare providers should be open and respectful of differences in each family's beliefs and values is considered which of the following?

A. Cultural competence
B. Cultural effectiveness
C. Cultural humility
D. Cultural sensitivity
E. Cultural awareness

64. You are putting together a workshop for hospital medicine fellows on the basics of medical education, including the concepts of assessment and evaluation, since you know people often confuse those terms. You plan to introduce the concepts with some real-life scenarios. Which of the following scenarios uses the terms correctly?

A. Giving a learner feedback about the technique they used for a lumbar puncture is evaluation
B. Assigning a grade to a medical student for their pediatrics rotation is assessment
C. Scoring residents on educational milestones every 6 months to inform their individualized curriculum is evaluation
D. Taking the pediatric hospital medicine boards at the end of fellowship is assessment
E. Using an entrustable professional activity (EPA)–based form to coach a resident on how they managed a specific patient admission is assessment

65. A pediatric hospitalist is reading a systematic review to determine the benefits of histamine-2 receptor antagonists (H2RAs) versus proton pump inhibitors (PPIs) in the acute management of gastroesophageal reflux disease. The review describes five articles on the subject as described in Table 3.3 below.

Based on the data, which is the biggest limit to performing meta-analysis on these studies?

A. Heterogeneity
B. Inadequate total number of subjects
C. Inclusion of observational studies

D. Incomplete outcome data
E. Selective reporting

66. You are nearing the end of your overnight shift, and your last admission is a 2-year-old boy born at 24 weeks' gestation admitted for pneumonia and hypoxia. He has had a cough and congestion for 3 days, and his parents brought him to the emergency department due to worsening work of breathing. A chest x-ray demonstrates a right lower lobe opacity, and he is started on ampicillin. His initial oxygen saturation is 87%, so he is placed on 0.5 L/min oxygen via nasal cannula, with improvement in his oxygen saturation to 95%. Since admission, his work of breathing has worsened, and he is now requiring 2 L/min via nasal cannula, with an oxygen saturation of 90%. You have ordered a repeat chest x-ray. You are preparing to hand off this patient to your colleague, who has just arrived. What is the best way to start this patient's handoff in order to reduce the chances of a handoff error?

A. "Please follow up on his x-ray as soon as possible"
B. "His symptoms started 3 days ago"
C. "He is an ex–24-week male with a right lower lobe pneumonia"
D. "He is our sickest patient, and I'm concerned he's getting worse"
E. "He has pneumonia and is on a nasal cannula at 2 L/min"

67. A pediatric hospitalist is serving on a hospital committee whose purpose is to improve the timeliness of morning laboratory results. By observing the process, the committee discovers that five phlebotomists each travel to multiple floors to perform laboratory draws. According to the principles of lean healthcare, this is an example of which type of waste?

A. Extra-processing
B. Inventory
C. Motion
D. Overproduction
E. Transportation

Table 3.3 SUMMARY OF LITERATURE REVIEW DATA

AGE	SCENARIO	OUTCOME	STUDY DESIGN	SUBJECTS	CONCLUSION
6–12 weeks	Reflux	Reported symptoms	Prospective cohort	150	No difference
12–17 years	Endoscopy	Bleeding	Randomized controlled trial	200	PPI is superior to H2RA
6–18 years	Peptic ulcer	Readmission	Retrospective cohort	80	H2RA is superior to PPI
12–17 years	Reflux	pH probe results	Case control	70	No difference
6–18 years	Nonsteroidal anti-inflammatory drug–induced gastritis	Bleeding	Prospective cohort	350	PPI is superior to H2RA

68. Your institution's chief executive officer has asked you to identify opportunities to increase high-value care and minimize healthcare waste. Which of these is unlikely to improve healthcare value?

    A. Implement a value-based payment model
    B. Create public reports of quality and cost
    C. Pay bonuses to providers based on highest relative value units (RVUs)
    D. Generate competition among healthcare systems to outperform each other
    E. Educate patients on what constitutes high-quality care at the lowest cost

69. In your division's journal club this month, you review a new study on disparities in pain control by race and ethnicity among children with fractures. Your group discusses the possibility of bias contributing to differences in pain management. Which of the following is a true statement about implicit biases?

    A. Implicit biases develop early in life and are a normal form of cognitive processing
    B. Healthcare professionals exhibit lower levels of implicit bias than the general population
    C. Implicit biases are defined as conscious attitudes or stereotypes that impact understanding, actions, and decisions
    D. Implicit biases are system-level factors contributing to health disparities
    E. Strategies to address implicit bias include focusing on patterns in groups of people and providing pro-group empathy

70. A physician at a children's hospital wants to know if children who take zinc supplements are less likely to be hospitalized for gastroenteritis (GE). They plan to review the medical records and survey the parents of all children admitted to their hospital with GE in the last year to ask if the children were taking zinc supplementation. Which of the following changes would improve the internal validity of the study?

    A. Calling the parents of all children with a prescription for zinc
    B. Excluding children who had traveled overseas
    C. Measuring blood samples to look for zinc levels
    D. Surveying the parents of all children in the city
    E. Testing the survey questionnaire prior to use

71. A 6-year-old patient with newly diagnosed asthma is ready for discharge. After reviewing the asthma action plan with the family, you ask the patient's father to tell you what symptoms should prompt an increase in the albuterol frequency. This is an example of which of the following?

    A. Discharge planning
    B. Discharge checklist
    C. Medication reconciliation
    D. Patient instructions
    E. Teach back

72. You are caring for a 3-year-old boy with right knee cellulitis at a community hospital. In the last few hours, the patient has had worsening swelling of the right knee. His temperature is 39.2°C, his heart rate is 150 beats per minute, his respiratory rate is 24 breaths per minute, he has a blood pressure of 90/50 mm Hg, and his oxygen saturation is 92%. His capillary refill time is 4 seconds. He is sleepy but awake, his lungs are clear to auscultation, and his breathing is nonlabored. You are concerned the patient has a septic joint and arrange for transfer to a pediatric intensive care unit 1 hour away. You broaden antibiotic coverage and order a bolus of 40 mL/kg of normal saline. A critical care transport team is en route and is 30 minutes away. While awaiting the transport team, what is the most appropriate next step?

    A. Begin bag-valve mask ventilation
    B. Place the patient on 100% nonrebreather face mask
    C. Place the patient on nasal cannula at 2 liters per minute
    D. Place the patient on a simple face mask
    E. Prepare for endotracheal intubation

73. The chief medical officer of your hospital recently attended your division meeting to discuss the hospital leadership's vision for patient safety and quality in the upcoming year. Her focus was on becoming an organization that will be preoccupied with failure, reducing variation of processes, providing timely feedback when processes are not performing, and allowing experts to design many processes throughout the hospital. She is hoping your group will be committed to these principles and assist in implementation. Which of the following best describes this hospital's approach to quality and safety?

    A. Human factors engineering principles
    B. Clinical operational principles
    C. High-reliability organization principles
    D. Just culture principles
    E. Situational awareness principles

74. You are teaching a course on high-value care to medical students. One of the students asks about the difference between charges and costs. Which is considered a charge and not a cost in healthcare?

A. Amount requested by the provider, displayed on the patient's hospital bill
B. Expense of delivering healthcare services to a patient
C. Amount an insurance company pays to a provider for services
D. Amount a patient pays for out-of-pocket services
E. Amount of a patient's hospital fees paid by a credit card

75. You are serving as a mentor for a junior faculty member in your department who is a person of color. She mentions that she has just been approached about helping lead a new diversity, equity, and inclusion (DEI) task force at your institution. She is debating whether to take on that role, especially given the other projects she is currently doing. How can your institution help prevent overburdening your mentee?

A. Ensure that mentoring students and residents to a publication remains the gold standard for evaluating trainee mentoring relationships
B. Develop rigorous requirements for what constitutes scholarly work to ensure that academic promotion remains meaningful
C. Promote a culture of service so that leading a task force that benefits the academic community is viewed as an honor
D. Ensure that protected academic time is given to physicians who serve on DEI committees
E. Advocate for the creation of an institution-wide statement of commitment to diversity, equity, and inclusion

76. A pediatric hospitalist is concerned that the overuse of cardiopulmonary monitoring is inappropriately increasing the length of stay among all pediatric inpatients. She performs a literature review and finds an article that describes a large, randomized, controlled noninferiority trial in which otherwise-healthy patients admitted to the hospital for cellulitis were randomized to receive either full cardiopulmonary monitoring or vital signs every 4 hours without further monitoring. The study's results showed no differences in transfers to the pediatric intensive care unit (PICU), and the length of stay was significantly lower for the group receiving vital sign monitoring only. Of the following, the hospitalist should be most concerned about which limitation of this study?

A. Causal inference
B. Generalizability
C. Internal validity

D. Power
E. Reliability

77. You are caring for a 5-year-old female with fever of unknown origin for 17 days. The patient continues to experience discomfort when febrile but does not have any additional symptoms. The hematologists have been consulted and are recommending a bone marrow biopsy. The rheumatologists have also been consulted, and they are recommending initiating a course of corticosteroids for a possible autoimmune disease. The infectious diseases team has been consulted as well, and they are recommending further testing for rare fungal infections prior to initiation of immunosuppression. Which of the following is the best next step?

A. Order the bone marrow biopsy as a malignancy is most likely to be deadly
B. Order corticosteroids as they are most likely to help the patient defervesce
C. Observe without further testing as a viral process is the most likely etiology
D. Engage the family in a conversation about the care options
E. Discuss the case at the hospitalist division case conference

78. A pediatric hospitalist is made aware of a serious safety event that occurred in the hospital in which a patient was inadvertently given a 10 times larger dose of a benzodiazepine than was intended. The patient developed apnea and required intubation and transfer to the pediatric intensive care unit. Of the following, which is the best quality improvement tool to employ in responding to this error?

A. Ask-request-concern-chain of command (ARCC)
B. Failure mode and effects analysis (FMEA)
C. Plan-Do-Study-Act (PDSA) cycle
D. Root cause analysis and actions (RCA2)
E. Situation-background-assessment-recommendation (SBAR) tool

79. A 20-month-old uncircumcised male presents with a fever of 39°C and pain when he urinates. On physical examination, he is healthy and well appearing. The urinalysis shows 2+ bacteria, 2+ leukocyte esterase, and 20 white blood cells per high-power field. The urine culture grows 100,000 colony forming units (CFU) per milliliter of *Escherichia coli*. He is started on oral cephalexin with resolution of his symptoms. What is the best next step in management for this patient?

A. No further intervention needed
B. Obtain a repeat urine culture

C. Obtain a renal and bladder ultrasound (RBUS)

D. Obtain a voiding cystourethrography (VCUG)

E. Stop oral cephalexin and administer intramuscular ceftriaxone

80. A hospitalist has noticed that children hospitalized for failure to thrive have increasingly been prescribed medium-chain triglyceride (MCT) oil. He wanted to investigate whether that treatment resulted in improved weight gain during hospitalization, shorter length of hospitalization, and improved weight gain 1 month posthospitalization. The hospitalist performed the study, with results as follows:

VARIABLE	MCT OIL N = 50	NO MCT OIL N = 50	P VALUE
Age in months (mean, SD)	4.2, 2.0	4.1, 1.9	.75
Prematurity (%, 95% CI)	60 (46, 72)	8 (3, 19)	<.001
Milk protein allergy (%, 95% CI)	36 (24, 50)	32 (21, 46)	.83
Male sex (%, 95% CI)	64 (50, 76)	68 (54, 79)	.83
Weight, in kilograms at admission (mean, 95% CI)	4.2 (3.8, 4.6)	5.1 (4.6, 5.6)	.02
Weight gain, in kilograms at 1-month follow-up (mean, 95% CI)	1.4 (0.6, 2.2)	0.3 (-0.5, 1.1)	.01
Length of stay in days (median, IQR)	5 (3, 7)	5 (3, 7)	.84

CI, confidence interval; IQR, interquartile range; SD, standard deviation.

The researchers concluded that the MCT oil did not affect length of stay but was associated with increased weight gain. Which of the following is a likely confounding variable in this study?

A. Age in months

B. Length of stay

C. MCT oil

D. Milk protein allergy

E. Prematurity

81. Which of the following is true of working with medical interpreters?

A. Requests for medical interpreters should come from patients, not from providers

B. Unlike medical translators, medical interpreters are trained to adapt what providers are saying in order to remove redundancies or inaccuracies and adjust for cultural nuances

C. For languages that are rarely spoken, hospitals can require patients and families to provide their own interpreter

D. Healthcare systems can provide testing options for providers to demonstrate fluency in order to be able to converse with families in that language without a medical interpreter

E. Certified deaf interpreters must demonstrate adequate hearing as part of their certification process

82. You are supervising a resident performing a lumbar puncture. She performs the time out, positions the child, locates appropriate landmarks, and prepares to insert the needle. You interrupt her and tell her to use the chlorhexidine prep to clean the skin before inserting the needle. She does this and completes the procedure. Which of the following "just culture" of patient safety behaviors best describes the resident's error during the procedure?

A. At-risk behavior

B. Lapse

C. Reckless behavior

D. Sentinel event

E. Slip

83. You are teaching an evidence-based medicine course for pediatric residents. Your curriculum consists of designing a clinical question, categories of evidence, validity of the evidence, and applying the evidence to specific patient populations. When evaluating a randomized controlled trial, which of the following is a threat to external validity?

A. Loss of subjects to follow-up, leading to missing data

B. Data collectors knowing random group assignments of study participants

C. Study participants not adhering to the assigned intervention

D. Lack of blinding of study participants to group assignments

E. Study sample is not representative of the general population

84. In a cohort study, researchers found that patients with asthma whose parents purchased air filtration systems have significantly lower pulmonary function tests than those whose parents have not. The researchers are concerned that filtration systems are causing worse pulmonary function in children with asthma. Which of the following would most conclusively disprove this idea?

A. Other studies have not demonstrated the same association

B. The researchers cannot think of a theory that would explain their results
C. The researchers were expecting the association to be in the opposite direction
D. The pulmonary function tests were performed prior to filtration purchase
E. There is only a weak association between filtration systems and pulmonary function

85. A third-year medical student is rounding with the inpatient pediatric team on his first day on the pediatric clerkship. What is the most effective and learner-centered way to engage this student?

A. Assign him a paper to read about a great bread-and-butter diagnosis that one of the patients on the team has
B. Have him shadow the first day so he is more comfortable with the routine and engage him by asking directed questions about pathophysiology
C. Encourage him to ask you and the senior residents questions about the different patients on the team and ensure there is time to do so during rounds
D. Ask him to prepare a 5-minute talk on a pediatric topic of his choice to share with the team tomorrow
E. Allow him the opportunity to demonstrate his competence by having him care for several medically complex patients

86. A pediatric hospital has incidentally discovered two separate serious safety events. It was found that neither event was reported within the hospital's error-reporting system. A pediatric hospitalist serving on the patient safety committee has been asked to investigate ways to increase timely identification of patient safety events. The change most likely to identify a broad range of specific errors is implementation of which of the following?

A. Automatic review of all patient deaths
B. Daily huddle with key questions to each unit
C. Easier error-reporting system
D. Education of clinical staff
E. Electronic trigger tool

87. A 5-year-old male presents to the emergency department (ED) after a bicycle accident about 15 minutes ago. He hit his head on the concrete while wearing a helmet. He has been acting normally and did not lose consciousness. On physical examination, he is well appearing, alert, talking, and moving normally with a normal neurologic examination. His skull has no signs of fracture, no hematoma, no retroauricular or periorbital bruising, and no hemotympanum. His Glasgow coma score is 15. His mother denies vomiting or headache. What would you recommend to the ED team?

A. Observe in the ED and monitor for worsening symptoms
B. Obtain computerized tomography (CT) of the head without contrast
C. Obtain a CT of the head with contrast
D. Admit for overnight monitoring
E. Obtain magnetic resonance imaging (MRI) of the brain

88. You work at a community hospital that has several pediatric rooms on floors with adults. In response to a surge in COVID-19 in the community, the hospital institutes a no visitor policy. You are called by the emergency department in the middle of the night to admit a 3-day-old breastfeeding infant with hyperbilirubinemia with a bilirubin of 22 mg/dL. The mother is not vaccinated against COVID-19 as she is concerned about what she has read online about the vaccine. She becomes tearful when she is told about the new visitor policy. Which of the following is the best action to take regarding this admission?

A. Admit the baby without the mother and provide a hospital-grade pump for her to use
B. Admit the baby without the mother and, with her permission, transition to donor breastmilk or formula for the duration of the hospitalization
C. Admit the baby to the hospital, allow the mother to stay with the infant if she screens negative for infectious symptoms, and plan to discuss the hospital policy with administration in the morning
D. Contact risk management to guide decision-making prior to agreeing to admit the infant
E. Use open-ended questions to explore the mother's concerns regarding the vaccine

89. A hospitalist on the intestinal rehabilitation co-management team is interested in reducing the number of central line–associated bloodstream infections (CLABSI) at their hospital. Table 3.4 below summarizes the chart review the hospitalist performed on patients with short-gut syndrome seen over the past year. What was the incidence rate of CLABSI in the study (per central line-year)?

A. 0.083
B. 0.105
C. 0.400
D. 1.000
E. 1.250

90. A pediatric hospitalist is hired to be the medical director of a six-bed general pediatrics unit within a community hospital. A team is convened to create the processes and policies for medication administration

Table 3.4 CENTRAL LINE INFECTIONS IN PATIENTS WITH SHORT GUT SYNDROME

PATIENT	JAN	FEB	MAR	APR	MAY	JUN	JUL	AUG	SEP	OCT	NOV	DEC	CENTRAL LINE INFECTIONS	MONTHS WITH CENTRAL LINE
1	X	X	X^a	X									1	4
2					X^a	X	X	X	X^a	X	X	X	2	8
3													0	0
4			X	X						X	X	X	0	5
5	X	X	X^a	Died									1	3
6					X	X	X						0	3
7		X					X	X	X	X	X	X	0	7
8	X	X	X	X	X	X	X	X	X	X	X	X	0	12
9		X^a											1	1
10				X	X	X	X	X		X	X		0	7
Total													5 infections 4 patients	48 (4 years)

X, Central line in place.

^a Central line infection.

within the new unit in order to prevent harm to patients. Which of the following quality improvement tools will best meet the needs of this administrative team?

A. Cause-and-effect diagram
B. Failure mode and effects analysis
C. Key driver diagram
D. Plan-Do-Study-Act cycle
E. Root cause analysis

91. You are working overnight at a tertiary care hospital during a winter storm. You receive a phone consultation from an adult emergency department (ED) physician at a community hospital 1 hour away who is seeing a 2-year-old male with 8 days of fever. His physical examination reveals an irritable child with a diffuse erythematous rash on the chest, unilateral cervical lymphadenopathy, and conjunctival injection. His temperature is 39.1°C, heart rate 110 beats per minute, respiratory rate 24 breaths per minute, blood pressure 100/65 mm Hg, and oxygen saturation 99%. Laboratory analysis reveals a C-reactive protein level of 3.1 mg/dL, white blood cell (WBC) count of 16.7 × $10^3/\mu L$, hemoglobin 12 g/dL, and platelet count of 665 × $10^3/\mu L$; additional laboratory tests are still pending. The ED physician asks whether the patient requires admission, and if so, whether they should be transferred to your hospital or be admitted to their small pediatric unit that is staffed by pediatric hospitalists, but does not have pediatric subspecialists or dedicated pediatric radiology capabilities. How should you advise the ED physician regarding this patient's disposition?

A. Admit the patient to their community hospital
B. Discharge the patient home with outpatient follow-up the next day
C. Transfer the patient to your tertiary care hospital via air ambulance
D. Transfer the patient to your tertiary care hospital via ground ambulance
E. Have the patient's parents drive him to your tertiary care hospital

92. A pediatric hospitalist is asked to consult on their state's newborn metabolic screening program. A new test is available for a genetic disease, and the state is trying to decide whether to add this test to the standard newborn screening performed. Of the following options, which would be a valid argument for incorporating this test?

A. Despite the mutated gene being present at birth, symptoms do not arise until adulthood
B. Diagnosis of the disease is subjective, without expert consensus

C. Patients with the mutated gene may or may not develop the disease in their lifetime
D. The test is highly specific, but has limited sensitivity
E. Treatment for the disease is primarily symptomatic

93. A pediatric hospitalist is caring for multiple patients on a busy clinical service. He accidentally orders computed tomography (CT) of the abdomen and pelvis for the incorrect patient. By the time he discovers the error, the incorrect patient has had the CT performed. After writing an order for the correct patient to receive the needed CT, he goes to the room of the patient who incorrectly received the scan. He tells the parents that the child had received a CT that was not intended and that there was unnecessary radiation due to the CT. Which of the following terms best describes the conversation between the pediatric hospitalist and the parents?

A. Apology
B. Disclosure
C. Remediation
D. Reporting
E. Trigger

94. You are preparing to discharge a hospitalized immigrant child with a new diagnosis of juvenile idiopathic arthritis (JIA). The child is uninsured and does not qualify for public insurance in your state because of his citizenship status. Which of the following are the key elements of healthcare access?

A. Coverage, cultural competence, value
B. Timeliness, services, workforce
C. Timeliness, cultural competence, workforce
D. Coverage, workforce, value
E. Timeliness, services, value

95. A fully immunized 8-month-old male is admitted for respiratory distress in the setting of respiratory syncytial virus (RSV) bronchiolitis. He is being supported with maintenance fluids and 2 liters per minute of oxygen delivered via nasal cannula. His lung examination initially had diffuse crackles throughout all lung fields. He is started on nebulized albuterol every 4 hours. What is the use of albuterol an example of?

A. Standard of care
B. Overtreatment
C. Overdiagnosis
D. High-value care
E. Adverse event

96. You sit down after rounds to give a senior resident feedback on how she supervised the interns and medical students. You highlight what worked well and make

suggestions about what she could do differently tomorrow. In addition, you ask her if there are ways you could better support her autonomy during rounds. Which term best describes the type of feedback you are giving?

A. Summative feedback
B. Self-feedback
C. Formative feedback
D. 360-degree feedback
E. Intrinsic feedback

97. In the setting of the SARS-CoV-2 pandemic, a pediatric hospitalist is attempting to recruit pediatric patients for a newly begun vaccine randomized controlled trial of children 6 months to 12 years of age. An otherwise healthy and developmentally normal 9-year-old female is admitted to the hospital for treatment of an abscess and cellulitis of the right leg. After approaching the family about the trial, the mother and father are excited and fervently sign the informed consent because "she might get a working vaccine sooner and be protected," but the girl does not want to be in the trial because "it will involve a lot of needles, and I might still need to get the COVID shot later." After a prolonged conversation, the child can state what the trial would entail and is consistent about her reasons for not wanting to participate. Of the following, which is the best approach?

A. Enroll the child in the randomized trial because the likely benefit outweighs the harm
B. Enroll the child in the randomized trial because the parents have provided informed consent
C. Enroll the child in the trial and ensure that she receives the vaccine instead of placebo
D. Not enroll the child in the randomized trial because as a child she is part of a vulnerable population
E. Not enroll the child in the randomized trial because she does not assent to participation

98. The local pediatric hospital has a safety committee that serves to review safety events and outline appropriate actions to take to address those events. It is also the responsibility of the committee to report sentinel events to the Joint Commission along with a response plan and measurable outcomes to prevent future occurrences. Which of the following safety events should the committee submit as a sentinel event to the Joint Commission?

A. A child was running around the hospital room, tripped over a toy, and fell to the ground. The injuries he sustained were limited to bruising.
B. A nurse brought an antibiotic to administer to a child. Prior to administration, she discovered that the antibiotic was intended for a different patient on her floor.

C. A patient received a medication that resulted in an acute kidney injury. The patient remained hospitalized for two extra days, but the acute kidney injury resolved without requiring intervention.

D. An admitted teenager received a portable chest radiograph that was intended for the patient in the room next door with the same last name.

E. An infant's peripheral intravenous line infiltrated and was not noticed immediately. The infant developed compartment syndrome and was taken to the operating room for debridement.

99. You are leading family-centered rounds (FCR) with a senior resident, intern, medical student, and nurse present. During rounds, a parent of a patient comments: "We were surprised to see the intern, Dr. Rogers, taking care of our child is Black, but we're impressed with how articulate and smart he is." Which of the following is the most appropriate response?

A. Agree with the parent that Dr. Rogers is a smart intern and you are proud of his contribution to the team

B. Pause to allow Dr. Rogers to respond

C. State that you are very confident in the team of doctors regardless of the color of their skin, then debrief with the team after leaving the room about next steps

D. Respond that racist comments like that will not be tolerated and that you will be filing a bias incident report

E. Ignore the comment and proceed with rounds

100. A 16-month-old male is diagnosed with Kawasaki disease and treated with intravenous immunoglobulin (IVIG) and aspirin with clinical improvement. He is ready for discharge home. On review of his immunizations, he is noted be due for diphtheria, tetanus, acellular pertussis vaccine (DTaP); *Haemophilus influenzae* B vaccine (HiB); pneumococcal conjugate vaccine (PCV13); inactivated poliovirus vaccine (IPV); measles, mumps, rubella (MMR) vaccine; varicella vaccine; and hepatitis A vaccine (HAV). Which of the following is true regarding future vaccination?

A. DTaP, HiB, PCV13, IPV, MMR, varicella vaccine, and HAV should be given

B. DTaP, HiB, PCV13, IPV, and HAV should be given, and MMR and varicella vaccine should be delayed

C. All vaccines should be delayed

D. MMR and varicella vaccine should be given, and DTap, HiB, PCV13, IPV, HAV should be delayed

E. DTaP and HiB should be given, and PCV13, IPV, MMR, varicella vaccine, and HAV should be delayed

101. A group of hospitalists on the quality and safety committee is reviewing patient outcome data. They note that the infants born to non-Hispanic Black women have a mortality rate that is 2.5 times higher than infants born to non-Hispanic White women in their hospital. This finding can best be described as which of the following?

A. Health disparity

B. Health inequity

C. Implicit bias

D. Discrimination

E. Social determinant of health (SDoH)

102. A pediatric hospitalist receives a call from the floor nurse about a patient who was recently accepted as a transfer from the pediatric intensive care unit (PICU). The patient was admitted directly to the PICU for respiratory failure; he spent 2 weeks on a ventilator in the PICU. The nurse, performing a skin assessment, noticed a skin finding that she needs you to evaluate. According to the Centers for Medicare and Medicaid Services (CMS), which of the following examination findings is a reportable hospital-acquired condition?

A. A 2-cm area of loss of skin with pink granulation tissue located over the left heel in the wound bed

B. A 3-cm area of skin loss over the child's occiput; the area shows fat tissue and a small, developing eschar

C. An area along the right arm near the elbow that is erythematous and non-blanching with no loss of skin

D. An area of skin around an infiltrated right antecubital fossa peripheral intravenous line that has minimal swelling but no redness or blistering and intact distal pulse

E. An eschar over the right scapula that was documented on admission to the PICU

103. A previously healthy 1-month-old female is presenting to the emergency room for spitting up with every breastfeeding. The spit-up is white in color. There is no projectile vomiting, difficulty feeding, or fevers. The newborn has about eight wet diapers per day and about two yellow seedy stools per day. She has otherwise been tracking along her growth curve at the 50th percentile. The baby is well appearing with a normal physical examination and vital signs. What is the best recommendation for this patient?

A. Obtain an esophageal pH study

B. Reassure the mother that this is normal and to follow up with the primary care provider

C. Prescribe famotidine

D. Recommend thickening feeds with cereal

E. Admit the patient for observation

104. You are reviewing a study on duration of antibiotics for community-acquired pneumonia (CAP). The authors failed to find a difference in complication rates between patients treated for 5 days compared to 7 days. Which statistical value gives the maximum probability of committing a type 2 error (false negative; failing to reject the null hypothesis when it is false)?

A. Alpha
B. Beta
C. *P* value
D. Effect size
E. Sample size

105. You are working on a curriculum and have been asked to write questions for a multiple-choice assessment. Which of the following is true about constructing effective multiple-choice tests?

A. The validity of a test is the degree to which it consistently measures a desired learning outcome
B. Questions that use negative phrasing—such as "all of the following except"—tend to have lower validity and reliability
C. Adding irrelevant information in the question stem as a distractor increases the reliability of the question
D. Answer choices such as "all of the above" or "none of the above" are effective ways to capture if a learner understands multiple aspects of a given topic rather than just one
E. Choosing multiple-choice assessments rather than essay or short-answer questions helps minimize inherent biases in the question stems

106. A newborn with neonatal abstinence syndrome has been requiring increasing doses of morphine to control his symptoms. The mother is at the bedside but quickly becomes frustrated when the baby cries, expressing difficulty in soothing him. Despite extensive counseling from the medical team about evaluation and treatment of neonatal abstinence syndrome, the mother is skeptical of their approach. She is opposed to neonatal abstinence scoring and does not believe the baby needs further treatment for withdrawal. Today on hospital day 2, the mother decides she will bring the baby home against medical advice. What is the best next step?

A. Provide the mother with "against medical advice" (AMA) discharge forms
B. Call Child Protective Services
C. Call the obstetric team to place a medical incapacity hold on the mother
D. Contact risk management
E. Call the father of the baby

107. A team of hospitalists is reviewing the process of placing medication orders in their new electronic medical record in order to identify steps in which errors may occur. This is an example of which of the following?

A. Root cause analysis
B. Adverse event
C. Failure mode and effect analysis
D. Trigger tool
E. Waste reduction

108. You are assessing a 1-hour-old newborn girl who is 39 weeks old and was born via spontaneous vaginal delivery to a first-time mother who is group B *Streptococcus* (GBS) positive. The mother received penicillin 4 hours prior to delivery, and her highest temperature was 98°F during labor. Rupture of membranes (ROM) occurred 5 hours prior to delivery. The infant's Apgar scores were 8 at 1 minute and 9 at 5 minutes.

On physical examination, the newborn is well appearing with a soft and flat anterior fontanelle. She is breathing comfortably without distress, and her lungs are clear to auscultation bilaterally. Her heart has a regular rate and rhythm without any murmurs, and she is warm and well perfused with 2+ femoral pulses bilaterally. Vital signs are within normal limits. What is the best next step in management of this patient?

A. Use an evidence-based sepsis risk calculator to determine management
B. Start ampicillin and gentamicin for presumed neonatal sepsis
C. Monitor the infant in the intermediate care nursery
D. Obtain blood for culture and laboratory tests
E. Obtain neonatal intensive care unit (NICU) consultation

109. Your hospital is implementing a quality improvement initiative to reduce unplanned hospital readmissions within 30 days. Which of the following areas of initial focus is likely to have the greatest effect on decreasing unplanned readmissions?

A. Monitoring all infants with fever for at least 48 hours while cultures are pending
B. Providing written asthma action plans for all asthma patients
C. Ensuring postoperative surgical patients have adequate pain control and hydration prior to discharge
D. Providing comprehensive written discharge instructions to each patient in their native language
E. Discharging patients with their filled prescription in hand from the hospital pharmacy

ANSWERS

1. ANSWER: E

Clinical practice guidelines attempt to reduce inappropriate variations in care by limiting harm and maximizing cost efficiency and optimal health outcomes for patients. CPGs help establish evidence-based practices.

The standards of CPG development include

1. Establishing transparency such as publishing the CPG in a publicly accessible place
2. Managing conflicts of interest such as disclosures or divesting participants from the GDP that may be affected by the CPG
3. Creating a multidisciplinary team that includes representation from all stakeholders, including patients
4. Using systematic reviews as the basis of evidence
5. Stating the evidence with a rating strength of recommendations
6. Articulating clinical practice recommendations
7. Having the CPG reviewed externally
8. Updating the CPG by monitoring for up-to-date and pertinent practices

A good CPG should have a plan to update the guidelines on a regular schedule so that it can incorporate new evidence. The GDP should determine the aggregate evidence quality for recommendations made in the CDP, evaluate the risk and benefits of the recommendations, and establish the strength of each recommendation. This helps to limit variation in practice and optimize the strongest evidence-based clinical care. A CPG, however, does not replace a physician's own clinical judgment.

Clinical practice guidelines should not be published on a private server as this prevents transparency and accessibility. The multidisciplinary team may not include all interested participants as participants may have significant conflicts of interest. CPGs should establish best practices based on systematic reviews rather than case reports.

[ABP 9.D. Principles of clinical guideline development and evaluation]

REFERENCE

1. American Academy of Pediatrics Steering Committee on Quality Improvement and Management. Classifying recommendations for clinical practice guidelines. *Pediatrics*. 2004;*114*(3):874–877.

2. ANSWER: C

Implementation of a standardized handoff model has been shown to decrease preventable adverse events without significant disruption in workflow. Recent changes in resident work hour restrictions, which may reduce the length of a clinical shift, have led to a compensatory increase in the number of handoffs that occur among trainees. Standardization of the order and content of a handoff, including both verbal and written components, allows for more consistency in the information that is transmitted. Several mnemonic devices have been studied and taught to residents. Ideally, handoff should include communication of illness severity, important events in the patient's hospital course, contingency planning, and an opportunity for the receiver to synthesize the information and ask questions.

Implementing separate handoffs for interns and senior residents may lead to an increase in communication errors as a result of parallel communication. Additionally, handoff should occur in a quiet location with minimal interruptions, making a nurses' station a nonideal location for handoff. Use of handwritten tools is not recommended as variability in handwriting quality may lead to communication errors. Finally, information presented during handoffs should be limited to what is most recent and salient for the receiving provider, so reviewing the patient's entire history of present illness is typically not recommended.

[ABP 7.A. Handoffs across the continuum of care]

3. ANSWER: D

Receiver operating characteristic curves are important to understand the specificity and sensitivity of a test at different cutoff values. The y-axis represents sensitivity (true positive rate), and the x-axis represents 1 - specificity (false-positive rate). The "best" cutoff to use depends on the purpose of the test. In this example, it is important for the test to detect all patients with the disease (100% sensitivity), even if it means patients without the disease may also have a positive test result (false positives). The best cutoff for this purpose is point D. Although a cutoff value at point E will also detect all patients with the disease, it will also have a much higher false-positive rate than point D. Point C may be the best test if the goal was to maximize both sensitivity and specificity. Point A would be the best cutoff if the goal was to maximize specificity, even if it means some patients with the disease will not test positive.

[ABP 13.A.7. Diagnostic tests (eg, ROC)]

4. ANSWER: B

The model for improvement is a method to guide improvement work within an organization. The first question in the model for improvement is, "What are we trying to accomplish?" The acronym SMART is an effective mnemonic to ensure aim statements are focused, are objective, and can be evaluated for success. An effective aim statement should be

S—Specific,
M—Measurable,

A—Achievable/Attainable,
R—Realistic/Relevant, and
T—Timely/Time bound

Although the draft aim statement meets the first four criteria, it is not time bound. Of the choices provided, choice B would add a time frame in which to accomplish the aim. Choices A and E describe possible interventions to achieve the aim, which should not be included in the aim statement. Choice C is a generic quality improvement statement that does not add to the effectiveness of the aim statement itself. Choice D is a potential balancing measure for the project, which should not be included in an aim statement.

[ABP 8.A. Model for improvement (eg, Plan-Do-Study-Act)]

REFERENCE

1. Resources. Institute for Healthcare Improvement. Accessed December 18, 2020. https://www.ihi.org/resources/Pages/default.aspx.

5. ANSWER: C

This infant presents with nonsevere, uncomplicated bronchiolitis. Bronchiolitis is a clinical diagnosis of a lower respiratory infection that results in inflammation of the bronchioles, which leads to wheezing and/or crackles in children less than 2 years old. This infant has no respiratory distress and no concerns for dehydration, and as such, there are no indications for further workup or treatment. The child should be discharged from the emergency department with return precautions.

Medical overuse is common and can lead to unnecessary costs, prolonged lengths of stay, and potential harm to patients. If a child is admitted with bronchiolitis and does not require supplemental oxygen, continuous pulse oximetry is not recommended. Routine administration of bronchodilators for nonsevere bronchiolitis is not recommended. The American Academy of Pediatrics and the Society of Hospital Medicine's "Choosing Wisely" campaign recommends against chest radiographs in children with uncomplicated bronchiolitis as it increases exposure to radiation. These guidelines strive to limit variation in practice, waste, financial cost, and medical harm. There is no indication for a complete blood count.

[ABP 9.A. Principles of value in healthcare for individuals and populations (e.g., reducing unwarranted variation, overuse, overtreatment, overdiagnosis)]

REFERENCES

1. Quinonez RA, Garber MD, Schroeder AR, et al. Choosing wisely in pediatric hospital medicine: five opportunities for improved healthcare value. *J Hosp Med.* 2013;8(9):479–485.
2. Coon ER, Young PC, Quinonez RA, Morgan DJ, Dhruva SS, Schroeder AR. Update on pediatric overuse. *Pediatrics.* 2017;139(2):e20162797.
3. Money NM, Schroeder AR, Quinonez RA, et al. 2019 update on pediatric medical overuse: a systematic review. *JAMA Pediatr.* 2020;174(4):375–382.

6. ANSWER: C

The main ethical issue of concern in this case is the principal of justice. This concept states that there should be an element of fairness in all medical decisions. The published Organ Procurement Transplant Network (OPTN) policy and the National Organ Transplantation Act require that only medical criteria be used in organ allocation decisions once a patient has been listed for transplantation. Criteria such as race, citizenship, and celebrity status are not permitted to play a role in transplant listing. Although likelihood of success is generally regarded as a legitimate criterion for allocating scarce organs, in both patients there is a significant psychosocial concern, and appropriate interventions and assessments should be made prior to the final decision of providing an organ. In the first part of the case, there is also a concern for the principle of autonomy, which refers to the right of the patient to retain control over his or her body. Given the patient's defiance, the child's autonomy comes into question, but the principle of justice better encompasses both cases. Beneficence refers to the moral obligation to act for the benefit of others. Nonmaleficence refers to inflicting the least harm possible to reach a beneficial outcome. Negligence is failure to act by a medical professional that deviates from the accepted medical standard of care.

[ABP 11.A. Ethical frameworks]

7. ANSWER: B

The Advisory Committee on Immunization Practices (ACIP) and the Centers for Disease Control and Prevention (CDC) recommend universal hepatitis B vaccination within 24 hours of birth for medically stable infants weighing 2000 g or more. Since the Hep B vaccination was issued, rates of acute hepatitis B virus (HBV) infections declined 88.5%. The complete Hep B series is a three-dose series, which achieves a protective antibody response in about 95% of all healthy infants. Hep B vaccination given within 24 hours is 75% effective in preventing perinatal HBV transmission in mothers who are HBsAg positive. Because of this efficacy and the possible rate of error with interpretation or documentation of maternal prenatal laboratory tests, a birth dose of Hep B vaccination provides a safety net for all babies regardless of maternal risk. If the mother's HBsAg is positive, it is recommended to give both the Hep B vaccination and hepatitis B immunoglobulin (HBIG) within 12 hours of life as this combination is 94%

effective in preventing perinatal HBV transmission. HBIG should not be given to an infant born to an HBsAg-negative mother.

In low-birth-weight infants weighing less than 2000 g, vaccine response at 1 month of age was 96% effective versus 68% efficacy if given within the first 3 days of life. Thus, the ACIP recommends waiting until 1 month of age for Hep B vaccination in these children. Gestational age is not a factor in determining vaccine timing.

[ABP 9.C. Identifying and addressing unmet healthcare needs (eg, preventive care)]

REFERENCE

1. Schillie S, Vellozzi C, Reingold A, et al. Prevention of hepatitis B virus infection in the United States: recommendations of the Advisory Committee on Immunization Practices. *MMWR Recomm Rep.* 2018;*67*(1):1–31.

8. ANSWER: E

In research studies, patient characteristics or outcomes are represented as data points with different values, known as variables. Variables fall into several common categories, including continuous, ordinal, nominal, and dichotomous. The kind of variable determines which statistical tests can be used to compare data between two or more groups. For statistical reasons, a researcher may choose to transform or represent the same data in one or more ways. In the example above, the PRS is a number on a 1-to-12 scale assigned to a patient in respiratory distress based on clinical factors (respiratory rate, retractions, dyspnea, auscultation). However, the researcher has chosen to break the PRS into three severity levels: mild, moderate, and severe. Because each severity level has a clear order from lowest to highest, PRS is considered ordinal data. If the categories are not related to each other by rank order, such as "White," "Black," "Asian," and "other" in the race variable, they are referred to as nominal data. Nominal data that only has two mutually exclusive categories, such as male versus female sex in the example, is considered a dichotomous variable. Continuous data are on a numerical scale where the separation between each number is the same amount. In the table, both age and the PEWS are represented as continuous variables regardless of whether they are reported using median, interquartile range, or mean ± standard deviation.

[ABP 13.A.1. Types of variables]

REFERENCE

1. Hulley SB, Cummings SR, Browner WS, et al. *Planning the Measurements: Precision, Accuracy, and Validity in Designing Clinical Research.* 4th ed. Lippincott Williams & Wilkins; 2013.

9. ANSWER: C

Pediatric hospitalists are often part of difficult conversations, including sharing unexpected news. It is important to recognize and reflect on implicit biases about particular diagnoses that may affect how the news is shared. Phrasing that remains open, such as, "I have some news which may be unexpected," is preferred (C) over phrasing that suggests that it is objectively bad news, such as, "I'm sorry to tell you this, but . . . " (A). In fact, research has shown that families ultimately tend not to see the diagnosis of Down syndrome as empirically bad and in fact would often change how they were told. Many parents cite the fact they were rarely congratulated on the birth of their child.

Regarding the postnatal management of infants with Down syndrome, the American Academy of Pediatrics' "Specialized Health Care Guidelines for Children with Down Syndrome" highlights that while certain workup should be performed (genetic testing, echocardiogram, thyroid function tests, etc.), they need not be done in a neonatal intensive care setting if the baby is feeding and breathing well and should be done while informing the family of the possible diagnosis (B, D, E).

[ABP 6.B. Patient/family-centered rounds]

REFERENCES

1. Carroll C, Carroll C, Goloff N, Pitt MB. When bad news isn't necessarily bad: recognizing provider bias when sharing unexpected news. *Pediatrics.* 2018;*142*(1):e20180503.
2. Skotko BG, Levine SP, Macklin EA, Goldstein RD. Family perspectives about Down syndrome. *Am J Med Genet A.* 2016;*170A*(4):930–941.

10. ANSWER: D

Neonatal abstinence syndrome (NAS) is the withdrawal of fetal exposure to opioids used during pregnancy and consists of neurologic, gastrointestinal, and musculoskeletal disturbances as described in this case. The American Academy of Pediatrics (AAP) report on NAS recommends first-line therapy to focus on nonpharmacological treatment such as demand feeding, swaddling, minimal stimulation, and manual rocking. More recently, many hospitals have adopted Grossman's novel method of treatment for babies with NAS, the "Eat, Sleep, Console" approach.

This method suggests that even the FNASS can disrupt and disturb a baby's comfort, leading to more pharmacological intervention. They recommend pharmacological intervention only when the baby is inconsolable for more than 10 minutes despite having been fed 1 ounce of formula or expressed breast milk (or breastfed for at least 10 minutes) or having slept 1 hour undisturbed. To give this baby methadone or morphine without having first attempted simple measures such as breastfeeding is an example of overtreatment, defined as a treatment that is without evidence of benefit or excessive in complexity, duration, or cost. The AAP no longer recommends avoiding breastfeeding for mothers who are taking methadone as the concentration in breast milk is very low and may actually help with withdrawal symptoms.

[ABP 9.A. Principles of value in healthcare for individuals and populations (e.g., reducing unwarranted variation, overuse, overtreatment, overdiagnosis)]

REFERENCE

1. Blount T, Painter A, Freeman E, Grossman M, Sutton AG. Reduction in length of stay and morphine use for NAS with the "Eat, Sleep, Console" method. *Hosp Pediatr.* 2019;9(8):615–623.

11. ANSWER: A

Patients with medical complexity and chronic medical conditions are at high risk for readmission following discharge from the hospital. It is crucial that hospital providers partner with caregivers to ensure their engagement and understanding of the patient's discharge plan. "Teach-back", or having the caregiver verbalize and/or demonstrate aspects of the patient's discharge plan, is an effective technique to ensure caregiver understanding of the patient's discharge plan and may prevent readmission.

While communication with the patient's PCP is important, providing excessive nonessential information, such as a complete medical record, may be counterproductive as it would dilute important information. Verbal communication of important hospital events and discharge plans is ideal. While a suction machine may benefit the patient, the patient's mother would require additional training to demonstrate competency in using this equipment. Additionally, home pulse oximetry machines are of varying quality and complexity and may be an exorbitant expense for the family to pay out of pocket and a source of unneeded stress. While a follow-up with the patient's PCP is important, this should occur sooner than 3 weeks to monitor the patient's resolution of their acute illness.

[ABP 7.D. Discharge coordination and communication]

12. ANSWER: D

To monitor the progress of a quality improvement effort, measures must be defined and followed over time. Measures optimally should be objective, action based, and standardized. Surveys and knowledge tests are often inadequate to measure what is occurring in the clinical setting. Proportions or rates rather than counts allow measures to be compared over time regardless of the number of opportunities measured. Measures are generally divided between outcome measures, process measures, and balancing measures. Outcome measures pertain to direct impacts on the patients or other customers of the process being measured and are typically related to the specific aims of the project. Process measures pertain to interim actions that are likely to affect the outcome of interest. In this case, handwashing is a process measure that is likely to impact the primary outcome of interest: nosocomial infections. Balancing measures are measures of other processes within the complex system that may be perturbed while trying to improve the process of interest.

[ABP 8.A. Model for improvement (eg, Plan-Do-Study-Act)]

REFERENCE

1. Establishing Measures. Institute of Healthcare Improvement. Accessed January 15, 2021. https://www.ihi.org/resources/Pages/HowtoImprove/ScienceofImprovementEstablishingMeasures.aspx.

13. ANSWER: D

An important part of team management includes establishing a process to openly deal with conflict, including expressing disagreement. It is recommended to establish GRPI in the following order: goals, roles, procedures/processes, and then interpersonal relationship principles. A clear and shared goal will help team members organize and coordinate their efforts. Although additional tasks will be created over time, establishment of roles and responsibilities should be established early and include defining each team member's authority, responsibility, and tasks in order to support the team goal. The procedures/processes principle provides guidance on decision-making, control, coordination, and communication in addition to conflict management to maintain an efficient team. Finally, interpersonal relationships are based on trust, support, and collegiality. They focus on the unique strengths and contributions of each team member. While interpersonal relationships do benefit from establishing a group culture, groupthink is discouraged. Groupthink can result in a loss of individual creativity or dysfunctional decision-making because of a group's desire for harmony or conformity. The GRPI principles can effectively be applied to clinical teams and may particularly be helpful for establishing expectations in clinical teams with frequent turnover.

[ABP 10.A. Principles of team leadership]

REFERENCE

1. Rocha M, Whitney S. Leading a team. In: Gershel J, Rauch D, eds. *Caring for the Hospitalized Child.* 2nd ed. American Academy of Pediatrics; 2017:353–356.

14. ANSWER: A

Sexually transmitted infections (STIs) are common in adolescents. Hospitalization presents an opportunity to deliver preventive care to adolescents, and this opportunity is often missed in the hospital setting. Clinician knowledge and comfort, lack of time, and concern for patient follow-up are barriers to screening of adolescent sexual health in the inpatient setting. A study by Guss et al. found that adolescents were interested in receiving reproductive-related health information and services in the inpatient setting. Part of preventive care for adolescents is screening for STIs and providing counseling and treatment when indicated. In this case, this patient is sexually active and not consistently practicing safe sex. She should be screened for STIs and pregnancy, as well as counseled on safe sex practices. Adolescents can self-consent for diagnosis and treatment of STIs; the hospitalist does not need consent from the patient's parents to perform these tests. While consent used to be required for HIV testing, this was found to be a barrier to testing, and now patients may elect to "opt out" rather than "opt in." Concerns about confidentiality and privacy are known barriers to adolescents seeking care for STIs. Laws pertaining to mandatory reporting are state specific but may include assault-related injuries and risk of harm to self or others. All 50 states require physicians to report suspected child abuse.

[ABP 9.C. Identifying and addressing unmet healthcare needs (eg, preventative care), ABP 11.C. Confidentiality]

REFERENCES

1. Guss CE, Wunsch CA, McCulloh R, Donaldson A, Alverson BK. Using the hospital as a venue for reproductive health interventions: a survey of hospitalized adolescents. *Hosp Pediatr.* 2015;5(2):67–73.
2. Masonbrink AR, Richardson T, McCulloh RJ, et al. Sexually transmitted infection testing in adolescents: current practices in the hospital setting. *J Adolesc Health.* 2018;63(3):342–347.

15. ANSWER: D

Thomas et al. described a six-step approach for designing a new curriculum. The first step is to identify the current approach used for teaching the curricular content as well as the ideal approach in part via a thorough literature search. The second step is to do a needs assessment of the targeted learners for the educational environment; in this case, it includes figuring out which topics and skills interns need to learn in order to manage cross-cover calls. Once that has been identified, the third step is to write goals and objectives for the curriculum. The fourth step is to select the educational strategies to use (e.g., simulation-based cases vs. lecture) that are the most effective approach for teaching the material. The fifth step is implementation of the curriculum, which includes identifying potential barriers, piloting the curriculum, and making modifications as needed. The sixth and final step is to perform evaluation, of both individual learners and the curriculum itself.

[ABP 12.A. Principles of adult learning theory]

REFERENCE

1. Thomas PA, Kern DE, Hughes MT, Chen BY. *Curriculum Development for Medical Education: A Six-Step Approach.* 3rd ed. Johns Hopkins University Press; 2016.

16. ANSWER: E

Various regulatory and accreditation agencies, including the Food and Drug Administration (FDA), the Joint Commission, and the Institute for Safe Medication Practices (ISMP) have published guidelines for safe ordering, documentation, and administration of medications. In the case above, an error was made in accidentally ordering a look-alike/sound-alike medication. Tall man lettering, the use of capital letters to accentuate the differences between similar medication names, should be used as broadly as possible, including within electronic order entry. For example, the ISMP tall man lettering for the medications mentioned in this case are metroNIDAZOLE and metFORMIN. Although admission medication reconciliation is an important process to prevent medical errors for ongoing home medications, this would not be relevant to a case in which the medication was started in the hospital. "Do not use" abbreviations are to be avoided due to potential misinterpretations and ambiguities, such as not knowing whether mg/kg/d refers to "per day" or "per dose." "Coined names" are jargon terms for procedures that are not official and may lead to confusion, such as ordering a "banana bag" rather than specifying the exact contents of the intravenous fluid ordered. Leading zeroes are helpful when dosing less than 1 unit of anything as the decimal point may not be clear otherwise, for example using 0.25 mg rather than .25 mg.

[ABP 8.H. Role of regulatory, accrediting, licensing, and other legal agencies impacting the practice of pediatric hospital medicine]

REFERENCES

1. Institute for Safe Medication Practices. ISMP develops guidelines for standard order sets. Published March 11, 2010. Accessed April 15, 2021. https://www.ismp.org/resources/ismp-develops-guidelines-standard-order-sets.
2. US Food and Drug Administration. FDA list of established drug names recommended to use tall man lettering (TML). Published April 28, 2020. Accessed April 15, 2021. https://www.fda.gov/drugs/medication-errors-related-cder-regulated-drug-products/fda-name-differentiation-project.

17. ANSWER: C

The choice of summary statistic(s) is dependent on the type and distribution of the underlying data. Median is most appropriate when a distribution is skewed, meaning that one side of the distribution is much wider than the other. The distribution shown in Figure 3.2 is an example of right skewness, with the right side of the distribution much wider than the left. In addition to the median (50th percentile), the interquartile range (25th percentile to 75th percentile) is often used to describe the variation in the distribution rather than the range (minimum and maximum) because it is less susceptible to change due to outliers. Three measures of central tendency are used: mean, median, and mode. The mean is defined as the average value (the sum of all values divided by the number of subjects). The median is defined as the 50th percentile value, which half of the subjects are at or below. The mode is the most common value. In general, mean is most appropriate only for symmetric distributions approximating a normal curve. Standard deviation can also be used to estimate the variation within the distribution. Mode is rarely used as a summary statistic except for categorical data.

[ABP 13.A.2. Distribution of data]

REFERENCE

1. Mishra P, Pandey CM, Singh U, Gupta A, Sahu C, Keshri A. Descriptive statistics and normality tests for statistical data. *Ann Card Anaesth*. 2019;22(1):67–72.

18. ANSWER: D

Family-centered rounds have become the standard of care in pediatric hospital medicine and has been shown to lead to better communication, care coordination, resource utilization, and patient satisfaction. While there are nuances and risks to consider, the benefits of FCR have been established to outweigh these risks, and they should be offered as the default mode of rounding for all patients. A language barrier is not a reason to forgo FCR, as interpreters (remote or in person) can be incorporated as part of the interdisciplinary team. Patients with mental health diagnoses may sometimes prefer not to have the entire team present; however, FCR should still be offered to these patients, and the benefits of having the family and nurses present for discussion of the medical management still holds. Likewise, even patients with very sensitive discussions for which not all of the discussion may be appropriate to take place in the room (e.g., child abuse concerns), the benefits of discussing the medical management of the patient in the FCR model remain. Patients whose families cannot be physically present in the room also benefit from having access to FCR even if done remotely. Finally, patients as well as their families should have access to the full interdisciplinary discussion taking place during FCR.

[ABP 6.B. Patient/family-centered rounds]

19. ANSWER: C

Transitions of care from pediatric to adult providers can be stressful for patients and families, particularly those with chronic medical conditions. Most children transition to adult providers around age 18 years, but some children with chronic conditions may take longer to transition. The transition should be a deliberate and collaborative process to ensure the family, patient, and providers all have adequate time and resources. The hospitalist should elicit and discuss the family's concerns about the transition and provide handoff to the patient's primary care pediatrician regarding that discussion. The hospitalist should avoid unilaterally advising or facilitating a transition to adult providers without input from all providers involved in the patient's care.

[ABP 7.A. Handoffs across the continuum of care]

20. ANSWER: D

The tool that would allow the team to explore all possible causes contributing to delay in patient laboratory results is a fishbone diagram. The "fishbone" diagram is also called a cause-and-effect diagram or Ishikawa. Its purpose is to display information in a format that shows all potential causes contributing to an effect or variation occurring in a process and allows identification of areas for improvement. A scatterplot is a quality improvement tool used to show the association between two measures. A Pareto chart is used in quality improvement to show which factors make the most impact on an effect from largest to smallest contribution. This can be used to prioritize improvement interventions. A key driver diagram is a tool that shows which contributing factors will impact a team's ability to achieve the aim for a quality improvement project. Finally, a process map is a visual representation of the steps of a process. It is used early in a quality improvement project to understand the current state.

[ABP 8.B. Quality improvement tools]

REFERENCE

1. Langley GJ, Nolan KM, Nolan TW, Norman CL, Provost LP. *The Improvement Guide*. 2nd ed. Jossey-Bass; 2009.

21. ANSWER: A

Clinical practice guidelines are defined by the Institute of Medicine as "statements that include recommendations intended to optimize patient care that are informed by a systematic review of evidence and an assessment of the benefits and harms of alternative care options." When considering patient safety and high-value care, healthcare practices should attempt to limit variation in practice by relying on evidence-based medicine. The American Academy of Pediatrics (AAP) recommends implementing clinical practice guidelines and monitoring adherence to guidelines in order to reduce pediatric patient harm.

The AAP recognizes five levels of evidence of quality, which are as follows:

> Level A. Well-designed and conducted trials, such as randomized controlled trials without limitations, meta-analysis
> Level B. Trials with minor limitations or consistent with multiple observational studies
> Level C. Single or few observational studies or multiple studies with inconsistent findings or major limitations
> Level D. Based on expert opinion, case reports, reasoning from principles
> Level X. Situations where validating studies cannot be performed and benefit or harm is clear

After comparing levels of evidence, guideline implementers should assess each study for benefit or harm. If benefit and harm are equivalent, then it is a weak recommendation or no recommendation can be made. A randomized controlled trial is level A and is therefore the highest quality of evidence.

Beyond level of evidence, there are other factors to consider when assessing an article's quality and applicability. One factor is search strategy, emphasizing use of highly comprehensive databases relevant to the topic (i.e., PubMed). Another is inclusion and exclusion criteria, which should be examined to ensure applicability of the work. When examining outcome measures in a given work, there is a hierarchy of importance in which tier 1 refers to health status (e.g., survival), tier 2 refers to the recovery process (e.g., length of illness), and tier 3 refers to sustainability of health (e.g., life expectancy). Lastly, recommendations should evaluate safety practices for efficacy, cost, and sensibility.

[ABP 9.D. Principles of clinical guideline development and evaluation]

REFERENCE

1. Leu M, ed. in chief; Alvarez F, ed. Evidence-based clinical practice guidelines. Development and implementation manual. American Academy of Pediatrics. Revised June 28, 2019. Accessed September 11, 2021. https://downloads.aap.org/DOCCSA/CPGManual20190 628.pdf.

22. ANSWER: D

Change management works through a series of steps to ultimately create a new changed culture. Step 1: Create a sense of urgency (rather than convenience) to help others see the importance of acting. Step 2: Pull together the guiding team, which should include members with credibility, communication skills, analytical skills, authority, and leadership skills. These members may or may not hold formal leadership positions as Kotter's steps do not speak to bottom-up or top-down approaches. Step 3: Develop the change vision and the strategy to achieve change. Step 4: Communicate the vision to ensure others understand and buy into it. Step 5: Empower others to work collectively to make the vision a reality. Step 6: Produce short-term wins that are visible and unambiguous to encourage continued progress. Step 7: Don't let up after the first successes. The team must institute change after change until the vision becomes a reality, and this may include reinvigoration with new projects. Step 8: Create a new culture over time with improved actions and behaviors. Steps 1–4 move away from the status quo, steps 5–7 introduce new practices and sustain momentum, and step 8 grounds the changes in a new culture to ensure sustainability.

[ABP 10.B. Principles of change management]

23. ANSWER: C

This vignette is based on a historical case in which a patient and his mother claimed that using chemotherapy violated their spiritual beliefs. The best answer is C because a multidisciplinary meeting may involve an ethics consultant, an alternative medicine practitioner, the patient's primary care provider, and the family's spiritual leader in addition to the attending hospitalist, oncologist, nurse, social worker, hospital interfaith chaplain, and language/cultural translator (as needed). The goal of the meeting is to provide a nonjudgmental and supportive environment to develop a shared understanding of the patient's medical condition and needs. An important goal is to develop an individualized care plan that does not foreclose decisions the patient may make in the future. The goal is always to obtain assent from minor children even if they cannot legally consent. The American Medical Association Code of Medical Ethics suggests: "Where there are questions about the efficacy or long-term impact of treatment alternatives, physicians should encourage ongoing collection of data to help clarify value to patients of different approaches to care." Recent evidence suggests that time-limited trials of potentially nonbeneficial treatment with regular, scheduled meetings can increase our ability to elicit family values and preferences and may cultivate alignment between clinicians, patients, and families.

While it would be reasonable to consult the Spiritual Care team to explore the family's religious traditions (B), multiple other justifications for refusal likely contribute and need to be explored and addressed. The remaining answer choices (A, D, and E) are premature, as collaborative efforts to improve communication and understanding between healthcare providers, patient, and family are needed at this early stage.

[ABP 11.B.2. Shared decision-making]

REFERENCE

1. Fisch MJ, Lee RT. When patients choose CAM over EBM—how to negotiate treatment. *Virtual Mentor*. 2011;*13*(6):336–341.

24. ANSWER: B

A Taxonomy for Learning, Teaching, and Assessing, informally known as Bloom's revised taxonomy, is an updated (2001) version of Bloom's original work that was published in 1956 (see Figure 3.5). The goal of the taxonomy is to classify learning objectives into six progressive levels that describe the different cognitive processes involved in learning. Each level of the taxonomy consists of a more sophisticated level of learning than the previous. From simplest to most complex, the levels are remember, understand, apply, analyze, evaluate, create. When applying Bloom's taxonomy, learning objectives should be written using active verbs. In this question, *define* and *describe* fall lower on the hierarchy, reflecting the taxonomy levels of *remember* and *understand*, respectively. *Implement* is an example of the *apply* level of the taxonomy, while *assess* maps to the *evaluate* level. Finally, *design* is an example of the most sophisticated level of learning, categorized in the *create* level of Bloom's taxonomy.

[ABP 12.A. Principles of adult learning theory]

REFERENCE

1. Mcdaniel R. Bloom's taxonomy. Vanderbilt University. Published June 10, 1970. Accessed June 1, 2021. https://cft.vanderbilt.edu/guides-sub-pages/blooms-taxonomy.

25. ANSWER: A

Understanding the statistical concepts that are used in testing a research hypothesis can help hospitalists design high-quality research studies and set up for success prior to collecting any data. In our example, the hospitalist is presuming that there is an association between the predictor (the nasal decongestant) and the outcome (the length of stay). Statistical tests can only be performed on the null hypothesis—that there is no association between the decongestant and length of stay. If we reject the null hypothesis when it was true (i.e., false positive), we have committed a type 1 error. The maximum probability of committing a type 1 error is called α (alpha), which is also called the level of statistical significance, and is usually set as .05. This means the investigator has a 5% chance of finding the decongestant changes length of stay when it actually does not. Beta (β) is associated with making a type 2 error (saying the decongestant does not change length of stay when it actually does). The quantity $[1 - \beta]$ is called power. Effect size is the minimum clinically significant difference between the two groups. The hospitalist can set any effect size they want for a study, but often use existing literature or clinical relevance to determine the exact number. For example, if the decongestant changes the length of stay but only by 30 minutes, the hospitalist probably doesn't care. They might want to set their effect size as a change of at least 1 day. A larger sample size, or the number of subjects in the study,

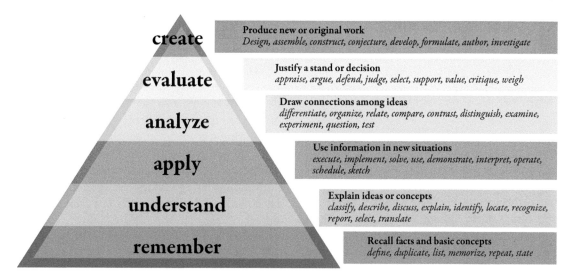

Figure 3.5 Blooms Taxonomy–*Available via creative commons from Vanderbilt University Center for Teaching: https://cft.vanderbilt.edu/guides-sub-pages/blooms-taxonomy/*

will always make your sample look more like the general population. Increasing sample size will reduce your chance of making a type 1 or type 2 error, but it can be expensive or time consuming. Providing a statistician with the α, β, effect size, and your study plan will allow calculation of the minimum number of patients you will need to recruit.

[ABP 13.A.3. Hypothesis testing]

REFERENCE

1. Guyatt G, Rennie D, Meade MO, Cook DJ. *Users' Guides to the Medical Literature: A Manual for Evidence-Based Clinical Practice.* 3rd ed. McGraw-Hill; 2014.

26. ANSWER: B

One of the questions in the Institute for Healthcare Improvement (IHI) model for improvement is: "What change can we make that will result in improvement?" One method for answering this question is to create a key driver diagram. A key driver diagram lists the factors that are likely preventing the process from achieving its aims. In the case above, one potential reason that patients may not vacate their room within 90 minutes is the need to wait for prescriptions to arrive. Key drivers such as this can help to divide a problem into smaller pieces that potential interventions can target. Choice C is an example of a global aim, and choice D is an example of a SMART (specific, measurable, attainable, relevant, and time-bound) aim. Another potential key driver might be "failure to begin discharge process early," for which one potential intervention is choice A. Readmission rate is an example of a measure, specifically one that likely would be used for balancing (i.e., determining if changes designed to improve one aspect of a system are causing new problems in another aspect of the system).

[ABP 8.B. Quality improvement tools]

REFERENCE

1. Resources. Institute for Healthcare Improvement. Accessed November 16, 2020. https://www.ihi.org/resources/Pages/default.aspx.

27. ANSWER: B

The patient had a significant decrease in his hyperbilirubinemia after phototherapy and has likely reached his bilirubin plateau. Now that the total bilirubin is 14 mg/dL at 98 hours of life, phototherapy should be discontinued. This newborn male has no risk factors for neurotoxicity such as hemolytic disease, glucose-6-phosphate dehydrogenase (G6PD) deficiency, asphyxia, significant lethargy, temperature instability, sepsis, acidosis, or hypoalbuminemia.

Since the baby is vigorous and eating well with supplementation, he can be safely discharged. Babies with a gestational age greater than 38 weeks who respond well to phototherapy treatment have a low probability of rebound hyperbilirubinemia; a repeat bilirubin test is not warranted and would prolong length of stay. For newborns older than 38 weeks, a decrease of 2 mg/dL from the initial bilirubin predicts that the probability of rebound bilirubinemia reaching the threshold for phototherapy is about 2.5%.

Since the start of universal bilirubin screening, there has been a significant decrease in severe hyperbilirubinemia (>30 mg/dL) and an increase in use of phototherapy. It is unclear whether phototherapy is associated with any long-term adverse effects, but some studies have demonstrated modest associations with childhood seizures, diabetes, autism, and cancer. Given the potential harms and costs associated with hospitalization for phototherapy, it is important to only provide phototherapy when it is indicated and to stop treatment when it is no longer needed.

There is no indication for exchange transfusion or additional laboratory tests as the patient improved with phototherapy and is not at high risk of hemolysis.

[ABP 9.A. Principles of value in healthcare for individuals and populations (e.g., reducing unwarranted variation, overuse, overtreatment, overdiagnosis)]

REFERENCES

1. American Academy of Pediatrics Subcommittee on Hyperbilirubinemia. Management of hyperbilirubinemia in the newborn infant 35 or more weeks of gestation. *Pediatrics.* 2004;*114*(1):297–316.
2. Chang PW, Newman TB. A simpler prediction rule for rebound hyperbilirubinemia. *Pediatrics.* 2019;*144*(1):e20183712.
3. Newman TB, Wu YW, Kuzniewicz MW, Grimes BA, McCulloch CE. Childhood seizures after phototherapy. *Pediatrics.* 2018;*142*(4):e20180648.

28. ANSWER: B

Kotter's change management approach describes errors that are common to organizational change. These include declaring victory too soon, allowing for complacency, failing to create a sufficiently powerful change team, not integrating the vision, allowing obstacles to block change, not celebrating short-term wins, and neglecting to anchor changes firmly in the culture. Culture change comes last, and declaring victory too soon may mean that there have not been sufficient shifts in norms and values to sustain the changes in the culture. Short-term wins should be celebrated to encourage progress. It is important to have a strong team leading change efforts. Although difficult, changing the culture may involve personnel turnover, including that of key people.

[ABP 10.B. Principles of change management]

29. ANSWER: E

It is well recognized that adolescents may have capacity for medical decision-making. As clinicians, we should look for evidence of stable values in adolescent medical decision-making that is reflective of the patient's maturity. This criterion forms the basis for the mature minor doctrine, which is recognized in some states. In the current vignette, the patient shows evidence of comprehending her medical condition and the risks and consequences of accepting or refusing treatment. She demonstrates a deep-seated religious conviction pre-dating her hospitalization. Minors who are deemed by their physician to be mature in their decision-making may be afforded legal authority to consent to or refuse medical treatment.

Consultation of social work for decision-making authority is unnecessary. In the current vignette, the patient's long estrangement from her parents casts doubt on their role in decision-making, and her aunt has only been her caregiver for a few years. In most states, the patient's prior pregnancy is only relevant to medical services relating to her pregnancy. The legal recognition of emancipated status for minors is based on known characteristics—living separately from parents and self-supporting, married, or on active duty with the armed forces—which are generally considered legal grounds for a person to make their own decisions and provide consent for medical care.

[ABP 11.B.1. Capacity to consent]

REFERENCES

1. Coleman DL, Rosoff PM. The legal authority of mature minors to consent to general medical treatment. *Pediatrics.* 2013;*131*(4):786–793.
2. Katz AL, Webb SA; Committee on Bioethics. Informed consent in decision-making in pediatric practice. *Pediatrics.* 2016;*138*(2):e20161485.

30. ANSWER: B

The sensitivity of a test calculates the probability that an individual with the disease will have a positive test. The specificity of a test calculates the probability that an individual without the disease will have a negative test. The first step in calculating sensitivity and specificity is creating a 2 × 2 table:

	DISEASE +	DISEASE -	
Test +	TP = 50	FP = 5	TP + FP = 55
Test −	FN = 10	TN = 35	FN + TN = 45
	TP + FN = 60	FP + TN = 40	TP + FP+FN + TN = 100

FN, false negative; FP, false positive; TN, true negative; TP, true positive.

Once the 2 × 2 table is complete, several calculations can be made:

Sensitivity: TP/(TP + FN) = 50/60 = 0.83
Specificity: TN/(TN + FP) = 35/40 = 0.88

The predictive value of a test determines the probability that a patient with a positive test has the disease (positive predictive value) and one with a negative test does not have the disease (negative predictive value). It is important to note that disease prevalence impacts the predictive value of the test.

Positive predictive value: TP/(TP + FP) = 50/55 = 0.91
Negative predictive value: TN/(TN + FN) = 35/45 = 0.78

[ABP 13.A.7. Diagnostic tests]

31. ANSWER: B

In the vignette above, the hospital is concerned for hospital-acquired infections (HAIs). These infections have been identified as a significant cause of preventable morbidity in hospitalized patients. HAIs include central line–associated bloodstream infections (CLABSIs), catheter-associated urinary tract infections (CAUTIs), surgical site infections (SSI), and ventilator-associated pneumonias (VAPs).

In terms of interventions, there is a hierarchy of error prevention tools. At the lower end of this hierarchy are interventions that are less powerful and less likely to be sustained, such as education, rules and policies, and checklists. Higher on the hierarchy are powerful, sustainable changes that include standard forms, automation, and forcing functions. By having a required form that asks whether a central line can be discontinued, it is highly likely that central lines will be discontinued quicker and that this practice will continue, especially if the form is within an electronic medical record. Because central line discontinuation is a complicated decision that must be made by an expert, automation after 7 days would likely lead to central lines being unsafely and inappropriately removed.

[ABP 8.G. Hospital-acquired conditions]

REFERENCE

1. Healthcare-associated infections. Centers for Disease Control and Prevention. Published March 4, 2016. Accessed March 16, 2021. https://www.cdc.gov/hai/.

32. ANSWER: E

Commercial cardiorespiratory monitoring devices have not been shown to decrease the incidence of SIDS. The safety and accuracy of these devices have also not been established. Home monitors may lead to detection of motion artifact, transient alterations in heart rate and oxygen saturation, or other clinically insignificant findings that can lead to overdiagnosis, where an abnormality is diagnosed but the abnormality requires no further treatment or management. These can lead to unnecessary costs in the form of subsequent extra health visits or diagnostic testing, as well as increased stress for caregivers.

Full-term newborns have a lower risk of extreme events, such as apnea lasting longer than 30 seconds or bradycardia with apnea lasting 20 seconds, when compared to preterm infants. Even in-hospital monitoring has not been found to identify infants at risk for SIDS.

The "Safe to Sleep" campaign should be recommended to all newborn parents as it has been found to reduce the risk of sleep-related infant deaths, including SIDS. This campaign emphasizes back to sleep, using a firm sleep surface, breastfeeding, room sharing with the infant in a separate sleep surface until at least 6 months of age, removing soft objects and loose bedding from the infant's sleep area, avoiding smoke exposure, avoiding drug use and alcohol during pregnancy and after birth, avoiding overheating, obtaining adequate prenatal care, and immunizing infants according to American Academy of Pediatrics and Centers for Disease Control and Prevention guidelines. The campaign also highlights not using home cardiorespiratory monitors as they do not reduce the risk of SIDS.

[ABP 9.A. Principles of value in healthcare for individuals and populations (e.g., reducing unwarranted variation, overuse, overtreatment, overdiagnosis)]

REFERENCES

1. Task Force on Sudden Infant Death Syndrome. SIDS and other sleep-related infant deaths: updated 2016 recommendations for a safe infant sleeping environment. *Pediatrics*. 2016;*138*(5):e20162938.
2. Hodgman JE, Hoppenbrouwers T. Home monitoring for the sudden infant death syndrome. The case against. *Ann N Y Acad Sci*. 1988;533:164–175.

33. ANSWER: D

Psychological safety is the concept that members of a team or organization—especially those who are not in positions of power—are able to speak up about their concerns or opinions without fear of retribution. Psychological safety is important in medical education. It has been shown that when learners perceive that there is psychological safety in the clinical learning environment, their overall learning experience improves. One example of providing psychological safety is an attending who tells her team at the beginning of the week that she wants people to speak up when they have questions or concerns about a case and who then responds to those comments in a positive way. Adhering to

a traditional hidden curriculum usually means deferring to hierarchy, which is the opposite of providing psychological safety. While encouraging debrief sessions and decreasing microaggressions might positively impact psychological safety, the definition is broader than either of those topics. De-escalation techniques are unrelated to psychological safety.

[ABP 12.B. Teaching strategies for multiple types and levels of learners, including patients and caregivers]

REFERENCE

1. Appelbaum NP, Santen SA, Aboff BM, Vega R, Munoz JL, Hemphill RR. Psychological safety and support: assessing resident perceptions of the clinical learning environment. *J Grad Med Educ*. 2018;*10*(6):651–656.

34. ANSWER: C

The choice of a statistical hypothesis test depends on the type of underlying data and, in many cases, its distribution. In looking for associations, it is important to compare the explanatory variable (also known as exposure or independent variable) with the response variable (also known as outcome or dependent variable). When both the explanatory and response variables are categorical, a chi-square test can be used to determine whether there are significant differences between groups. When the explanatory variable is continuous, regression is typically used. The specific type of regression is dependent on the type and distribution of the response variable. When the explanatory variable (e.g., resident number) is categorical and the response variable (e.g., test score) is continuous, multiple tests may be appropriate, depending on other factors. If, as in the case above, both groups of data belong to the same individual, a paired t test is most appropriate if the data are normally distributed versus a signed rank test if not. When there are two independent groups (e.g., if the pretest were performed on 2019 residents and the posttest were performed on 2020 residents), a two-group t test is most appropriate if the data are normally distributed versus a rank sum test if not. One-way ANOVA is most appropriate if there are more than two groups in the explanatory variable.

[ABP 13.A.4. Common statistical tests]

REFERENCE

1. Soyemi K. Choosing the right statistical test. *Pediatr Rev*. 2012;*33*(5):e38–e44.

35. ANSWER: D

Assessing health literacy—the degree to which people have the capacity to obtain, process, and understand basic health-related decisions—is an essential part of hospital care. There are several validated single questions that can be used to assess health literacy, including (1) "How often do you have someone help you read hospital materials?" (2) "How often do you have problems learning about your medical condition because of difficulty with written information?" and (3) "How confident are you filling out forms by yourself?" Answers of any frequency besides "never" are considered failed screens for health literacy.

One cannot make assumptions about a patient or family member's ability to comprehend medical information based on their education level (A) or preferred mode of learning or reading (B). Additionally, one's ability to decode a specific instance of jargon or an acronym does not equate to high health literacy (C). Health numeracy is the ability to access, use, and communicate basic mathematical information and ideas to make effective health decisions; while low numeracy and literacy are often found together, this is not always the case.

[ABP 6.D. Health literacy]

REFERENCES

1. Institute of Medicine (US) Committee on Health Literacy; Board on Neuroscience and Behavioral Health. Nielsen-Bohlman L, Panzer AM, Kindig DA, eds. *Health Literacy: A Prescription to End Confusion.* Washington, DC: National Academies Press; 2004.
2. Chew LD, Griffin JM, Partin MR, et al. Validation of screening questions for limited health literacy in a large VA outpatient population. *J Gen Intern Med.* 2008;23(5):561–566.

36. ANSWER: C

Autism spectrum disorder (ASD) is a neurodevelopmental disorder with a reported prevalence of 1 in 59 children in the United States. It is characterized by deficits in social interactions and communication as well as repetitive behavioral and activity patterns. Standard screening for ASD occurs at 18 and 24 months. Children with concern for ASD should have initial hearing, vision, and lead screening. Hospitalists should be aware of resources available for children with suspected or confirmed ASD in their communities and should refer children to these services as indicated. Zuckerman et al. found that children with ASD in Latino families with limited English proficiency had fewer therapy hours and more unmet needs than children with ASD in non-Latino White families, highlighting disparities in this patient population.

An EEG is not the first line in evaluating children with concern for ASD but may be indicated in certain cases, such as if there is concern for Landau-Kleffner syndrome in children with language regression. Neuroimaging in children with concern for ASD generally has low yield in children with no other neurologic findings. Testing for immunodeficiency or heavy metals other than lead is not indicated as the first-line workup when there is concern for autism.

[ABP 9.C. Identifying and addressing unmet healthcare needs (eg, preventative care)]

REFERENCES

1. Hyman SL, Levy SE, Myers SM; Council on Children with Disabilities, Section on Developmental and Behavioral Pediatrics. Identification, evaluation, and management of children with autism spectrum disorder. *Pediatrics.* 2020;145(1):e20193447.
2. Zuckerman KE, Lindly OJ, Reyes NM, et al. Disparities in diagnosis and treatment of autism in Latino and non-Latino White families. *Pediatrics.* 2017;139(5):e20163010.

37. ANSWER: C

Verbal handoffs are a crucial part of hospital-to-hospital transfers. It is important to ensure key pieces of information are conveyed clearly and succinctly. One helpful strategy is to ask the receiver to "read back" critical information, which has been shown to reduce handoff errors. In this case, the antibiotics and fluids are important details of the patient's hospital course that will be crucial to the ongoing care of the patient. The patient's bedside is not an ideal location for a telephone handoff, as it is important to minimize distractions and interruptions. During handoff, it is important to allow the receiver to ask clarifying questions throughout the exchange. Additionally, an assessment of the patient's illness severity should be stated at the beginning of the handoff, as it helps provide the receiver with the appropriate context of their clinical course. While providing detailed written documentation is important, a verbal handoff that emphasizes high-yield details is a more effective transfer of care.

[ABP 7.A. Handoffs across the continuum of care]

38. ANSWER: C

The model for improvement asks three questions: (1) What are we trying to accomplish? (2) How will we know that a change is an improvement? and (3) What change can we make that will result in improvement? The third question paves the way for performing rapid tests of change on a small scale before adopting that change. A test of change is performed using the Plan-Do-Study-Act (PDSA) cycle. The plan phase of a PDSA cycle consists of planning the test, making predictions about the results, and planning how data will be collected. The do phase of the PDSA cycle consists of carrying out the test on a small scale while collecting data and documenting observations. Each of these first two phases is described in the vignette, making the study phase the best next step. Studying consists of reviewing the data collected and comparing the results to the predictions made during planning. Finally, in response to the information gained from the study phase, the act phase consists of choosing in general terms what the next PDSA cycle will consist of, typically either scaling up a previous test or modifying it in some logical way. Spreading an improvement is a process by which a successfully implemented change is modified and implemented in a different setting.

[ABP 8.A. Model for improvement (eg, Plan-Do-Study-Act)]

REFERENCE

1. Resources. Institute for Healthcare Improvement. Accessed January 11, 2021. https://www.ihi.org/resources/Pages/default.aspx.

39. ANSWER: C

This patient has moderate-to-severe uncomplicated community-acquired pneumonia (CAP), which is defined by respiratory distress, hypoxemia, and an abnormal lung examination. It is distinguished from hospital-acquired (nosocomial) pneumonia, which should be considered in patients who were admitted to a hospital or other residential healthcare setting in the past 3 months.

The recommended treatment for an uncomplicated CAP in a hospitalized fully immunized child over 12 months of age is intravenous ampicillin or penicillin G given that the most typical invasive pathogen for CAP is *Streptococcus pneumoniae*. If the patient is not fully immunized, the Infectious Disease Society of America recommends considering ceftriaxone. The use of broad-spectrum antibiotics such as ceftriaxone has not been shown to reduce length of stay, costs, readmissions, or transfers to the intensive care unit in immunized children over 12 months old with uncomplicated CAP.

The Institute of Medicine defines high-value care as "the best care for the patient, with the optimal result for the circumstances, delivered at the right price." Given a narrow antibiotic provides no difference in clinical outcomes and no difference in costs, pediatric patients presenting with uncomplicated CAP should be started on narrow-spectrum antibiotics (i.e., amoxicillin or ampicillin). Children on appropriate therapy should demonstrate signs of clinical improvement within 48–72 hours. The recommended duration of combined parenteral and oral antibiotics is 7 to 10 days; however, there are few data to support duration of treatment, and evidence is emerging for shorter courses.

Routine chest radiographs are not necessary for confirmation of the diagnosis of CAP in children with mild, uncomplicated lower respiratory tract infections who are well enough to be treated as outpatients. Chest radiography is recommended in patients requiring admission. Repeat imaging is not required in children who clinically improve as expected.

[ABP 9.A. Principles of value in healthcare for individuals and populations (e.g., reducing unwarranted variation, overuse, overtreatment, overdiagnosis)]

REFERENCES

1. Bradley JS, Byington CL, Shah SS, et al. The management of community-acquired pneumonia in infants and children older than 3 months of age: clinical practice guidelines by the Pediatric Infectious Diseases Society and the Infectious Diseases Society of America. *Clin Infect Dis*. 2011;53(7):e25–e76.
2. Williams DJ, Hall M, Shah SS, et al. Narrow vs broad-spectrum antimicrobial therapy for children hospitalized with pneumonia. *Pediatrics*. 2013;132(5):e1141–e1148.

40. ANSWER: A

Social determinants of health include age and conditions in the environments in which people are born, live, learn, work, and play that affect a wide range of health, functioning, and quality-of-life outcomes and risks. Access to healthcare services is a social determinant of health. Other examples of social determinants of health are community resources, access to transportation, quality of housing conditions, access to food resources, language, literacy, and quality of education. The other answer choices, including exposure to toxic substances (and other physical hazards), contact with green spaces, type of school setting, and housing and community design are physical determinants of health. While the conditions of the physical environment are social determinants of health, the environment itself is a physical determinant of health.

[ABP 10.C.2. Social determinants of health]

41. ANSWER: A

Many states require mandatory reporting of names of persons newly diagnosed with HIV to local or state health departments. However, the father has not established a patient-doctor relationship with you and has not provided formal laboratory results. Therefore, his HIV status remains hearsay and is not reportable by you. Laws pertaining to mandatory reporting are state specific but may include various infectious diseases, assault-related injuries, and risk of harm to self or others. All 50 states require physicians to report suspected child abuse. While physicians may feel an ethical obligation to warn partners of possible HIV exposure, case law and legal statutes enforce only reporting to public health authorities. Furthermore, because the mother has not established a patient-doctor relationship with you either, it is not within the scope of practice to order laboratory tests for the mother. Therefore, the most correct answer is to explain that unusual causes of failure to thrive need to be evaluated, given the clinical context. Stating that HIV testing is part of standard workup violates the physician's obligation to communicate truthfully.

[ABP 11.C. Confidentiality]

REFERENCE

1. Schleiter KE. Testing newborns for HIV. *Virtual Mentor.* 2009;*11*(12):969–973.

42. ANSWER: A

Successful educational scholarship requires attention to study design, including an awareness of the levels of educational outcomes that are used to demonstrate the effectiveness of an intervention. The most popular framework used to describe these outcomes is the Kirkpatrick model of educational outcomes. The highest level of outcome (level 4) is called the "results" level and requires a demonstration that the intervention led to the intended results in the real world. This level is considered the "holy grail" of educational scholarship and is often difficult to achieve. In the handwashing example, a demonstration that postintervention there were fewer nosocomial infections among the patients who took the course versus those who did not would reach level 4. Level 3 is the "behavior" level and requires demonstration that learner behavior in the real-world setting has changed. Among the answer choices, choice A describes an observed behavior change in a clinical setting and is therefore the highest level among the answer choices. Level 2 is called the "learning" level and requires demonstration that learning of new knowledge or skills occurred. This level is often assessed using comparisons of pre- and post-knowledge tests. Adding time to the post-assessment, as in choice D, shows that knowledge has been retained and thus the intervention offers durability, but this still remains a level 2 outcome. The presence of a control group, as in choice E, is helpful, but again the outcome level remains an assessment of knowledge gain only, and thus it also remains level 2. The lowest level of outcomes for an educational intervention are the learners' reactions. These can include metrics such as how satisfied a learner was with a session or any other self-reported reaction, including their perceived change in confidence. Choices B and C both describe reaction level results, and while the higher response rate in choice B is nice, it does not change that the result is a low-tier outcome.

[ABP 12.A. Principles of adult learning theory]

REFERENCE

1. Kirkpatrick DL, Kirkpatrick JD. *Evaluating Training Programs: The Four Levels.* 3rd ed. Berrett-Koehler; 2008.

43. ANSWER: C

The pediatric hospitalist in this question is trying to determine if an exposure (prophylaxis) alters the probability of an outcome (DVT) or, in other words, if it changes the patient's risk. Risk refers to the probability of developing a disease over a set amount of time and is sometimes referred to as incident risk; for example, if 10 out of 100 patients without a disease develop it in the course of the study, this would be equivalent to 10% risk. Relative risk (RR) is the ratio of the risk in the exposed group to the risk in the unexposed group. In the example above, this is 10/(10 + 90) ÷ 30/(30 + 70) = 0.33. Since our RR is less than 1, events are significantly less likely in the treatment than in the control group. Absolute risk reduction, on the other hand, is the difference in the risks, in this case 0.30 - 0.10 = 0.20. Because the study was based on exposure and followed patients over time, such as in a cohort or randomized controlled trial, it was possible to calculate risk and therefore to calculate relative risk. In case-control studies, risk cannot be calculated because the groups are chosen based on already having or not having the disease in question rather than exposure. In cross-sectional studies, risk cannot be calculated because data are gathered at only one point in time and assessment of risk requires longitudinal data over time. If risk and relative risk cannot be calculated, odds ratios can be used instead. Odds are a ratio between those who do and do not have a disease, for example, 10 patients with DVT to 90 patients without DVT = 1:9 odds. Odds ratios can be calculated by the ratio of positive to negative outcomes in each group; in this case, 10/90 ÷ 30/70 = 0.26. It is important to set up the comparison such that it is the risk within the experimental exposure group divided by the risk in the control group.

[ABP 13.A.5. Measurement of association and effect]

REFERENCE

1. Sheldrick RC, Chung PJ, Jacobson RM. Math matters: how misinterpretation of odds ratios and risk ratios may influence conclusions. *Acad Pediatr.* 2017;*17*(1):1–3.

44. ANSWER: C

Patient-physician cost conversations can reduce costs. Zafar et al. showed 57% of patients with cancer who discussed cost with their physicians reported lower out-of-pocket costs. Healthcare spending in children in the United States increased from $149.6 billion in 1996 to $233.5 billion in 2013; spending was greatest in children under 1 year of age. Creating an awareness of costs and value in healthcare for both providers and families increases transparency and drives change, as demonstrated by the "Choosing Wisely: A Special Report on the First Five Years," which encourages patient-physician discussions about high-value care and has seen physicians "more likely to report reducing the numbers of unnecessary tests or procedures in the past 12 months."

Reducing nonclinical support staff is generally not an effective way to reduce costs because the nonclinical tasks must then be done by physicians, whose time is much more expensive. Reducing the number of operating rooms leads to more idle time spent by surgical teams waiting for rooms to be cleaned and readied for the next case. Limiting variation in practice is an effective way to reduce unnecessary costs. Limiting clinic visits in order to increase the number of patient encounters will likely increase profits in the short term. However, this is likely to increase healthcare costs in the long term as it limits time for counseling and other preventive care services that can save costs over the course of an individual's lifetime.

[ABP 9.B. Commonly used terms and metrics (eg, length of stay, readmissions, costs and charges)]

REFERENCES

1. Zafar SY, Chino F, Ubel PA, et al. The utility of cost discussions between patients with cancer and oncologists. *Am J Manag Care*. 2015;*21*(9):607–615.
2. Choosing Wisely: a special report on the first five years. Choosing Wisely. Published October 26, 2017. Accessed June 6, 2021. https://www.choosingwisely.org/choosing-wisely-a-special-report-on-the-first-five-years/.

45. ANSWER: D

Availability bias is the tendency to diagnosis a patient with the same disease that has been encountered recently in another patient. Thus, in this case, the residents are at risk of misdiagnosing this patient with bronchiolitis (when, in fact, the child may have reactive airway disease or a foreign body in their airway) because three other children have recently presented with bronchiolitis. Omission bias is the tendency to favor inaction over action (e.g., "watchful waiting" rather than starting antibiotics). Visceral bias happens when a clinician's feelings about a patient/family impact the diagnoses that are considered (e.g., assuming that if a patient's parent is a smoker, they are not using their child's asthma medications correctly). Outcome bias results in clinicians making diagnoses with good outcomes over those with poor outcomes. Finally, aggregate bias happens when clinicians do not believe that aggregate data apply to their patient and make diagnostic decisions accordingly (e.g., refusing to use evidence-based clinical guidelines even though the patient meets inclusion criteria).

[ABP 7.A. Handoffs across the continuum of care]

REFERENCE

1. Croskerry P. The importance of cognitive errors in diagnosis and strategies to minimize them. *Acad Med*. 2003;*78*(8):775–780.

46. ANSWER: B

Patients who are discharged with feeding tubes require close monitoring in the outpatient setting. It is crucial to engage the patient's PCP on the discharge plan both to provide handoff and to collaborate on what additional services or referrals need to be made for the patient. You should discuss what resources they have in their office or nearby community (e.g., nutritionist or occupational therapy) before making your own referral to another provider. While the patient may ultimately require a gastrostomy tube, this is not an emergent need if they are doing well with the nasogastric tube, and a surgery referral can be made by the primary care provider.

[ABP 7.D. Discharge coordination and communication]

47. ANSWER: B

The Institute for Healthcare Improvement (IHI) framework for improvement work includes four types of plan-do-study-act (PDSA) cycles: design a change, test a change, implement a change, and spread an improvement. "Incorporat(ing) feedback from multiple providers" is an example of a design-a-change PDSA cycle, in which a potential change is improved outside of the clinical setting where it is ultimately intended to be used. Implementing a change is the process of putting a sustainable change into widespread, permanent practice. Spreading an improvement is the process of adapting a proven innovation for use in an additional setting.

The project described is now in the test-a-change phase, and the innovator has attempted to use the new template in the clinical setting. Initial testing should be limited to "1 physician, 1 patient, 1 time." After successful tests of change, a rule of thumb is to scale up one of these factors by three to five. A next reasonable step would be to repeat the small-scale test (three to five patients) with someone who did not create the template. Pitfalls in the test-a-change phase include waiting for buy-in (choice A), testing only using innovators (choice E), moving too quickly to implementation (choice D), and waiting for technological change (choice C).

[ABP 8.A. Model for improvement (eg, Plan-Do-Study-Act)]

REFERENCE

1. Resources. Institute for Healthcare Improvement. Accessed November 16, 2020. https://www.ihi.org/resources/Pages/default.aspx.

48. ANSWER: A

This patient is presenting with a brief resolved unexplained event (BRUE). A BRUE is defined by the American Academy of Pediatrics as "an event occurring in an infant younger than 1 year when the observer reports a sudden, brief, and now resolved episode of ≥1 of the following: (1) cyanosis or pallor; (2) absent, decreased, or irregular breathing; (3) marked change in tone (hyper- or hypotonia); and (4) altered level of responsiveness" and occurs without an alternative explanation.

Low-risk patients are defined by the following criteria: "(1) age >60 days; (2) gestational age ≥32 weeks and postconceptional age ≥45 weeks; (3) occurrence of only 1 BRUE (no prior BRUE ever and not occurring in clusters); (4) duration of BRUE <1 minute; (5) no cardiopulmonary resuscitation by trained medical provider required; (6) no concerning historical features; and (7) no concerning physical examination findings." This patient is considered a low-risk patient because although he was premature, he was born at 33 weeks' gestation and is now post-conceptual age 47 weeks. The event also lasted less than 60 seconds, was a first occurrence, and the patient did not receive CPR from a trained medical provider.

The guidelines recommend educating caregivers about BRUE and offering resources for CPR training for the caregiver. A provider can consider monitoring briefly with pulse oximetry and obtaining a pertussis test and 12-lead electrocardiogram but neither is mandatory. Laboratory testing is not recommended as most patients with BRUEs will have unremarkable findings. Medications should also not be considered without further history suggestive of gastroesophageal reflux disease. Last, a low-risk patient should not be admitted to the hospital to observe for cardiorespiratory monitoring. These guidelines have been found to be safe and cost-effective and have been shown to reduce testing and admissions.

[ABP 9.A. Principles of value in healthcare for individuals and populations (e.g., reducing unwarranted variation, overuse, overtreatment, overdiagnosis)]

REFERENCES

1. Tieder JS, Bonkowsky JL, Etzel RA, et al. Brief resolved unexplained events (formerly apparent life-threatening events) and evaluation of lower-risk infants: executive summary. *Pediatrics.* 2016;*137*(5):e20160591.
2. Colombo M, Katz ES, Bosco A, Melzi ML, Nosetti L. Brief resolved unexplained events: retrospective validation of diagnostic criteria and risk stratification. *Pediatr Pulmonol.* 2019;*54*(1):61–65.

49. ANSWER: C

Health in all policies refers to a strategy that focuses on the goal of improving health and health equity by addressing health in all areas of government. It recognizes that complex interrelated factors impact health and health equity. For example, when legislatures and government officials make decisions on schools, transportation, and neighborhood resources, the resulting policies can have several downstream effects on health. Health in all policies is not specific to children. While health may not always be the primary consideration, policymakers should consider the impact of policies on health at all levels and be accountable for the consequences of public policies on health systems, determinants of health, and well-being. Health policy refers to the decisions, plans, and actions that are undertaken to achieve specific healthcare goals within a society. Health policy is not part of all policies.

[ABP 10.C.1. Health care access, ABP 10.C.2. Social determinants of health]

50. ANSWER: D

The most reasonable choice is to discharge this patient home as requested. In this situation, the parents demonstrate full understanding of the diagnosis and prognosis, and given that they continue to hold the child's best interest, it is reasonable to follow their wishes. In general, it is preferred to disclose a terminal diagnosis and allow a teenage child to participate in the decision to withhold potentially life-saving or life-extending treatment. While parents have the authority to make decisions in the interests of their children, children approaching adulthood are increasingly recognized to exhibit decision-making abilities sometimes equivalent to adults. It is always preferable to seek a child's assent to treatment even if they cannot legally consent. However, given her mental instability and ongoing stress and anxiety regarding her illness, it is reasonable to follow the parents' wishes to minimize that patient's suffering; thus, A and B are incorrect. Importantly, physicians should let parents know that deception is counter to core medical ethics and professional integrity (E). Tissue biopsy is not routinely necessary when multiple sites of recurrence are confidently identified on imaging (C).

[ABP 11.B.2. Shared decision-making, ABP 11.D. Professional integrity]

REFERENCE

1. Friebert S. Nondisclosure and emerging autonomy in a terminally ill teenager. *Virtual Mentor.* 2010;*12*(7):522–529.

51. ANSWER: A

Simple linear regression is the statistical method of describing the relationship between a single predictor variable and an outcome of interest. Linear regression assumes that there is a linear relationship (i.e., that each additive change in the predictor causes the same additive change in the expected value of the outcome). The regression line itself is typically summarized by the slope (in this case 5.73 mm Hg per gram/day Na) and the y-intercept (in this case 108.7 mm Hg). The slope is the marginal increase in expected value of the outcome for each unit of increase for the predictor variable. In this case, an increase of 1 g/d Na intake increases the expected SBP by 5.73 mm Hg, and the theoretic SBP of someone who does not take in any Na would be 108.7 mm Hg (choice B). One cannot directly calculate the marginal slope of the predictor for each unit increase in outcome (choice C). In addition to the best-fit line itself, the goodness of fit is usually summarized by r^2, which is defined as the proportion of variation in the outcome variable that is explained by the predictor variable (choice A). Statistical significance (choices D and E) can also be calculated for simple linear regression, but the r^2 does not directly inform this calculation.

[ABP 13.A.6. Regression]

52. ANSWER: D

Discharge coordination and communication for a patient with medical equipment can be challenging for both providers and caregivers. It is important to maintain consistent, open communication with all multidisciplinary team members. In this instance, a meeting to discuss the patient's care and the parents' concerns may help minimize conflict between the family and the team and can elucidate barriers in the parents' tracheostomy education and their financial worries. Transferring the patient to a different physician team or RT would be disruptive and create an additional handoff that could worsen communication. While it is important for the parents to engage in self-care, leaving the hospital for several days would not fix communication issues with the care team. A referral to CPS is also premature and would only worsen distrust between the parents and the care team.

[ABP 7.D. Discharge coordination and communication]

53. ANSWER: B

A run chart is a tool that can be used to track data over time when performing a quality improvement project. It consists of an x-axis, typically representing a timescale, and the y-axis, representing the quality indicator that is being measured. As data are plotted, the median is calculated, which indicates the point where half of the data points fall above the line and half of the data points fall below the line. This median is sometimes referred to as the centerline. The median is used to determine if the quality interventions are causing "signals" in the data that indicate either improvement or degradation of a process. Signal changes can be defined by three probability-based rules that allow for a run chart to be analyzed. The first rule is a shift, which is defined as six or more consecutive points either all above or all below the median line (choice E). The second rule is a trend, which is defined as five or more consecutive points

going all up or all down. A trend can cross the median. The trend in the data above is represented by choice B, which is demonstrating eight consecutive data points going down and is the correct answer. The third rule is an astronomical point, represented by choice D, which is a point that is distinctively different from all the rest of the points on the run chart. Choices A and C do not represent signals of special cause variation.

[ABP 8.B. Quality improvement tools]

REFERENCE

1. Perla RJ, Provost LP, Murray SK. The run chart: a simple analytical tool for learning from variation in healthcare processes. *BMJ Qual Saf.* 2011;*20*(1):46–51.

54. ANSWER: D

The most appropriate next step to consider is early transition to oral cephalexin. Although there is no consensus on the duration of intravenous (IV) antibiotic treatment for osteomyelitis, many consensus guidelines agree that oral antibiotics should be considered early in treatment, especially if the inflammatory markers are down-trending, there is lack of fever, and the patient is clinically improving. The 2021 Choosing Wisely campaign recommendations for pediatric hospital medicine specifically emphasize not prescribing IV antibiotics for predetermined durations for hospitalized patients with infections such as osteomyelitis.

In a large cohort of children and adolescents with osteomyelitis, there was no association between treatment failure and mode of antibiotic treatment, and the patients with central lines for IV antibiotics had increased risk of adverse outcomes, such as central line complications. IV antibiotics have also been associated with higher cost of treatment and longer hospital stays.

Furthermore, this patient has been identified to have MSSA osteomyelitis, and antibiotic treatment should be narrowed accordingly. MSSA is best treated with an antistaphylococcal β-lactam such as oxacillin, nafcillin, cefazolin, and cephalexin. Clindamycin can be considered in patients with a penicillin or cephalosporin allergy, but it is not the best option for this patient.

[ABP 9.A. Principles of value in healthcare for individuals and populations (e.g., reducing unwarranted variation, overuse, overtreatment, overdiagnosis)]

REFERENCES

1. Pediatric hospital medicine—SHM, AAP, APA: Five things physicians and patients should question. Choosing Wisely. Published January 11, 2021. Accessed January 29, 2021. https://www.choosingwisely.org/societies/pediatric-hospital-medicine-shm-aap-apa/.

2. McMeekin N, Geue C, Briggs A, et al. Cost-effectiveness of oral versus intravenous antibiotics (OVIVA) in patients with bone and joint infection: evidence from a non-inferiority trial. *Wellcome Open Res.* 2019;4:108.

55. ANSWER: D

Although live professional interpretation services are preferred, remote video and phone interpretation services are acceptable forms of communication. In particular, for less common languages, phone services may be the only available option. The Joint Commission requires that a patient's race/ethnicity, preferred language, and any communication needs be documented in the chart. Having the pediatric patient or patient's sibling provide translation services is not a recommended practice as they may lack sufficient understanding, provide selective interpretation, or be placed in a difficult position. Members of the medical team who are fluent in a language may undergo hospital translation service certification to communicate with patients and families in that language without requiring a translator. Recommended practice when working with an interpreter includes giving the interpreter a brief introduction to the patient and discussing what will be covered during the visit prior to the start of the encounter. During the encounter, the provider should address the patient directly, speak slowly, avoid medical jargon, and provide pauses throughout the conversation for the interpreter to translate.

[ABP 10.C.4. Culturally effective healthcare and cultural humility]

56. ANSWER: A

While therapeutic privilege was widely practiced in medicine decades ago, its application has largely given way to informed consent, in which information is shared openly to allow for autonomous patient decision-making. However, in severe anorexia nervosa (AN), body image disturbances are known to fluctuate and may be "triggered" by multiple cues during hospital encounters. Comments about a patient's weight, calories taken in, or appearance can exacerbate the psychological disturbance of AN, worsening clinical outcomes. As such, patients with AN undergoing refeeding are well served by entrusting their nutrition to a physician, who is expected to exercise therapeutic privilege to avoid exacerbating body image disturbances.

While nonmaleficence, to "do no harm," may be the ethical basis for physicians to withhold clinical information that may trigger psychological distress, therapeutic privilege is what patients expect when relinquishing informed consent for a refeeding protocol. Capacity to consent is generally defined by an ability to use information about one's illness to make decisions in line with one's values. It is often defined by four principles: understanding, expressing a choice, appreciation of how the information applies to

oneself, and reasoning to understand consequences. The patient described in the above scenario clearly demonstrates capacity. Although respect for persons is a core value of medical practice, it does not specifically address the withholding of information in the patient-physician relationship.

[ABP 11.A. Ethical frameworks, 11.B.1. Capacity to consent]

REFERENCE

1. Richard C, Lajeunesse Y, Lussier MT. Therapeutic privilege: between the ethics of lying and the practice of truth. *J Med Ethics.* 2010;36(6):353–357.

57. ANSWER: D

The best approach to working with a struggling learner is to first approach them with kindness and compassion and work with them to diagnose what the specific issues are that are impacting the learner's ability to meet expectations. For example, is this student's knowledge base below average? Does he suffer from social anxiety? Does he struggle with organization? In addition, be aware that for many learners, stress outside of work can have marked impact on their clinical performance.

While documenting performance concerns using statements of fact is important, it is not the first step in working with a struggling learner. Ensuring expectations are clear is critical, but since the senior resident has already given feedback, more intervention is needed in this case. Public praising of learners is a nice practice, but it is unlikely to resolve the problems of a struggling learner. Finally, while it is always important to create psychological safety, taking away all patient care responsibilities risks undermining a learner's confidence and does not allow the opportunity to learn through practice.

[ABP 12.C. Principles of effective assessment and feedback]

58. ANSWER: D

When a hospitalist gets a test result back as "positive" or "negative," it is important to understand the underlying characteristics or accuracy of that test in order to interpret its result and apply it to an individual patient. Sensitivity is defined as the proportion of patients with a disease who test positive. The example above shows that the biomarker was positive in 20 and negative in 30 of the 50 patients with meningitis, and therefore sensitivity is 0.4 (20/[20 + 30]). Specificity is defined as the proportion of patients without a disease who test negative. The example above shows that the biomarker was positive in 5 and negative in 45 of the 50 patients without meningitis and therefore the specificity is 45/(45 + 5) = 0.9. The proportion of patients with the disease out of those who test positive in a particular population is defined as the positive predictive value. The proportion of patients without the disease who test negative in a particular population is defined as the negative predictive value. Both the positive and negative predictive value can only be calculated if the prevalence of the disease in the population is known. The prevalence cannot be calculated from the presented data because the study has a case-control design, selecting patients based on their diagnosis, rather than from the population at large.

[ABP 13.A.7. Diagnostic tests]

REFERENCE

1. Guyatt G, Rennie D, Meade M, Cook D. *Users' Guides to the Medical Literature: A Manual for Evidence-Based Clinical Practice.* 3rd ed. McGraw-Hill Education; 2015.

59. ANSWER: A

Communicating on rounds also includes how we communicate *about* our patients. Person or people-first language is the intentional effort to emphasize the person rather than their disease, disability, or diagnosis. The person should be put before the diagnosis by describing what the person "has" rather than what the person "is." For example, describing a patient as an "autistic child" or "cystic fibrosis patient" or "CF-er" places their disease as their first defining characteristic, whereas a "child with autism" or a "child with cystic fibrosis" underscores their personhood first. Using people-first language about and with our patients conveys dignity and respect. The other answer choices are all best practices in communicating during family-centered rounds, including setting an agenda, involving the child in the decision-making, and incorporating nurse and family information, but these are not examples of the linguistic strategy of person-first language.

[ABP 6.B. Patient/family-centered rounds]

60. ANSWER: D

The patient has indirect hyperbilirubinemia above the recommended phototherapy threshold given his gestational age. In this case, admission to a general pediatrics floor for intensive phototherapy is indicated. A home biliblanket may not be sufficient to treat this degree of hyperbilirubinemia. Admission to the NICU is not necessary as the patient does not require critical care services at this time. Transferring the patient to a nearby ED is also not necessary as it would not change the need for admission and may incur an unnecessary cost to the family. Similarly, obtaining a CBC and Coombs test in the rural clinic is not immediately necessary and would only delay the initiation of phototherapy.

[ABP 7.B. Triage within the health care system]

61. ANSWER: C

Statistical process control (SPC) charts are an advanced mathematical methodology of displaying and analyzing quality improvement data over time. Based on the assumed underlying distribution of the data, specific SPC charts can be used to monitor stability of a process over time. Common-cause variation is the natural variation that occurs despite data being consistent over time and does not signal any change (choice B). Special-cause variation, on the other hand, occurs when data behave in a way that is highly unlikely if the process were consistent over time. In the case of the data presented, a shift has occurred, defined as a certain number (typically eight or more) points in a row that are either all above or all below the center line. The red points illustrate 15 consecutive points above the baseline centerline, which would only happen once every $2^{14} = 16,384$ times randomly. When special-cause variation occurs, one must next determine whether it is an improvement and whether it is explained. Because it is an upward shift of a measure the team is aiming to increase, this is an improvement and not a worsening. In the case above, the shift began a full 6 months prior to the quality improvement effort and is therefore not explained. Had it occurred at or shortly after the intervention, then it would more likely have been explained by the intervention. While any point occurring outside of the control limits (defined as three standard deviations above and below the mean) is considered special-cause variation, there are multiple ways in which special-cause variation can occur that do not require data to be outside the control limits.

[ABP 8.B. Quality improvement tools]

REFERENCE

1. Johnson DP, Patterson BL. The natural order of time: the power of statistical process control in quality improvement reporting. *Hosp Pediatr.* 2018;8(10):660–662.

62. ANSWER: E

Patients with diabetes mellitus are more susceptible to *Streptococcus pneumoniae* and influenza infections, likely due to the harmful effects of hyperglycemia on the immune system and pulmonary function. As such, the Centers for Disease Control and Prevention (CDC) and American Diabetes Association recommend all patients with diabetes mellitus receive an annual influenza vaccine and all patients older than 2 years receive the PPSV23. Vaccination can help decrease the risk of infection and thus prevent hospitalization.

The PPSV23 should be given at least 8 weeks after the PCV13 series is complete, which is typically finished at the 12- to 15-month well-child visit in a fully immunized child. Other populations who should receive PPSV23 include patients with sickle cell disease or other hemoglobinopathies; anatomic or functional asplenia; congenital or acquired immunodeficiency; human immunodeficiency infection; chronic renal failure or nephrotic syndrome; iatrogenic immunosuppression, including radiation therapy; multiple myeloma; generalized and metastatic malignancies; and solid-organ transplant. A second dose is required at least 5 years after the first dose.

[ABP 9.C. Identifying and addressing unmet healthcare needs (eg, preventive care)]

REFERENCES

1. Korbel L, Easterling RS, Punja N, Spencer JD. The burden of common infections in children and adolescents with diabetes mellitus: a Pediatric Health Information System study. *Pediatr Diabetes.* 2018;*19*(3):512–519.
2. Pneumococcal vaccination summary: who and when to vaccinate. Centers for Disease Control and Prevention. https://www.cdc.gov/vaccines/vpd/pneumo/hcp/who-when-to-vaccinate.html. Published August 2, 2020. Accessed January 29, 2021.

63. ANSWER: C

Cultural humility is the premise that healthcare providers should be open to and respectful of differences in each family's beliefs and values. Although the medical team may not see the benefit of the mother praying over her child with an egg, the mother is compliant with the medical team recommendations and is using this prayer as an adjunct to care. Cultural sensitivity and cultural awareness are terms that are sometimes used interchangeably to describe the awareness that cultural similarities and differences exist without assigning a value to these cultural differences. Cultural competence is the ability of healthcare providers and organizations to understand the cultural and language needs of a patient. Cultural effectiveness is the delivery of care within the context of cultural competence and appreciation of all cultural distinctions leading to optimal health outcomes. Cultural effectiveness and cultural humility are considered to be the goal as they go beyond awareness, sensitivity, and competence.

[ABP 10.C.4. Culturally effective healthcare and cultural humility]

64. ANSWER: E

While the terms *assessment* and *evaluation* are sometimes incorrectly used as synonyms, they are two distinct entities used when working with learners. Both assessment and evaluation require clear criteria and measurement. Evaluation tests what has been learned and happens at the end of an identified period of learning (e.g., board certification examination at the end of fellowship or a grade at the end of medical student's rotation). Evaluation is intended to identify weaknesses and is judgmental in that it results in a final score or grade that is measured against a specific benchmark.

In contrast, assessment is an ongoing process. Rather than making a judgment, assessment is a diagnostic process, aimed at determining how learning is going and identifying areas for improvement. Assessment happens during the learning process and provides feedback for the learner and teacher. Thus, all of the examples above that are intended to give a learner real-time feedback or identify growth areas (e.g., feedback after a lumbar puncture, completing milestone assessments, using EPAs to coach learners on a specific encounter) rather than giving a final score or grade are examples of assessment.

[ABP 12.C. Principles of effective assessment and feedback]

65. ANSWER: A

Systematic review and meta-analysis are at the peak of the levels-of-evidence pyramid. While they can powerfully summarize the current state of evidence across multiple studies, the conclusions reached are dependent on the quality of both the systematic review methodology and the underlying studies. Although sometimes mentioned interchangeably, systematic review and meta-analysis have distinct differences. Systematic review refers to the process of collecting and summarizing all studies on a given topic. The systematic review then attempts to determine the quality and risk of bias of the various studies involved. A meta-analysis is a statistical method (typically performed within a systematic review) in which the data from multiple studies are combined, effectively creating a single, larger trial. The most important requirement for performing meta-analysis is homogeneity, meaning similarities in the population, scenario, and outcome of interest in the studies being analyzed. In the example above, there is significant heterogeneity as no two studies are on the same clinical scenario or outcome. This heterogeneity prevents pooling data as part of a larger meta-analysis. Although an increased number of studies and subjects allows for more powerful meta-analysis, the number of patients in the above studies would not preclude meta-analysis. Although observational and experimental studies are often separated in meta-analysis, the inclusion of observational studies does not itself prevent meta-analysis. There is no mention of limited outcome data or selective reporting in the vignette, although these factors would limit the validity of the conclusions of the meta-analysis.

[ABP 13.A.8. Systematic review and meta-analysis]

REFERENCE

1. Ahn E, Kang H. Introduction to systematic review and meta-analysis. *Korean J Anesthesiol.* 2018;*71*(2):103–112.

66. ANSWER: D

Utilizing a structured handoff tool, such as IPASS (illness severity, patient summary, action list, situational awareness, synthesis by receiver), has been shown to reduce serious safety events that result from handoff errors. As part of this tool, the handoff should start with a statement about the patient's illness severity. This allows the receiver to appropriately contextualize the information that follows and inform the questions they may ask. The other answer choices communicate important information that should be conveyed after discussing the patient's illness severity.

[ABP 7.A. Handoffs across the continuum of care]

67. ANSWER: C

Lean healthcare is a version of the Toyota Manufacturing System (Lean), specifically designed for healthcare organizations. A major goal of lean healthcare is to identify and eliminate "waste," defined as actions that do not add value to stakeholders. Table 3.5 lists the eight types of waste, often summarized with the mnemonic DOWNTIME, with definitions and examples. In the example above, employees are traveling to multiple floors when it might be possible to have local assignments, limiting unnecessary motion.

[ABP 8.C. Waste and variation reduction (eg, Lean, Six Sigma)]

REFERENCE

1. Graban M. Eight types of waste in healthcare. *Lean Blog.* Published December 27, 2015. Accessed November 17, 2020. https://www.leanblog.org/eight-types-of-waste-in-healthcare/.

68. ANSWER: C

Paying bonuses to providers based on highest RVUs does not optimize value to the patient but rather to the hospital or healthcare provider. Healthcare value is most commonly defined as the best health outcome at the lowest cost, or the output of healthcare per unit of cost. The value equation typically is Value = [Quality + Service (or Experience)] ÷ Cost. In most models, the value equation is patient centered as the patient perspective is the most unifying among patient, payer, and provider value.

Primary drivers of increasing healthcare value include increased transparency and public reporting of quality and cost; encouraging healthcare systems to compare relative performance; educating patients about value and costs (including financial, physical, psychological, etc.); reporting additional measures of quality care; and encouraging the transition from traditional fee-for-service models to value-based payment models.

[ABP 9.B. Commonly used terms and metrics (eg, length of stay, readmissions, costs and charges), ABP 13.B.7 Cost benefit, cost effectiveness, and outcomes]

Table 3.5 TYPES OF WASTE SEEN IN HEALTHCARE WITH DEFINITIONS AND EXAMPLES[a]

WASTE	DEFINITION	EXAMPLE(S)
Defects	Errors that do not produce the desired outcome	Misdiagnosis, medication errors
Overproduction	Doing/creating more than what is needed by the patient	Delivering meals to patients who are not allowed to eat by mouth
Waiting	Delay in service provided	A patient not being discharged until 5 PM when they were clinically ready at noon
Not using talent	Failing to utilize individuals' potential or assigning them to jobs below their maximum ability	Having a charge nurse serve as the one-to-one sitter when there is a patient under suicide precautions
Transportation	Unnecessary movement of materials or patients within the system	A patient is brought to and from a centralized electrocardiography room rather than performing the procedure in their room
Inventory	Extra supplies that may not be used, may expire, and take up space	Printing 1000 copies of a form that is then replaced after only 200 have been used
Motion	Unnecessary movement by employees within the system	Phlebotomists traveling to multiple floors rather than having local assignments
Extraprocessing	Performing additional tasks or making existing tasks more complex than necessary	Requiring a complex form to be completed that includes unnecessary information

[a] Adapted from Reference 1.

REFERENCES

1. Scheurer D, Crabtree E, Cawley PJ, Lee TH. The value equation: enhancing patient outcomes while constraining costs. *Am J Med Sci*. 2016;*351*(1):44–51.
2. Defining value: connecting quality and safety to costs of care. In: Shah N, Arora V, Moriates C, eds. *Understanding Value-Based Healthcare*. McGraw-Hill; 2015.

69. ANSWER: A

Implicit biases are a normal form of social cognitive processing and occur early in life in response to repeated exposure and reinforcement of stereotypes. These unconscious attitudes can impact understanding, actions, and decisions. The Implicit Association Test is an established measure of implicit bias, and studies have shown that healthcare professionals exhibit the same levels of implicit bias as the general population. Biases are provider-level factors that contribute to health disparities. In order to improve health equity, it is critical to recognize that implicit biases exist and to consciously work to mitigate their effects. Strategies include stereotype replacement, individuation, understanding patient perspectives, and individual patient empathy. Notably, empathy biases also exist, and if a provider experiences empathy toward one group over another, this can worsen disparities in care.

[ABP 10.C.3. Implicit bias]

REFERENCE

1. Raphael JL, Oyeku SO. Implicit bias in pediatrics: an emerging focus in health equity research. *Pediatrics*. 2020;*145*(5):e20200512

70. ANSWER: E

When designing a study, a researcher must accept that most study designs are imperfect. It can be too expensive, too time consuming, or unethical to recruit the optimal number of subjects or use the most accurate test. Therefore, the researcher designs the best study they can and then draws inferences from their findings that they apply to both their study population (internal validity) and the world at large (external validity). Testing and validation of a survey tool (choice E) is a necessary process to ensure that the results represent the actual exposure of the patients and will help the internal validity of the study. While an objective measure such as blood zinc levels (choice C) may help ensure internal validity in some cases, it would be inappropriate in this study because the study is retrospective and zinc levels would only measure exposure after admission. In the example above, surveying a broader population (choices A and D) could improve external validity by ensuring that the study population is as representative of all children who have the exposure or outcome. Limiting the types of gastroenteritis by excluding patients with recent travel (choice B) will also primarily affect the external validity of the study, but in this case would limit generalizability to a single subset of patients with GE. This may be appropriate to ensure a consistent, homogeneous population, but it may also inadvertently introduce selection bias.

[ABP 13.B.1. Study design, performance, and analysis]

REFERENCE

1. Hulley SB, Newman TB, Cummings SR. Planning the measurements: precision, accuracy, and validity. In: Hulley SB, Cummings SR, Browner WS, et al., eds. *Designing Clinical Research*. 4th ed. Lippincott Williams & Wilkins; 2013:37–50.

71. ANSWER: E

The technique described is known as teach back, in which a patient or caregiver explains the newly learned information back to the physician. This is an important teaching method to ensure the learner, in this case a patient or caregiver, understands the information received. Discharge planning is the process of preparing for transitioning a patient out of the hospital, taking into consideration their anticipated healthcare needs such as medications, medical equipment, and disposition. A discharge checklist is a tool usually used by provider teams to systematically ensure all aspects of the discharge process are completed. Medication reconciliation involves comparing a patient's discharge medication list to their list before admission to identify any changes. In this case, reviewing all of the new asthma medications that were started during this admission would be an example of medication reconciliation. The asthma action plan itself is an example of written and verbal patient instructions.

[ABP 6.E. Patient/family education, ABP 12.B. Teaching strategies for patients and caregivers]

72. ANSWER: B

The patient is developing a septic joint and subsequent septic shock requiring transfer to a tertiary care children's hospital for further evaluation and potential surgical intervention. Patients with septic shock are at risk for tissue hypoxia due to impaired perfusion. In this case, it is important to maximize the patient's fraction of inspired oxygen (FiO_2) in preparation for the 1-hour transport. A nonrebreather is the best way to provide this in a noninvasive fashion and can be continued during transportation. Neither a nasal cannula nor a simple face mask provides significant supplemental FiO_2. Neither bag-valve mask ventilation nor intubation is indicated as the patient is not currently displaying signs of respiratory failure, and both of these interventions would make transport more challenging.

[ABP 7.C. Transport facilitation and risk mitigation]

73. ANSWER: C

The chief medical officer is describing high-reliability organization principles. Many healthcare organizations have adopted these principles, better known outside the healthcare industry, as they work to develop failure-free processes. The primary principles of high-reliability organizations are as follows: preoccupation with failure (i.e., thinking about and planning for the ways a process could go wrong); a reluctance to accept variation as the norm, especially when an adverse event has occurred; an awareness of common ways that daily processes can result in failure; leadership commitment to timely feedback about processes and outcomes, using data to report these outcomes, and learning from underperformance; allowing experts with the appropriate skill set to design processes. Human factors engineering principles focus on the interaction between humans and the system and how those interactions lead to adverse events. Clinical operations focus on the day-to-day running of the organization, including staffing and supplies. Just culture principles include an approach to evaluating errors by looking at the system and promoting a safe environment to discuss errors without fear of retribution. Situational awareness is an awareness of what is going on around you in order to anticipate future actions or events that may occur and lead to adverse events.

[ABP 8.D. Principles of patient safety and high reliability organizations (HROs)]

74. ANSWER: A

A charge is the amount asked by a provider for a service rendered; it is usually a combination of the actual cost of the healthcare service rendered plus a markup. This is the hospital's "asking price" and is often determined by rate setting. Rate setting consists of assessing resource consumption to cost per unit of service provided and often factors in extra costs, such as future hospital expansion.

Cost finding consists of measuring cost by resource consumption, including time, effort, and money. The expense of delivering healthcare to the patient is a cost to the provider. The amount an insurance company pays to a provider is a cost to the payer. Out-of-pocket services are a cost to the patient. Cost is not only financial cost but also physical harm, adverse effects, psychological effects, and other unanticipated harms to both the provider and patient, such as an acquired acute kidney injury secondary to medication. Charges have no relationship to the form of payment by the patient. Since there is often a discrepancy between charges and costs, there is usually an agreement on rates between provider and payer.

[ABP 9.B. Commonly used terms and metrics (eg, length of stay, readmissions, costs and charges)]

REFERENCE

1. Finkler SA. The distinction between cost and charges. *Ann Intern Med.* 1982;96(1):102–109.

75. ANSWER: D

The minority tax is a significant issue impacting Black/Indigenous/people of color (BIPOC) physicians in academic medicine. Broadly speaking, the minority tax is the additional responsibilities and obligations shouldered by BIPOC physicians (compared with their White colleagues) in the name of advancing DEI efforts. In their commentary, *Paying a Penny for Our Thoughts and Then Asking for Our 2 Cents*, Drs. Mustapha and Eyssallenne outlined institutional changes that can help reduce the minority tax. Given the significant amount of time many BIPOC faculty spend mentoring BIPOC colleagues and learners to help promote retention, a key step is to recognize the value of that mentoring with protected academic time. Another step is for an institution to commit to supporting community-based research at the same level it supports bench research, given the disproportionate amount of health disparities research done by BIPOC faculty. Broadening the definition of scholarly work (e.g., publication of a reflective piece of the experience of being a BIPOC physician) and ensuring that service for DEI work is acknowledged with protected time to do that work (rather than just praise) are other important steps to reduce the minority tax.

[ABP 12.D. Principles of mentorship]

REFERENCE

1. Mustapha T, Eyssallenne T. Paying a penny for our thoughts and then asking for our 2 cents. *Acad Med.* 2020;95(12):1788.

76. ANSWER: B

Generalizability refers to the ability of a study to be applied to the clinical population of interest. In the case above, the study is limited to patients with cellulitis, who are unlikely to represent the patients for whom cardiopulmonary monitoring may be most helpful. As such, the fact that there were no increased PICU transfers may not apply to all patients on an acute care unit. There is no evidence that the results here are not internally valid, meaning that the results of the study represent the reality within that study and are not significantly affected by bias and/or confounding. Because the study is a randomized controlled trial, one can reasonably assume causal inference, meaning that changes in the variable of interest directly led to the differences in outcomes seen. This study should also have sufficient power due to the large sample size. Power, the ability of a study to find differences if they exist, is increased as the sample size increases. Reliability refers to the results remaining consistent if measured by multiple observers. In this case, both PICU transfers and length of stay are objective measurements that should have good reliability.

[ABP 13.B.2. Generalizability]

REFERENCE

1. Plake BS, et al. Validity. In: Plake BS, Wise LL, Cook LL, et al., eds. *Standards for Educational and Psychological Testing*. American Educational Research Association; 2014:11–32.

77. ANSWER: D

Shared decision-making is a critical aspect of patient-centered care. This process involves clinicians and patients working together to make decisions based on both physician expertise and evidence-based medicine as well as patient experience and values. In all situations, but particularly circumstances where there is no clear "right" answer, shared decision-making is a valuable tool for reaching a consensus and is the approach generally preferred by patients. As leaders of multidisciplinary teams, hospitalists are well positioned to aid in the shared decision-making process. Patients and caregivers should be invited to participate in decision-making and should be told the risks and benefits of each option. Then, the hospitalist can help guide a conversation about what the patient or family's values are and help them to feel comfortable making a decision. Choosing the bone marrow biopsy in order not to miss a malignancy or the corticosteroids to provide comfort are not the best options because the physician would be deciding the patient's priorities. While the most common cause of fever in pediatric patients is viral infection, observation alone is unlikely to be sufficient after a prolonged period of fever. Discussing the case in the hospitalist care conference may be helpful, but it is not the best option as it does not engage the patient or caregiver in the decision-making process.

[ABP 6.A. Shared decision-making and conflict resolution]

78. ANSWER: D

Root cause analysis and actions is a technique that seeks to find the underlying hidden causes of an error after one has occurred. In the case above, this would be the most effective method to discover which causes can be targeted by improvement. While also aiming to prevent errors, FMEA is a proactive process aimed to prevent errors due to a new system before they occur. PDSA cycles are efforts to implement improvements, but they cannot function in isolation before root causes are identified.

ARCC and SBAR are communication methods that can be used during a critical moment to attempt to prevent an error, but they are not tools to respond to an error once one has occurred.

[ABP 8.E. Safety processes and tools]

79. ANSWER: C

This patient has a confirmed febrile urinary tract infection (UTI). A UTI is diagnosed by the presence of both a urinalysis that suggests infection and at least 50,000 CFU/mL of an organism in a catheterized urine culture. The American Academy of Pediatrics (AAP) clinical practice guideline for the diagnosis and management of the initial UTI in febrile infants and young children 2–24 months of age recommends an RBUS. The RBUS should evaluate for renal scarring, hydronephrosis, or other signs of vesicoureteral reflux (VUR). It is estimated that about 15% of cases in this age group will have an abnormal RBUS. This may be deferred to the end of treatment as reversible infection-mediated dilation may be misdiagnosed as hydronephrosis.

A VCUG should not be routinely obtained for a first febrile UTI unless the RBUS is abnormal. The majority of infants with a first febrile UTI will not have treatable VUR; thus, a VCUG would lead to overdiagnosis and expose infants to unnecessary radiation. However, the AAP does recommend monitoring for future recurrences of UTIs as this may suggest the need for further evaluation to prevent renal scarring.

This patient is well appearing and can be trialed on oral antibiotics. Intramuscular or intravenous antibiotics should be reserved for infants requiring hospital admission. There is also no evidence for a "test-of-cure" repeat urine culture unless the patient fails to respond to treatment.

[ABP 9.A. Principles of value in healthcare for individuals and populations (e.g., reducing unwarranted variation, overuse, overtreatment, overdiagnosis)]

REFERENCE

1. Subcommittee on Urinary Tract Infection. Reaffirmation of AAP clinical practice guideline: the diagnosis and management of the initial urinary tract infection in febrile infants and young children 2–24 months of age. *Pediatrics*. 2016;*138*(6):e20163026.

80. ANSWER: E

Most research is intended ultimately to identify causal relationships between variables. While randomized controlled trials can more directly identify causal relationships, it is important to ensure that the associations found in observational studies are not due to other unidentified factors. A confounding variable is a factor that is associated with both the exposure variable (choice C) and the outcome variable (choice B) and has a direct causal relationship on both the exposure and outcome. This often leads not only to incorrectly identifying associations where there are none but also can mask true associations that exist. In the case above, patients who were premature (choice E) were both more likely to be taking MCT oil and more likely to have larger weight gain after 1 month as they "caught up" with their nonpremature counterparts. Therefore, the MCT oil itself may have had no direct benefit. Because age in months (choice A) and milk protein allergy (choice D) are not significantly associated with the outcome variable, as evidenced by p values greater than .05, they are not candidates for confounding variables. To remove the effect of a confounder, investigators can control for the potential confounder (e.g., with a randomized controlled trial) or perform a stratified analysis.

[ABP 13.B.3. Bias and confounding]

REFERENCE

1. Normand SL, Sykora K, Li P, Mamdani M, Rochon PA, Anderson GM. Readers guide to critical appraisal of cohort studies: 3. Analytical strategies to reduce confounding. *BMJ*. 2005;*330*(7498):1021–1023.

81. ANSWER: D

Patients and providers must be able to communicate effectively with each other to optimize care. While hospital systems can provide testing options for providers to demonstrate competency to communicate with patients in a given language (D), federal law requires hospitals and clinics that receive any federal reimbursement (e.g., Medicare, Medicaid, etc.) to provide language services, including navigating access for languages that are rarely spoken (C). This includes access to languages used by the deaf or hard of hearing, which may include sign language interpreters or certified deaf interpreters who themselves are deaf or hard of hearing (E). The request for interpreters may be made by either party (patient/family or providers) when there is a concern for limited English proficiency (A). Medical interpreters work with verbal communication, whereas medical translation is the act of transcribing the written word from one language to another (e.g., discharge summaries and informed consent). According to the National Standards of Practice for Interpreters in Health Care, medical interpreters should "render all messages accurately and completely, without adding, omitting, or substituting . . . repeat[ing] all that is said, even if it seems redundant, irrelevant, or rude" (Rushke) (B).

[ABP 6.C. Cultural competency (language, cultural factors)]

REFERENCE

1. Rushke K, Bidar-Sielaff S. National standards of practice for interpreters in health care. Published September 2005. Accessed September 15, 2021. https://www.ncihc.org/assets/documents/publications/NCIHC National Standards of Practice.pdf.

82. ANSWER: B

Within healthcare organizations, the just culture approach is one that focuses on addressing systems issues that lead to patient harm and improving those systems in a way that reduces an individual's likelihood to perform an unsafe task. A just culture is one where individuals are held accountable for abiding by rules and procedures; however, there is acknowledgment that most errors are a result of fallible humans working in a complex system that increases the risk of making an error. In the vignette above, the chlorhexidine step was forgotten, a lapse. Simple human errors, such as lapses (forgetting to do something that was intended) or slips (inadvertently performing a task incorrectly, e.g., pouring salt in one's coffee instead of sugar), are inevitable, and the system should work to protect patients from harm when they do occur. The response to these errors should involve training the person who has made the error, but the mainstay of response should be to improve the system's processes and design. At-risk behavior, on the other hand, occurs when someone purposely breaks a rule due to underestimation of the risk. An example of this outside of medicine is texting while driving. Such behaviors can be addressed by increasing situational awareness and by shifting incentives. Reckless behaviors involve conscious disregard for risk and within the just culture framework warrant disciplinary action and remediation. Sentinel events are specifically defined errors that need to be reported depending on an organization's accreditation and jurisdiction. Generally, these are errors that result in permanent or severe harm or death.

[ABP 8.E. Safety processes and tools]

REFERENCE

1. Ulrich B. Just culture and its impact on a culture of safety. *Nephrol Nurs J*. 2017;*44*(3):207–259.

83. ANSWER: E

External validity refers to the degree to which results of the study apply to patients outside of the study. It is also known as generalizability. If a study sample population is not representative of the general population, this is a threat to external validity as the results may not be applicable to the patient population of a practitioner deciding whether or not to implement study results for his or her patient. Internal validity is the extent to which the results of the study demonstrate a true cause-and-effect relationship. Bias and chance threaten the internal validity of a study. Bias is an error that can produce a conclusion that is different from true effect. Randomized controlled trials are designed to minimize bias, but it is difficult and costly to avoid all forms of bias. Loss of subjects to follow-up leading to missing data, data collectors knowing random group assignments of study participants, study participants not adhering to assigned intervention, and lack of blinding of study participants to group assignments are all examples of sources of bias in randomized trials that can affect the internal validity of a study.

[ABP 9.E. Principles of evidence evaluation (source and strength), ABP 13.B.8. Measurement (eg, validity, reliability)]

REFERENCE

1. Crowne SS. Research and statistics: generalizability and how it relates to validity. *Pediatr Rev.* 2010;*31*(8):335–336.

84. ANSWER: D

Observational studies can demonstrate associations but not causation, while controlled experiments can provide evidence of causality. Association, the opposite of independence, means that having information about one variable provides some predictive information about another variable. On the other hand, causality requires a direct and directional effect of some exposure variable on an outcome. Said another way, if there is a causal relationship from variable A to variable B, then changing variable A will lead to changes in variable B. In addition to the results of direct experimentation, the likelihood of a causal relationship between two variables is bolstered by the Bradford-Hill criteria, which include

1. The strength of the empirical association (choice E)
2. Consistent association in multiple study settings (choice A)
3. The exposure occurring prior to the outcome (choice D)
4. The existence of a plausible mechanism of causation (choices B and C)

Although each of the answer choices above would relatively weaken the evidence for a causal link, the reversed time order (choice D), is an absolute contradiction because a cause must precede an effect.

[ABP 13.B.4. Causation]

REFERENCE

1. Lucas RM, McMichael AJ. Association or causation: evaluating links between "environment and disease." *Bull World Health Org.* Published October 2005. Accessed September 15, 2021. https://www.who.int/bulletin/volumes/83/10/792.pdf.

85. ANSWER: C

While all of these approaches are routinely used with learners in medical education and each can be valuable when used appropriately, one of the most effective things to do when beginning with any learner is to assess their current knowledge base and skill level. Doing so allows for teaching to be targeted at the edge of their knowledge (their "zone of proximal development"), which is the most effective way to promote learning. By encouraging a student to ask questions about patients on rounds, you will be able to begin developing an understanding of what they do and do not know. Assigning an article (A) or a teaching topic (D) is a fine way to build their knowledge base, but it does not add to your understanding of their current knowledge level. Participatory learning (B) is generally more effective than observation, but directed questioning (i.e., "pimping") can be overly stressful for some students. While assigning a full load of patients (E) may allow for assessment of the student's knowledge base, it is less learner centered than option C.

[ABP 12.B. Teaching strategies for multiple types and levels of learners, including patients and caregivers]

86. ANSWER: E

Identification of patient safety events and near misses is a difficult process that often relies on members of the healthcare team having the awareness and time to utilize a hospital's error-reporting system. While voluntary error reporting is an important component of the capture of events, a system that utilizes information from multiple sources is more robust and more likely not to miss important learning opportunities. Trigger tools, such as the Global Assessment of Pediatric Patient Safety (GAPPS) tool, utilize the processing power of the electronic medical record to automatically identify key adverse events. Because trigger tools are automated, their implementation is more reliable and sustainable than most approaches that rely on human effort and attention, such as the voluntary error-reporting system and daily huddles. However, both approaches are integral to casting as wide a net as possible to capture potential patient safety events. Focus on severe events, especially patient deaths, is also necessary for both patient safety and required reporting reasons, but these are thankfully rare and will miss many near-miss events as well as minimal harm events.

[ABP 8.E. Safety processes and tools]

REFERENCE

1. Stockwell DC, Bisarya H, Classen DC, et al. Development of an electronic pediatric all-cause harm measurement tool using a modified delphi method. *J Patient Saf.* 2016;12(4):180–189.

87. ANSWER: A

This patient is presenting with a minor head injury without neurologic signs or high-risk factors as defined by the Pediatric Emergency Care Applied Research Network (PECARN). The Choosing Wisely campaign promotes high-value care that is centered on evidence, truly necessary, not duplicative of care already received, and does not cause harm. The Choosing Wisely campaign recommends following the PECARN prediction rule.

The prediction rule for children older than 2 years includes normal mental status, no loss of consciousness, no vomiting, nonsevere injury mechanism, no signs of a basilar skull fracture (e.g., retroauricular or periorbital bruising or hemotympanum), and no severe headache. The rule has a negative predictive value of 99.95% and a sensitivity of 96.8% for diagnosing a clinically important traumatic brain injury.

For this case, PECARN recommends observing in the ED and monitoring for worsening symptoms. This patient does not need admission overnight if there are no worsening symptoms after a time period of observation in the ED. A head CT and brain MRI are not warranted in this case as there is a less than 1% risk of a significant traumatic brain injury.

[ABP 9.A. Principles of value in healthcare for individuals and populations (e.g., reducing unwarranted variation, overuse, overtreatment, overdiagnosis), ABP N.5. Trauma (including head trauma)]

REFERENCES

1. American Academy of Pediatrics. AAP—CT scans for minor head injuries. Choosing Wisely. Published October 29, 2018. Accessed April 18, 2021. https://www.choosingwisely.org/clinician-lists/american-academy-pediatrics-ct-scans-to-evaluate-minor-head-injuries/.
2. Kuppermann N, Holmes JF, Dayan PS, et al. Identification of children at very low risk of clinically-important brain injuries after head trauma: a prospective cohort study *Lancet.* 2009;374(9696):1160–1170.

88. ANSWER: C

During the peak of the COVID-19 pandemic, hospital-based clinicians had the difficult task of keeping track of constantly evolving hospital policies ranging from use of personal protective equipment to screening and testing protocols. Most hospitals across the country instituted strict zero-visitation policies, and while children's hospitals tended to consider the nuances of these policies for children, some hospitals did not provide distinctions. The American Academy of Pediatrics (AAP) swiftly released a policy statement calling for at least one family member to be present at the bedside during the hospital stay of a child if the family member screened negative for symptoms.

One of the challenges a hospitalist must face is how to best advocate for their patients within the confines of occasionally unclear hospital policies. In this case, separating the infant from the asymptomatic breastfeeding mother is not an appropriate medical decision or the best decision for the patient and mother's well-being. Given the risk-benefit ratio of separating the family or delaying admission, the baby should be admitted to the hospital to receive the necessary medical care and the mother should be allowed to continue to breastfeed, which is consistent with AAP best practices. In the morning, the hospitalist should discuss the case with relevant administrators to justify the clinical decision-making.

While the hospitalist should aim to use their therapeutic alliance with the mother to broach a discussion about vaccination, this conversation should wait until the patient is safely admitted and the logistics of visitation have been sorted out.

[ABP 6.F. Patient and caregiver resiliency and well-being]

REFERENCE

1. Family presence policies for pediatric inpatient settings during the COVID-19 pandemic. American Academy of Pediatrics. https://services.aap.org/en/pages/2019-novel-coronavirus-covid-19-infections/clinical-guidance/family-presence-policies-for-pediatric-inpatient-settings-during-the-covid-19-pandemic/. Published 2020. Accessed April 24, 2021.

89. ANSWER: E

It is often beneficial for researchers to measure the frequency of disease in a population to determine the burden and quantify the benefit of prevention or treatment. The most common measures of frequency are incidence and prevalence. Incidence is a measure of the number of new cases among patients at risk over time. Because incidence is a rate, a time component must be noted (in this case, CLABSIs per central line-year). Because CLABSIs only occur in patients with central lines, only the months in which a patient had a central line count (4 years total). In addition, because CLABSIs can recur, a given patient may count multiple times if they still have a central line and develop an additional infection. The incidence in this case is five CLABSIs in 4 central line-years, or 1.25 CLABSIs per central-line year. It would be incorrect to only count the four patients with infections (choice D). In addition, it is important to use the correct time unit, as not doing so can lead to large over- or underestimation of incidence; for example, five CLABSIs per 48 months (0.105, choice B) or four patients per 48 months (0.083, choice A). Prevalence is the proportion of the population at risk that has the disease at a given point in time. As a proportion, prevalence must be between 0 and 1. None of the choices in the question is truly a prevalence, although the cumulative incidence, 4 out of 10 patients = 0.400 (choice C) is the closest.

[ABP 13.B.5. Incidence and prevalence]

REFERENCE

1. Noordzij M, Dekker FW, Zoccali C, Jager KJ. Measures of disease frequency: prevalence and incidence. *Nephron Clin Pract.* 2010;*115*(1):c17–c20.

90. ANSWER: B

Failure mode and effects analysis is the best tool for the team's purpose. This tool allows a team to map a process and proactively identify risks where harm might occur within that process. The team would (1) list the steps in the process, (2) identify failure modes (ways in which each step could go wrong), (3) determine the causes of the potential failure, and (4) what would be the effects of that failure occurring. This tool allows a team to correct processes before implementation to prevent harm. A key driver diagram is a tool that is used in quality improvement to identify the changes that may result in an improvement. A Plan-Do-Study-Act cycle is a quality improvement tool that allows a team to methodically test a change to see if it leads to improvement. Typically, a team will engage in several Plan-Do-Study-Act cycles before achieving their improvement goals. A root cause analysis is a tool used after an error has occurred to explore the factors that may have led to the error. A cause-and-effect diagram, also known as a fishbone diagram, is a specific type of root cause analysis tool primarily used to explore the multiple causes that contributed to an outcome that already occurred.

[ABP 8.E. Safety processes and tools]

REFERENCE

1. Resources. Institute for Healthcare Improvement. Accessed March 25, 2021. https://www.ihi.org/resources/Pages/default.aspx.

91. ANSWER: D

This patient's history, physical examination, and laboratory findings are concerning for incomplete Kawasaki disease, which requires hospital admission. The patient may require additional workup, such as an echocardiogram, and specialty consultation that may not be available at the local community hospital. In this case, transportation via ground ambulance to a tertiary care hospital would be the most appropriate. Transporting the patient via private vehicle would carry considerable risk due to the weather conditions and the need for monitoring during transport. The patient is not far away or unstable enough to justify an air ambulance, which also carries a significant risk during these conditions and may result in a significant charge to the family.

[ABP 7.B. Triage within the healthcare system]

92. ANSWER: A

Test screening as an epidemiologic tool needs to follow certain principles. The traditional list of principles, created by Wilson and Jungner, includes

1. The condition sought should be an important health problem
2. The natural history of the condition, including development from latent to declared disease, should be adequately understood (opposite of choice C)
3. There should be a recognizable latent or early symptomatic stage (choice A)
4. There should be a suitable test or examination (opposite of choice D)
5. The test should be acceptable to the population
6. There should be an agreed policy on whom to treat as patients (opposite of choice B)
7. There should be accepted treatment for patients with recognized disease (opposite of choice E)
8. Facilities for diagnosis and treatment should be available
9. The cost of case finding (including diagnosis and treatment of patients diagnosed) should be economically balanced in relation to possible expenditure on medical care as a whole
10. Case finding should be a continuing process and not a "once-and-for-all" project

The goal of screening in general is to find potential cases from a general population, limiting false negatives. Confirmatory testing may be necessary. As a result, in general, sensitivity (opposite of choice D) is much more important than specificity.

[ABP 13.B.6. Screening]

REFERENCE

1. Dobrow MJ, Hagens V, Chafe R, Sullivan T, Rabeneck L. Consolidated principles for screening based on a systematic review and consensus process. *CMAJ.* 2018;*190*(14):E422–E429.

93. ANSWER: B

Disclosure is communication that is directed toward patients or their family that informs them of a medical error or adverse event that occurred. Disclosure is considered a legal and ethical duty for physicians, promotes a positive therapeutic relationship, and likely decreases the risk of litigation. In the vignette above, the hospitalist has explained that an error has occurred and the likely risks from that error, which constitute a disclosure. Unlike an apology, disclosure does not hypothesize about the root cause or attempt to assign blame or fault. The difference between disclosure and apology is important, as most medical errors are multifactorial and associated more with problems within the system than any individual. Error reporting, on the other hand, is the process by which a clinician informs an organization and regulators about an error and is separate from communication with the patient or family. Triggers are intended to identify potential adverse events and medical errors automatically to augment error reporting. Remediation is a process through which physicians who have shown negligence or a pattern of consistent error are supported to improve.

[ABP 8.F. Patient safety regulations (eg, mandatory reporting, disclosure, never events)]

REFERENCE

1. Committee on Medical Liability and Risk Management, Council on Quality Improvement and Patient Safety. Disclosure of adverse events in pediatrics. *Pediatrics*. 2016:*138*(6):e20163215.

94. ANSWER: B

Healthcare access is composed of four key elements: coverage, services, timeliness, and workforce. Coverage refers to insurance status and facilitates a patient's access to the healthcare system in the United States. Services include having a usual source of care for screening, prevention, and follow-up. Timeliness is the ability to receive healthcare when needed. Workforce is the access to capable and qualified providers. Cultural competence is part of the workforce element but is not one of the key elements in itself. Value can be defined by quality of outcomes for the cost of care. Although value is fundamental in healthcare, it is not one of the four elements of healthcare access.

[ABP 10.C.1. Health care access]

REFERENCE

1. Chartbook on Access to Healthcare. Agency for Healthcare Research and Quality. Accessed September 16, 2021. https://www.ahrq.gov/research/findings/nhqrdr/chartbooks/access/elements.html.

95. ANSWER: B

The American Academy of Pediatrics clinical practice guideline for bronchiolitis does not recommend the use of albuterol as there has been no effect on infants hospitalized with bronchiolitis, and albuterol can be associated with significant tachycardia. As such, the use of albuterol for this patient is considered overtreatment.

Overuse is defined as the provision of medical services that are more likely to cause harm than good or the provision of medical services that a fully informed patient does not want. Direct measurement of overuse is when scientific evidence or consensus dictates what is appropriate and there is a deviation from the standard. Indirect measurement of overuse is when there is unexpected variation in healthcare utilization that is not attributable to population differences.

Overtreatment is a type of overuse that is defined as a treatment where there is no evidence of benefit, such as any treatment that is futile or excessive in complexity, duration, or cost.

Overdiagnosis is closely related to overuse and can lead to overtreatment. It is defined as the over-detection and over-definition of a disease. This is different from a misdiagnosis, for which there is an incorrect identification of disease. Overdiagnosis identifies a true abnormality, but the abnormality will not bring harm to the patient. An example is the use of pulse oximetry in bronchiolitis, which detects transient desaturations, prolonging hospitalizations despite the patient not requiring additional respiratory support.

[ABP 9.A. Principles of value in healthcare for individuals and populations (e.g., reducing unwarranted variation, overuse, overtreatment, overdiagnosis)]

REFERENCES

1. Ralston SL, Lieberthal AS, Meissner HC, et al. Clinical practice guideline: the diagnosis, management, and prevention of bronchiolitis. *Pediatrics*. 2014;*134*(5):e1474–e1502.
2. Coon ER, Quinonez RA, Moyer VA, Schroeder AR. Overdiagnosis: how our compulsion for diagnosis may be harming children. *Pediatrics*. 2014;*134*(5):1013–1023.

96. ANSWER: C

Providing feedback is a critical part of working with learners. There are many types of feedback, and the type highlighted in this scenario is best described as formative feedback. Formative feedback is given during or after a particular encounter or task, with the goal of helping the learner make timely adjustments to improve their performance in that area. The feedback is concrete and focuses on specific behaviors or skills. It is a "low-stakes" type of evaluation in that it generally does not count toward a grade or final performance rating. In contrast, summative feedback is a comprehensive assessment of a learner's performance at the end of a course or clinical rotation. Self-feedback involves reflection and can involve self-rating. Feedback can be obtained from multiple perspectives using 360-degree feedback (e.g., from attendings, peers, nurses, and patients' families).

Finally, intrinsic feedback is what a learner experiences as they perform a task (e.g., feeling a needle running into a spinous process during a lumbar puncture attempt).

[ABP 12.C. Principles of effective assessment and feedback]

REFERENCE

1. Kelly E, Richards JB. Medical education: giving feedback to doctors in training. *BMJ*. 2019;366:l4523.

97. ANSWER: E

It is vitally important for medical research to maintain the public trust and promote public good by adhering to ethical standards. The Belmont Report laid out the principles of ethical research as respect for persons, beneficence, and justice. Within pediatric research, respect for persons is particularly important as children are a vulnerable population that might not have full control over their ability to volunteer. Informed consent is the most common application of the respect-for-persons principle and states that "subjects, to the degree that they are capable, be given the opportunity to choose what shall or shall not happen to them." In pediatrics, this is complicated by the fact that children cannot legally consent to most procedures. Starting at an intellectual age of 7, a child should be given the opportunity to understand and affirmatively assent to participation in a research study. In the case presented, the child has adequate understanding and decision-making capacity, and the circumstance is not an emergency; hence, the child's failure to assent should lead to non-enrollment. It would be unethical to enroll the child despite her lack of assent and even more so to tamper with the randomization process. Although all children are considered a "vulnerable" population, not enrolling any children would lead to a lack of evidence basis for this population and would harm the care of children.

[ABP 13.C.1. Professionalism and misconduct in research; ABP 13.C.2 Principles of research involving human subjects; ABP 13.C.3 Principles of consent and assent]

REFERENCE

1. Department of Health, Education, and Welfare; National Commission for the Protection of Human Subjects of Biomedical and Behavioral Research. The Belmont Report. Ethical principles and guidelines for the protection of human subjects of research. *J Am Coll Dent*. 2014;81(3):4–13.

98. ANSWER: E

Sentinel events are defined as an event not related to the natural course of a patient's illness that results in death, permanent harm, or severe temporary harm to a patient.

"Severe temporary harm" is considered a potentially life-threatening harm that lasts for a limited time but may require transfer to a higher level of care or additional surgery or procedure to resolve the condition. Of the choices above, choice E is a sentinel event because the injury (a) occurred due to the care provided and (b) led to surgery, with the potential for permanent harm.

Healthcare organizations, including hospitals, typically receive oversight for healthcare delivery from an accrediting body such as the Joint Commission, Det Norske Veritas (DNV), and others. These accrediting bodies partner with healthcare organizations to evaluate serious patient safety events, with the goal of preventing future harm. Sentinel events require immediate investigation with a planned response and method to measure that response. Hospitals are generally mandated to report sentinel events to their respective accreditation program. A subset of sentinel events, "never events" are clearly identifiable, are preventable, and result in serious harm. Examples of "never events" include surgery on the wrong body part and discharging an infant with the wrong parent; these events are thought to be so egregious that they should never happen under any circumstances.

Although a fall (choice A) would be considered a sentinel event if it resulted in a broken bone or other injury requiring surgery, in this case the child only had minor injuries. Choice B is considered a close call, or near miss, because the patient safety event did not reach the patient. The patient in choice C experienced an adverse event because the medication caused an acute kidney injury, but the injury was not severe or permanent. Choice D is a no-harm event, defined as a patient safety event that reaches the patient but does not cause harm. The placement of two patients with the same last name in adjacent rooms is considered a hazardous condition, a situation that increases the chance of an adverse event occurring.

[ABP 8.F. Patient safety regulations (eg, mandatory reporting, disclosure, never events)]

REFERENCE

1. Sentinel event. Joint Commission. Accessed March 31, 2021. https://www.jointcommission.org/-/media/tjc/documents/resources/patient-safety-topics/sentinel-event/camh_se-chapter.pdf.

99. ANSWER: C

Hospitalists are charged with not only keeping their patients safe and cared for, but also ensuring that the members of the care team have a safe learning environment. This includes safety from overt racist, sexist, or harmful language, as well as a space where microaggressions—brief environmental indignities that communicate derogatory or negative attitudes toward marginalized groups, regardless of intention—are dealt with. In this example, the family member's "surprise" that their doctor was Black followed with the statement "but we're impressed with how articulate and smart he is" both provide examples of this type of harmful language that reinforces hurtful stereotypes, even when the speaker may feel they are paying a compliment.

While there is no single correct way to handle these types of encounters, what is clear is the need to be prepared for when they happen. In this example, it is essential that the hospitalist leverage their position as the leader of the team to immediately make clear that they hear the microaggression, do their best to combat the hurtful stereotype surrounding it, and provide an opportunity for those affected to debrief and strategize how to best move forward (C). While it is essential to get Dr. Rogers's perspective as part of a debrief regarding what would be most helpful for him, demonstrating allyship in real time is important, and the burden should not be placed on the marginalized to speak up against a microaggression or be the first to respond (B).

While it may be tempting to simply pivot (A) or ignore (E) these types of comments, both allow the microaggression to remain without addressing it head on. Additionally, it can be tempting to confront the speaker aggressively in real time to highlight the racist language (D). Balancing the challenge of providing optimal care for the hospitalized child with a psychologically safe work environment often requires nuanced restraint. Providers should aim to maintain the therapeutic alliance with patience and explore comments as objectively as possible without responding with negative emotion. In this example, it may be ideal to circle back with the family to provide feedback, especially if this is an action step deemed appropriate as part of a debrief after the event.

[ABP 6.B. Patient/family-centered rounds]

REFERENCE

1. Wheeler DJ, Zapata J, Davis D, Chou C. Twelve tips for responding to microaggressions and overt discrimination: when the patient offends the learner. *Med Teach*. 2019;*41*(10):1112–1117.

100. ANSWER: B

Intravenous immunoglobulin started within the first 10 days of fever onset in children with Kawasaki disease reduces the risk of coronary aneurysms from approximately 25% to less than 5%. With timely IVIG treatment, only 1% of children develop giant aneurysms. The administration of live-virus vaccines should be postponed for children treated with IVIG and other blood products. This is due to antibodies in blood products potentially affecting the immunogenic response to live-virus vaccine administration.

The recommended length of delay is dependent on the product and the dose given. In this case, given that the child received high-dose IVIG, live-virus immunizations need to be delayed by at least 11 months. However, non-live vaccines should be administered. Yearly influenza vaccines are strongly recommended to decrease the risk of Reye syndrome for children on aspirin.

Admission to the hospital is an opportunity to review the overall health of a child. Pediatric hospitalists should know the immunization history of hospitalized children, as well as contraindications and side effects of vaccines. In this case, the MMR and varicella vaccines need to be delayed for at least 11 months. The plan of care for the child, including catch-up vaccinations, should be communicated to the child's outpatient physician during hospitalization and at discharge.

[ABP 9.C: Identifying and Addressing Unmet Healthcare Needs (e.g. preventative care)]

REFERENCE

1. Son MBF, Newburger JW. Kawasaki disease. *Pediatr Rev*. 2018;*39*(2):78–90.

101. ANSWER: A

The observed higher infant mortality rate in babies born to non-Hispanic Black women is a health disparity. A health disparity is a health difference that adversely affects groups of people who have systematically experienced obstacles to health or disadvantages based on any characteristic historically linked to discrimination, such as race/ethnicity, gender, religion, disability, sexual orientation or gender identity, and geographic location. When these health disparities or differences are avoidable, unfair, or unjust, they are considered a health inequity. In this vignette, all that is known is that there is a health difference associated with race. It is unclear why this disparity is occurring. Once health disparities are discovered, it is important to investigate avoidable factors contributing to the observed disparity, such as implicit bias (attitudes, feelings, or perceptions that may unconsciously influence a person's actions toward others) or discrimination (unequal, adverse, or unfair treatment based on physical characteristics or social group assignment). SDoH may also be contributing to the observed health disparity in this vignette. SDoH include age and conditions in the environment in which people are born, live, learn, play, and grow that affect health outcomes. Implicit bias, discrimination, and SDoH are factors that can be addressed by hospitalists in the healthcare setting in order to make progress in achieving health equity.

[ABP 10.C.2. Principles of change management, ABP 10.C.3. Health equity and health disparities]

102. ANSWER: B

The skin finding that is reportable is described in choice B. A 3-cm full-thickness loss of skin with visible adipose tissue and developing eschar describes a stage 3 pressure injury. Pressure injuries, previously called pressure ulcers, are damages to the skin typically occurring over a bony prominence or involving a medical device. The injury can involve just the skin or also the underlying soft tissue. Pressure injuries are staged as follows:

- Stage 1 pressure injury: non-blanchable erythema of intact skin (choice C)
- Stage 2 pressure injury: partial-thickness skin loss with exposed dermis (choice A)
- Stage 3 pressure injury: full-thickness skin loss with adipose tissue visible in the ulcer; sloughing and eschar may be visible (choice B)
- Stage 4 pressure injury: full-thickness skin and tissue loss; injuries expose fascia, muscle, tendon, ligament, cartilage, and/or bone.

Of the pressure injuries listed, those that are reportable as hospital-acquired conditions according to CMS guidelines are stage 3 and stage 4 pressure injuries. Choice D describes a peripheral intravenous line infiltration that does not meet criteria for a moderate or serious infiltration and thus is not a hospital-acquired reportable condition. Choice E describes an unstageable pressure injury due to the presence of an eschar obscuring the view. Unstageable pressure injuries are defined as obscured full-thickness skin and tissue loss with inability to stage the ulcer. Most eschars, if removed, will reveal a stage 3 or 4 pressure injury. This pressure injury would not be reportable as a hospital-acquired condition as it was documented on admission to the PICU.

[ABP 8.G. Hospital-acquired conditions]

REFERENCE

1. Quick safety 25: preventing pressure injuries. Joint Commission. Published July 2016. Accessed May 3, 2021. https://www.join tcommission.org/resources/news-and   multimedia/newsletters/ newsletters/quick-safety/quick-safety-issue-25-preventing-pressure-injuries/preventing-pressure-injuries/.

103. ANSWER: B

This patient presents with gastroesophageal reflux (GER) with no associated complications or adverse effects. The Montreal international consensus defines gastroesophageal reflux disease (GERD) in pediatric patients as reflux that causes troublesome symptoms or complications that have an adverse effect on the well-being of the patient. Since the patient is growing well and has no complications from these episodes of spitting up, reassurance is appropriate. The

other answer choices would contribute to overtreatment as they are unlikely to provide benefit to the patient and may increase cost of care and risk of harm. The American Academy of Pediatrics recommendations included in the Choosing Wisely campaign recommend specifically to "avoid using acid blockers and motility agents for physiologic gastroesophageal reflux (GER) that is effortless, painless, and not affecting growth. Do not use medication in the so-called 'happy-spitter.'"

[ABP 9.A. Principles of value in healthcare for individuals and populations (e.g., reducing unwarranted variation, overuse, overtreatment, overdiagnosis)]

REFERENCES

1. American Academy of Pediatrics. AAP—acid blockers for GER in infants: Choosing Wisely. Choosing Wisely. Published April 14, 2015. Accessed May 7, 2021. https://www.choosingwisely.org/ clinician-lists/american-academy-pediatrics-acid-blockers-motility-agents-for-gastroesophageal-reflux-in-infants/.
2. Lightdale JR, Gremse DA, Heitlinger LA, et al. Gastroesophageal reflux: management guidance for the pediatrician. *Pediatrics*. 2013;*131*(5):e1684–e1695.

104. ANSWER: B

This study's null hypothesis is that there is no difference in complication rates between patients with CAP treated with antibiotics for 5 days versus 7 days. The study has failed to reject the null hypothesis; in other words, they could not detect a difference in complication rates. If this finding was in error and there was in fact a true difference between these two groups in the population at large, the authors would have committed a type 2 error (i.e., false negative). The maximum probability of committing a type 2 error is called beta (β). This number can be adjusted but is often set at .20, which means the investigator accepts a 20% chance they will miss a true difference in complication rates between the two groups. The quantity [1 - β] is called power. With a .20 β, a power of 0.80 means there is an 80% chance of correctly finding an association between the duration of antibiotics and complication rates.

If we reject the null hypothesis when it was true (i.e., false positive), we have committed a type 1 error. The maximum probability of committing a type 1 error is called alpha (α), which is also called the level of statistical significance (or p value) and is usually set as .05. Effect size is the minimum clinically significant difference between the two groups, which will vary depending on the outcomes under consideration. A larger sample size, or the number of subjects in the study, will always make your sample look more like the general population. Increasing sample size will reduce your chance of making a type 1 or type 2 error.

[ABP 13.A.3. Hypothesis testing]

105. ANSWER: B

Multiple-choice questions are often a part of an educator's assessment toolkit and can be an effective (and efficient) way to assess learning outcomes. There are several best practices in question writing that if not adhered to can decrease both the test's validity (i.e., the degree to which a test measures the learning outcomes it intends to measure) and its reliability (i.e., the degree to which a test *consistently* measures a learning outcome). For example, questions that have negative phrasing, such "Which of the following does NOT . . ." or "All of the following EXCEPT" tend to be easier to write as the writer need only come up with one wrong answer, but they have been shown to cause greater difficulty for test takers and accordingly minimize a test's reliability and validity, making choice B the correct answer. Choice A is incorrect as the definition provided is for reliability, not validity.

Adding irrelevant information to the question stem decreases (not increases) the reliability of the question (C). As each possible answer should be free of clues to which response is correct, both "all of the above" and "none of the above" questions should also be avoided (D). When "all of the above" is a choice, test takers who can correctly identify two of the answers as correct are able to eliminate the other choices even when unsure, and conversely test takers who can eliminate a single option of a "none of the above" by knowing it is true, are able to eliminate the "none of the above" choice.

We must be aware that all forms of assessment and evaluation are prone to potential biases in both choosing what to include on a test and how question stems are written. Multiple-choice tests eliminate bias in how scores are calculated compared to more subjective assessments: The answer is either right or wrong, and scoring is not open to interpretation, which can introduce bias about a given learner. However, the construction of multiple-choice questions is prone to reflect our biases. Examples include using gender, racial, or cultural stereotypes in a question stem, or a given question requiring a shared cultural lens, which often assumes a shared lived experience to be able to arrive at the correct answer. Effective test writing requires applying an intentional lens to analyzing questions and answers for possible biases.

[ABP 12.A. Principles of adult learning theory]

106. ANSWER: B

In view of the baby's increasing morphine needs, it would be detrimental to the infant to be discharged at this time, especially given that opiate withdrawal symptoms can be seen up to 5 days after birth. As most pediatric patients are unable to consent for themselves, parents are obliged to make medical decisions that do not harm their children. As the mother's autonomy is not absolute, her decision must be judged on several factors: (1) the high risk to the child of significant adverse consequences from refusal of care, (2) the high probability of success of the treatment, (3) the minimal burden of the treatment on the patient/family, and (4) lack of significant adverse effects of treatment. As such, the mother's refusal to consent to treatment in this case constitutes medical neglect. Child Protective Services should be involved to allow the state to intervene and make medical decisions in place of the parent. The baby should not be allowed to leave the hospital given the high risks of adverse effects like feeding difficulties, fever, insensible fluid losses, failure to thrive, and seizures if the baby were untreated. Contacting the father could potentially be helpful in this case, but given lack of participation in care since delivery and acuity of the situation, it would not be the best answer. Contacting risk management could yield helpful advice but will not protect the child from imminent discharge. The mother's refusal of care does not lead to a medical incapacity hold because she is not the patient of concern, but rather in this case acts in the role of guardian and decision-making authority for the child.

[ABP 11.B. Consent and assent]

REFERENCE

1. Black L. Limiting parents' rights in medical decision making. *Virtual Mentor.* 2006;8(10):676–680.

107. ANSWER: C

Failure mode and effect analysis (FMEA) is a systematic approach of prospectively identifying potential problems or failures in a process in order to prevent them from occurring. This differs from root cause analysis, which retrospectively reviews an event to identify areas for improvement. An adverse event is one that caused harm to a patient as a result of medical management. FMEA attempts to prevent adverse events from occurring. Trigger tools may also be used to retrospectively identify adverse events by searching the medical record for clues that may indicate that an adverse event occurred, such as searching for naloxone orders to determine potential errors in opiate prescribing. Waste reduction is a method of maximizing output while minimizing steps or services that do not add value or improve outcomes.

[ABP 8.E. Safety processes and tools]

108. ANSWER: A

The American Academy of Pediatrics (AAP) in partnership with the Choosing Wisely campaign recommends not starting intravenous antibiotic therapy on "well-appearing newborn infants with isolated risk factors for sepsis such as maternal chorioamnionitis, prolonged rupture of membranes, or untreated group B streptococcal colonization. Use clinical tools such as an evidence-based sepsis risk calculator to guide management."

Based on the Kaiser Permanente neonatal early-onset sepsis (EOS) calculator, the EOS risk for this patient is 0.03 per 1000 births, taking into consideration the gestational age, maternal temperature, ROM duration, and adequate intrapartum antibiotics. Thus, after using the calculator, the recommendation for this well-appearing newborn is to continue with routine vitals without culture and without antibiotics.

This calculator was based on 204,485 infants and found no statistical difference between infants assessed with or without the EOS calculator in terms of readmissions and adverse clinical outcomes such as mechanical ventilation, meningitis, and death. The EOS risk calculator did, however, lead to fewer blood cultures and less empiric antibiotic administration in the first 24 hours. Overtreatment with antibiotics has been associated with risks such as higher cost, increased length of stay, and disruption in the gut microbiome. Given the low risk for EOS in this case, antibiotics should not be started, and laboratory tests are not indicated. The infant should not be monitored in the intermediate care nursery as the baby is low risk for EOS, and rooming-in is recommended by the AAP to encourage the parent-infant bond. NICU consultation is not necessary at this time.

[ABP 9.A. Principles of value in healthcare for individuals and populations (e.g., reducing unwarranted variation, overuse, overtreatment, overdiagnosis)]

REFERENCES

1. Do not start IV antibiotic therapy on well-appearing newborn infants with isolated risk factors for sepsis such as maternal chorioamnionitis, prolonged rupture of membranes, or untreated group-B streptococcal colonization. Choosing Wisely. Published January 11, 2021. Accessed May 10, 2021. https://www.choosingwisely.org/clinician-lists/phm5-do-not-start-iv-antibiotic-therapy-on-well-appearing-newborn-infants-with-isolated-risk-factors-for-sepsis-such-as-maternal-chorioamnionitis-prolonged-rupture-of-membranes-or-untreated-group-b/.
2. Puopolo KM, Benitz WE, Zaoutis TE; Committee on Fetus and Newborn; Committee on Infectious Diseases. Management of
neonates born at ≥35 0/7 weeks' gestation with suspected or proven early-onset bacterial sepsis. *Pediatrics*. 2018;*142*(6):e20182894.
3. Neonatal early-onset sepsis calculator. Northern California Kaiser-Permanente. Accessed April 5, 2021. https://neonatalsepsiscalculator.kaiserpermanente.org.

109. ANSWER: C

There has been an increased focus on hospital readmissions as a metric in pediatrics, with many reimbursement models implementing financial repercussions for hospitals with unplanned readmissions. Hospitalists should be at the forefront of addressing safe and effective discharges. This requires an understanding of the common reasons patients are readmitted and demonstration of best practices in patient and family discharge education. The most common cause for pediatric patients to be readmitted to the hospital within 30 days of discharge is complications from surgical procedures, most commonly pain or dehydration. As many as one in four adolescents, for example, is readmitted after a tonsillectomy, and nearly all (98%) of readmissions after an appendectomy are thought to be preventable. Ensuring postoperative patients have adequate pain control (after operative anesthetics wear off) and can tolerate oral intake prior to discharge is thus most likely to provide the highest yield in reducing readmissions.

Using asthma action plans and optimizing the filling of prescriptions have all been shown to improve outcomes, including resource utilization for various conditions, but their impact is less direct on unplanned readmissions. Some efforts, such as prolonging observation while cultures are pending, may improve one metric such as hospital readmissions, but negatively impact other balancing measures, such as length of stay or risk for errors.

[ABP 9.B. Commonly used terms and metrics (readmissions)]

REFERENCE

1. Payne NR, Flood A. Preventing pediatric readmissions: which ones and how? *J Pediatr*. 2015;*166*(3):519–520.

4.

QUICK FACTS

Deepa Kulkarni, Audrey Kamzan, and Charles Newcomer

NEUROLOGY

Infant with brief, frequent, "jackknifing" seizures especially in the morning	Infantile spasms
What does sixth cranial nerve palsy indicate?	Elevated ICP (if normal imaging, think pseudotumor cerebri)
Infant with poor feeding and constipation	Think botulism
Evidence of a CNS infection and focal neurologic findings. What imaging study is needed?	Head CT with contrast (brain abscess)
Erratic behavior progressing to altered mental status with CSF pleocytosis	Anti-NMDA encephalitis (in teen girls, think ovarian teratoma)
Newborn with bounding pulses, widened pulse pressure, and pulsatile fontanelle	Arteriovenous malformation
Most accurate imaging study for stroke?	MRI with DWI (if can be done ASAP)
Patient with progressive weakness who had a diarrheal illness a month ago?	Guillain-Barré syndrome (triggered by *Campylobacter jejuni* infection)

HEAD AND NECK

Warm, tender neck mass in the anterior triangle	Think infected branchial cleft cyst
Febrile child with hot-potato voice and inability to extend neck	Retropharyngeal abscess
Cyanosis that improves with crying	Choanal atresia
Nasal polyps	Think cystic fibrosis
Management of nasal septal hematoma	Needs urgent drainage to prevent ischemia of the septal cartilage
Nontender unilateral lymphadenopathy with violaceous overlying skin?	Nontuberculous mycobacteria (can cure with excision alone)
Cause of parotitis in unvaccinated patient	Mumps (if vaccinated, other viral causes)
Neonate with fever and swollen parotid gland	Acute suppurative parotitis due to *Staphylococcus aureus*
Most common source of orbital cellulitis	Ethmoid sinusitis
Tearing, pain, and foreign body sensation in eye	Corneal abrasion

PULMONARY

Delayed passage of newborn's first meconium is concerning for	Cystic fibrosis
Stridor in a neonate that resolves after intubation	Laryngeal web
Stridor in a neonate that appears after prolonged intubation	Subglottic stenosis
2-year-old with sudden-onset wheeze that doesn't respond to albuterol	Think foreign body aspiration (get decubitus chest films)
How to manage rising CO_2 levels in a mechanically ventilated patient?	Increase the respiratory rate or tidal volume
High fevers, drooling, and respiratory distress in an unvaccinated child: what is the management?	Intubate in the operating room ASAP and don't upset the child (epiglottitis)
What is the most common etiology and timing of stridor?	Extrathoracic obstruction and inspiratory
What is the most common etiology and timing of wheeze?	Intrathoracic obstruction and expiratory
Preferred imaging to evaluate parapneumonic effusion	Ultrasound
Unilateral pleural effusion after thoracic surgery	Think chylothorax
Tachypneic patient with normal $PaCO_2$?	Impending respiratory failure (should have low $PaCO_2$)
Most common organism in bacterial tracheitis?	*S. aureus*

CARDIOVASCULAR

Murmur worsens after standing up	Sit back down! Think hypertrophic cardiomyopathy
Most common cause of myocarditis in kids	Coxsackie B
Diffuse ST segment elevations	Pericarditis
Boot-shaped heart on chest x-ray	Tetralogy of Fallot
Egg-on-a-string shaped mediastinum on chest x-ray	Transposition of the great arteries
Snowman-shaped mediastinum on chest x-ray	Total anomalous pulmonary venous return
Cardiac defect associated with Down syndrome	Endocardial cushion defect (atrioventricular canal defect)
Reversible causes of cardiac arrest	*H*'s: hypovolemia, hypoxia, hydrogen (acidosis), hypoglycemia, hypo-/hyperkalemia, hypothermia *T*'s: tension pneumothorax, tamponade (cardiac), toxins, thrombosis (pulmonary or coronary)
Patient in shock that worsens after normal saline bolus	Cardiogenic shock
Which rhythms require an unsynchronized shock?	Ventricular fibrillation and pulseless ventricular tachycardia
What is the first-line medication for supraventricular tachycardia?	Adenosine

GASTROINTESTINAL

Patient has liver disease and low albumin but high total protein	Autoimmune hepatitis (high protein due to elevated IgG)
2-month-old infant has projectile vomiting and hyperbilirubinemia	Pyloric stenosis (icteropyloric syndrome)
Intussusception in a 10-year-old should prompt an evaluation for	A lead point (e.g., lymphoma or Meckel's)
Neonate with bilious emesis: what imaging is gold standard for diagnosis?	Upper GI series (malrotation/volvulus; time is bowel!)
What is the test for protein-losing enteropathy?	Stool alpha-1 antitrypsin
Well-appearing 3-month-old with bloody stools: what is the treatment?	Hydrolyzed formula or maternal cow's milk elimination diet if breastfed
Painless bright red blood per rectum	Meckel's diverticulum
Neonate with direct hyperbilirubinemia and high ferritin	Neonatal hemochromatosis
Fever, abdominal pain, jaundice	Cholangitis (Charcot triad)
Patient with ulcerative colitis presents with pruritis	Primary sclerosing cholangitis
Diarrhea and seizures	*Shigella*
Signs of toxin-mediated infectious diarrhea	Watery, nonbloody, and symptoms come on within hours not days (*S. aureus*, *Bacillus cereus*, etc.)

RENAL/GENITOURINARY/GYNECOLOGY

Urinalysis with + blood but no RBCs	Think rhabdomyolysis
Kidney disease with low C3 and normal C4	Postinfectious glomerulonephritis
Kidney disease with low C3 and low C4	Lupus glomerulonephritis
Persistent microscopic hematuria with a family history of stones	Hypercalciuria (get a urine Ca:Cr ratio)
Bilateral hydronephrosis in a male infant	Posterior urethral valves
Which stones are radiopaque?	Anything with mineral: calcium oxalate, calcium phosphate, mag-ammonium-phos (struvite)
What do WBC casts indicate?	Tubular disease (e.g., acute tubular necrosis)
Patient with nephrotic syndrome develops fever and abdominal tenderness	Spontaneous bacterial peritonitis (likely *S. pneumoniae*)
Testicular pain relieved by lifting testicle	Epididymitis
Sexually active female with pleuritic right upper quadrant pain	Fitz-Hugh-Curtis syndrome (gonorrhea)
Thrombocytopenia, microangiophatic hemolytic anemia, and acute kidney injury	Hemolytic-uremic syndrome

ORTHOPEDICS

Patient on chronic steroids develops hip pain	Osteonecrosis of femoral head
Radiographic evidence of supracondylar fracture	Anterior sail sign and/or posterior fat pad
2-year-old with osteomyelitis not improving on vancomycin, what organism should you consider?	*Kingella kingae* (give a cephalosporin)
Fever and refusal to bear weight	Septic joint (vs. transient synovitis can bear weight)

RHEUMATOLOGIC/VASCULITIS

Joint pain with daily, transient fever and rash	Think systemic JIA; treat with NSAIDs first line
Henoch-Schonlein purpura develops worsening abdominal pain	GI complications (intussusception, ischemia)
Newborn presents with heart block	Neonatal lupus; check anti-Ro (SS-A) and anti-La (SS-B) antibodies
How long after high-dose IVIG should you wait to give live vaccines?	11 months
Most specific marker of SLE flare	Anti-dsDNA

ENDOCRINE/METABOLIC

Hypoglycemia, omphalocele, and hemihypertrophy	Beckwith-Wiedemann syndrome
Blood test to confirm congenital adrenal hyperplasia (21-hydroxylase deficiency)	17-Hydroxyprogesterone
Delayed fontanelle closure	Think congenital hypothyroidism
Hyperammonemia with acidosis	Think organic acidemias
Hyperammonemia with alkalosis	Think urea cycle disorders
Positive urine reducing substances	Think galactosemia
Organism causing sepsis in neonate with galactosemia	*Escherichia coli*
Hypoglycemia without ketones	Hyperinsulinism versus fatty acid oxidation disorder
A patient on long-term prednisone presents with sepsis: what treatment to consider?	Hydrocortisone for adrenal insufficiency

CHILD MALTREATMENT

Frenulum injury	Think forced feeding or forced pacifier
Bruise in a baby that doesn't yet cruise	Think abuse
Most common cause of death from child abuse	Neglect
Other diagnosis to consider with subdural hematomas	Glutaric aciduria
Other diagnosis to consider with multiple fractures	Osteogenesis imperfecta
Fractures that are more likely to be from abuse	Posterior rib, scapular, sternal, spinous process, and metaphyseal avulsion
Most common physical examination finding in sexual abuse	Normal examination
Parent seeking unnecessary or harmful medical interventions	Medical child abuse

DERMATOLOGIC

Beard distribution of hemangiomas is concerning for	Internal or airway hemangiomas
Infection associated with recurrent erythema multiforme	HSV
Most common cause of necrotizing fasciitis	Group A strep
Rashes associated with IBD	Erythema nodosum > pyoderma gangrenosum
Skin and mucosal blistering a few weeks after new medication exposure	SJS/TEN
Eczema and absent thymic shadow	SCID
Eczema and thrombocytopenia	Wiskott-Aldrich syndrome

HEMATOLOGIC/ONCOLOGIC

Common organism in osteomyelitis in sickle cell patients	*Salmonella*
Hemolysis after cotrimoxazole	Glucose-6-phosphate dehydrogenase deficiency
Peripheral smear with schistocytes	Intravascular hemolysis
Peripheral smear with spherocytes	Extravascular hemolysis or spherocytosis
Peripheral smear with Howell-Jolly bodies	Asplenia
Peripheral smear with target cells	Thalassemia
Whose platelets should be transfused into a baby with neonatal alloimmune thrombocytopenia?	Mother's
GI bleed at 2–7 days of life	Think classic vitamin K deficiency bleeding
Patient with recent chemotherapy, fever, and acute abdomen	Think typhlitis
Clotting factors in the common pathway	1, 2, 5, 10 (think small bills $)

ALLERGY AND IMMUNOLOGY

Omphalitis, severe leukocytosis	Leukocyte adhesion deficiency
Dextrocardia on chest x-ray: what infections is the patient at risk for?	Encapsulated organisms (heterotaxy syndrome; associated with polysplenia)
Skin infections, deep organ abscesses, and inflammatory bowel disease	Chronic granulomatous disease
Fever, rash, lip swelling, diffuse lymphadenopathy after a medication	DRESS syndrome; check eosinophils
Foods most likely to cause fatal/near-fatal allergic reactions	Peanuts, tree nuts, soy, cow's milk, fish, and shellfish
Toddler with recurrent respiratory tract disease and absent lymph nodes/tonsils	X-linked agammaglobulinemia
Toddler with no response to vaccines with multiple, life-threatening infections	SCID

INJURIES AND EXPOSURES

Activated charcoal is not indicated for which ingestions?	Alcohol, caustics, heavy metals, lithium, hydrocarbons
Which coin is the most corrosive when swallowed?	Penny (has zinc)
Which type of snakebite always requires antivenom?	Coral snakes (vespid) because they release neurotoxins
Cherry red lips, headaches, and malaise	Carbon monoxide poisoning
Raccoon eyes, hemotympanum, and cerebrospinal fluid leaking from the nose	Basilar skull fracture
Facial trauma, can't look up, and decreased sensation over cheek	Orbital blowout fracture
Teenager with episodes of nausea and vomiting relieved by hot baths	Cannabinoid hyperemesis syndrome
Organism associated with puncture wound in the foot	*Pseudomonas*
Hyperthermia, agitation, and clonus in patient with depression	Serotonin syndrome
Acetaminophen overdose	Give *N*-acetylcysteine
Ethylene glycol or methanol overdose	Give fomepizole
Iron overdose	Give deferoxamine
Anticholinergic overdose	Give physostigmine
Cholinergic (i.e., organophosphate) overdose	Give atropine, pralidoxime
Calcium channel blocker overdose	Give calcium gluconate
Tricyclic antidepressant or salicylate overdose	Give sodium bicarbonate
Opiate overdose	Give naloxone
Benzodiazepine overdose	Give flumazenil

OTHER CONDITIONS

"Should dos" for low-risk BRUE	Educate about BRUE, offer CPR training
Most common cause of failure to thrive	Insufficient intake
Electrolyte abnormalities in cystic fibrosis	Hyponatremic hypochloremic alkalosis
First step in management of hyperkalemia	Give calcium (doesn't lower K+ but prevents life-threatening arrhythmias)
Management of refractory opiate induced constipation	Methylnaltrexone

BEHAVIORAL AND MENTAL HEALTH CONDITIONS

When feeding a severely malnourished patient, what electrolyte abnormalities are expected?	Hypophosphatemia, hypokalemia, hypomagnesemia, and hypocalcemia
Pharmacological treatment of delirium	Atypical antipsychotics (avoid benzodiazepines)
Patient with lupus develops psychosis that worsens with treatment	Think steroid-induced psychosis
Melanosis coli	Think laxative abuse
Patient started on antipsychotics develops trismus and torticollis: how to treat?	Benztropine or diphenhydramine (for acute dystonia)

NEWBORN CARE

Newborn with severe thrombocytopenia	NAIT (maternal antibodies to newborn's platelets containing paternal antigens)
TORCH most likely to cause hearing loss	CMV
TORCH with cardiac defects	Rubella
Opisthotonus (neck/trunk arching) and high-pitched cry	Think severe bilirubin encephalopathy
Caput succedaneum versus cephalohematoma on examination?	Caput crosses suture lines (like "putting on a cap"); cephalohematoma does not
How do you manage respiratory distress in a newborn with congenital diaphragmatic hernia?	Intubate (do not bag-mask ventilate!), place NG tube for decompression
Abdominal wall defect to the right of umbilical cord	Gastroschisis
Corrective steps if neonate not responding to PPV in delivery room	MRSOPA (mask, reposition airway, suction, open mouth, increase pressure, advanced airway)
Risk factors for neonatal hypoglycemia	Small for gestational age, late preterm > large for gestational age, diabetic mother
Drug exposures that improve with time	Toxicities (methamphetamines, cocaine) versus withdrawals that worsen with time (opiates, barbiturates)
Newborn conjunctivitis within hours	Chemical conjunctivitis
Newborn conjunctivitis within days	Gonococcal conjunctivitis
Newborn conjunctivitis within weeks	Chlamydial conjunctivitis
First-line treatment for neonatal abstinence syndrome	"Eat, sleep, console"

MEDICAL PROCEDURES

Contraindications to NG tube placement	Esophageal strictures, facial or basilar skull fracture
Contraindications to GT replacement	First 4–6 weeks postplacement, peritonitis
Contraindication to ketamine for sedation	Increased ICP
Contraindication to etomidate for sedation	Septic shock
Contraindication to arterial puncture	Lack of collaterals to hand (do Allen test)
Contraindication to bladder catheterization	Urethral trauma (history of pelvic fracture or blood at meatus)
What is the best way to assess if bag-valve-mask technique is effective?	Look for chest rise
Complication of UVC placement	Liver damage (accidental placement in portal venous system)
Which interspace should be targeted during lumbar puncture?	L4-L5 or L3-L4
Proper location for needle thoracentesis?	2nd intercostal space, midclavicular line

QUALITY IMPROVEMENT, PATIENT SAFETY, AND SYSTEMS-BASED IMPROVEMENT

The best way to prevent avoidable medical errors	Create a no-blame system for reporting
Unexpected occurrence involving death or serious physical or psychological injury or risk thereof	Sentinel event
Potential adverse event places patient at risk of injury but does not result in harm	Near-miss event
An injury caused by medical management rather than the underlying disease/condition	Adverse event
What makes for a strong goal or aim statement?	SMART (specific, measurable, attainable, relevant, time bound)
Difference between run chart and control chart?	Control chart has upper and lower control limit lines

CORE KNOWLEDGE IN SCHOLARLY ACTIVITIES

Test with high sensitivity	Patient with disease will have positive test
Test with high specificity	Healthy patient will have negative test
The positive or negative predictive value of any test depends on this measurement	Prevalence of the condition in the population being tested
Correlation coefficient interpretation	1 = strong positive association; 0 = no association; -1 = strong negative association
When to use a *t* test	Comparing two groups with continuous variables (e.g., IQ score)
When to use a paired *t* test	To compare the same patients (i.e., before and after)
When to use a Fisher exact test or chi-squared test	Comparing two groups with categorical variables (e.g., insured or uninsured)
Type I error in hypothesis testing	False positive; *p* value = chance of type I error
Type II error in hypothesis testing	False negative; prevent it with a power calculation
What percentage of data on a normal curve falls within 2 standard deviations (SD)?	95% (68% within 1 SD, 99.7% within 3 SD)

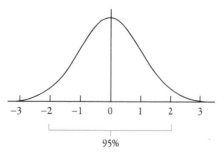

INDEX

Tables, figures, and boxes are indicated by *t*, *f*, and *b* following the page number.

macrophage activation syndrome (MAS), 27, 90

magnesium, intravenous, 54, 133

magnetic resonance arteriography (MRA), 44–45, 118

magnet ingestion, 34, 101

malar rash, 108

malrotation with midgut volvulus, 18, 78

mature minor doctrine, 221

McLaren method, 127–128, 128f

measures, in quality improvement, 215

mechanical insufflation-exsufflation (MIE), 138, 160

Meckel diverticulum, 37, 105

meconium aspiration syndrome (MAS), 172

medical child abuse, 5, 26, 63, 90

medical interpreters, 201, 206, 229, 236

medical misconnection, 142, 166

medical neglect, 8, 66, 211, 244

medical procedures. *See specific procedures*

medical procedures quick facts, 252

medication errors, 193, 216

meningitis, bacterial, 6, 65

mental health conditions. *See specific conditions*

mental health conditions quick facts, 251

mentorship, 205, 234

meta-analysis, 203, 231

metabolic quick facts, 249

methylmalonic acidemia (MMA), 46, 120

micafungin, 21, 82

microaggressions, 210, 241–242

micronutrient deficiency, 140, 162–163, 163t

migraine headache, 28, 92–93

Miller Fisher syndrome, 85

minimal change disease, 83

minority tax, 205, 234

mitochondrial myopathy, 85

mitral valve prolapse (MVP), 48, 123

model for improvement
    aim statement, 190–191, 212–213
    measures in, 192, 215
    PDSA cycle, 197, 199, 223–224, 226

modified Duke criteria, 46, 120–121, 121t

Moore method, 128

morphine administration, 145, 172

morphine milligram equivalents (MMEs), 40, 111, 111t

motion waste, 203, 232, 232t

mucocutaneous lesions, in systemic lupus erythematosus, 38–39, 108

multidisciplinary family meeting, 194, 218–219

multiple-choice tests, 211, 244

mumps, 2, 58

myasthenia gravis, 85

myocarditis
    in Epstein-Barr virus infections, 6, 65
    gold standard for diagnosis, 25, 88

naloxone, 25, 88

naproxen, 5, 63–64

nasogastric tube placement
    complications in, 143, 168
    discharge communication, 198–199, 226
    medical misconnection, 142, 166

nebulized hypertonic saline, 4, 61

needle thoracentesis, 147–148, 176

neonatal abstinence syndrome (NAS)
    ESC approach, 148, 176
    exposure to SSRIs, 154–155, 187
    medical neglect in, 244
    overtreatment in, 192, 214–215

neonatal herpes simplex virus (HSV) infection, 67

neonatal hyperbilirubinemia
    Bhutani nomogram, 144, 169–170
    discharge in, 137, 158–159
    phototherapy for, 155, 187, 195, 202, 220, 230

neonatal hypoglycemia, 141, 164–165

neonatal infections. *See* infections, neonatal

neonatal lupus syndrome (NLS), 36, 104

neonatal opioid withdrawal syndrome, 136–137, 158

neonatal resuscitation. *See* resuscitation, neonatal

nephritis, in systemic lupus erythematosus, 38–39, 108

nephrolithiasis, 31, 41, 97, 111

nephrotic syndrome, 2, 5, 22, 59, 63, 83

neuroleptic malignant syndrome (NMS), 117

neurology quick facts, 246

neuropathic pain, 52, 131

neuropsychiatric manifestations of lupus, 153, 184

neutropenia, 21, 44, 82, 117

never events, 241

newborn care quick facts, 252

newborn weight loss, 140, 163–164

non–anion gap metabolic acidosis, 115

nondisclosure in terminal illness, 199–200, 227

nongap metabolic acidosis, 55, 135

non–IgE-mediated food allergies, 16, 75

noninvasive ventilation (NIV), 49, 125–126

nonrebreather face mask, 204, 233

nonsteroidal anti-inflammatory drugs
    in Henoch-Schönlein purpura management, 5, 63–64
    in JIA management, 24, 86–87
    in pericarditis management, 27–28, 92
    in transient synovitis management, 2–3, 59

nontuberculous mycobacteria (NTM), 89

obstructive sleep apnea (OSA), 155–156, 188–189

occult spinal dysraphisms (OSDs), 182–183

odds ratios, 225

odontogenic infections, suppurative, 47, 122

oncologic quick facts, 250

opiate use disorder (OUD), 136–137, 158

opioids
    neonatal abstinence syndrome, 136–137, 148, 158, 176, 192, 214–215
    Prescription Drug Monitoring Programs, 38, 107
    toxicity, 25, 88, 98

oppositional defiant disorder (ODD), 143, 148–149, 168, 177, 188

oral Kayexalate, 10, 69

oral rehydration therapy (ORT), 49–50, 126

orbital cellulitis, 40, 110, 110t

organic acidemias, 147, 175–176, 176t

organophosphate toxicity, 9–10, 68

ornithine transcarbamylase (OTC) deficiency, 48–49, 125

orthopedic quick facts, 248

osteomyelitis, 70, 200–201, 228

osteopenia, 17, 77

otitis media, 57t

ovarian cysts, 26–27, 33–34, 90, 100

ovarian torsion, 33–34, 100

overdiagnosis, 240

overtreatment, 209, 240
    in neonatal abstinence syndrome, 192, 214–215
    in neonatal hyperbilirubinemia, 195, 220

overuse, 191, 213, 240

oxygen administration, in asthma, 19–20, 79–80

oxygen saturation, neonatal, 139, 161

paired *t* test, 196, 222

palivizumab, 95–96

pancreatic islet autoantibodies, 5, 63

pancreatitis, 16, 75

parainfluenza virus, 31, 96

parapneumonic effusions, 45, 118–119

parathyroid adenoma, 53, 132

Pareto chart, 217

Parkland formula, 125

parotitis
    acute suppurative, 17, 77
    due to stone, 20, 80
    in mumps, 2, 58

paroxysmal sympathetic hyperactivity, 155, 187

patient-physician cost conversations, 198, 225–226

patient safety quick facts, 253

Pediatric Emergency Care Applied Research Network (PECARN) prediction rule, 238

Pediatric Respiratory Score (PRS), 191, 213–214

pelvic fracture, 148, 177

pelvic inflammatory disease (PID), 17–18, 77–78

percutaneous endoscopic gastrostomy (PEG) tubes, 139, 153, 162, 162f, 185

pericarditis, 27–28, 92

periodic fever, aphthous stomatitis, pharyngitis, and cervical adenitis (PFAPA), 34, 100–101

peripheral hypotonia, 103

peripheral intravenous placement, 136, 147, 157–158, 175

peripherally inserted central catheter (PICC), 142, 154, 166, 186, 186t

peristomal leakage, 139, 162

peritonitis, 49, 125

peritonsillar abscesses (PTAs), 73

person-first language, 202, 230

pertussis, 52, 55, 129–130, 135

PHACE (posterior fossa anomalies, hemangioma, arterial lesions, cardiac abnormalities/coarctation of the aorta, eye anomalies) syndrome, 29–30, 94

pharyngitis, 4, 10, 62, 69

phenobarbital, 32, 98

phototherapy, 155, 187, 195, 202, 220, 230

physical abuse
    burn injury, 20, 81
    fractures, 77
    frenulum laceration, 22, 83

physical aggression. *See* aggressive behaviors

physical therapy, 33, 100

physician's order for life sustaining treatment (POLST), 199–200, 227

physostigmine, 6, 64–65

Pierre Robin sequence, 155, 188

plain radiographs, 11–12, 70

Plan-Do-Study-Act (PDSA) cycle, 197, 199, 223–224, 226

pneumococcal 23-valent polysaccharide vaccine (PPSV23), 202, 230–231

pneumonia
    bronchoalveolar lavage analysis, 43, 116, 116t
    community-acquired, 40, 109–110
    in foreign body aspiration, 10, 68
    hospital-acquired, 42, 113
    parapneumonic effusions in, 45, 118–119

pneumothorax, 147–148, 176

polycythemia, 182

port wine stain, 10, 68–69, 104–105

positional deformation, 149, 177

positive pressure ventilation, 143, 144, 169, 170–171

posterior reversible encephalopathy syndrome (PRES), 45, 119

postexposure prophylaxis (PEP) for rabies, 113

postrenal acute kidney injury, 86

poststreptococcal glomerulonephritis (PSGN), 44, 118

postural orthostatic tachycardia syndrome (POTS), 49, 125

Pott puffy tumor (PPT), 42, 113–114

Prader-Willi syndrome (PWS), 35, 102–103

prerenal acute kidney injury, 86

Prescription Drug Monitoring Programs (PDMP), 38, 107

preseptal cellulitis, 110, 110t

pressure injuries, 149, 178, 210, 243

prevalence of disease, 239

primary sclerosing cholangitis (PSC), 41, 94–95, 112

principle of justice, 191, 213

procedural sedation, 149, 151, 178–179, 182

process map, 217

prochlorperazine, 28, 92–93

propranolol, 94

prostaglandin E$_1$ (PGE$_1$), 9, 68

PRSS1 gene, 16, 75

psychogenic nonepileptic seizure (PNES), 144, 170

psychological safety, 196, 222

psychosis, lupus, 153, 184

psychosomatic disorders
    abdominal migraines, 140, 163
    complex regional pain syndrome, 138–139, 161
    conversion disorder, 146, 154, 174, 187
    psychogenic nonepileptic seizure, 144, 170
    somatic symptom disorder, 154, 185–186

pulmonary edema, 23, 84

pulmonary embolism (PE), 16, 50, 75, 127

pulmonary insertion of NGT, 143, 168

pulmonary quick facts, 247

pyelonephritis, 43, 115

QTc prolongation, drug-induced, 143, 169

quality improvement
    aim statement, 190–191, 212–213
    failure mode and effect analysis, 207–208, 239
    fishbone diagram, 194, 217
    key driver diagram, 195, 220
    measures in, 192, 215
    PDSA cycle, 197, 199, 223–224, 226
    quick facts, 253
    root cause analysis and actions, 205, 235
    run charts, 200, 228

Index by American Board of Pediatrics Content Domain

CONTENT SPECIFICATION	RELEVANT QUESTIONS (LISTED AS CHAPTER # : QUESTION #)
8. Quality Improvement, Patient Safety, and Systems-Based Improvement	2:32, 3:4, 3:12, 3:16, 3:20, 3:26, 3:31, 3:38, 3:47, 3:53, 3:61, 3:67, 3:73, 3:78, 3:82, 3:86, 3:90, 3:93, 3:98, 3:102, 3:107
9. Evidence-Based High-Value Care	3:1, 3:5, 3:7, 3:10, 3:14, 3:21, 3:27, 3:32, 3:36, 3:39, 3:44, 3:48, 3:54, 3:62, 3:68, 3:74, 3:79, 3:83, 3:87, 3:95, 3:100, 3:103, 3:108, 3:109
10. Advocacy and Leadership	3:13, 3:22, 3:28, 3:40, 3:49, 3:55, 3:63, 3:69, 3:94, 3:101
11. Ethics, Legal Issues, and Human Rights	3:6, 3:14, 3:23, 3:29, 3:41, 3:50, 3:56, 3:106
12. Teaching and Education	3:15, 3:24, 3:33, 3:42, 3:57, 3:64, 3:71, 3:75, 3:85, 3:96, 3:105
13. Core Knowledge in Scholarly Activities	3:3, 3:8, 3:17, 3:25, 3:30, 3:34, 3:43, 3:51, 3:58, 3:65, 3:68, 3:70, 3:76, 3:80, 3:83, 3:84, 3:89, 3:92, 3:97, 3:104

ADAPTED from: Pediatric Hospital Medicine Content Outline. American Board of Pediatrics website https://www.abp.org/sites/abp/files/pdf/hospital_medicine_content_outline.pdf. Accessed March 1, 2022.